**W9-AGR-686**

# MAYO CLINIC
## ON HEALTHY AGING

**Edward T. Creagan, M.D., FAAHPM**
Medical Editor

Mayo Clinic
Rochester, Minnesota

*Mayo Clinic on Healthy Aging* provides reliable information about dealing with the common physical, emotional and lifestyle-related changes that occur with aging. Much of the information comes directly from the experience of health care professionals at Mayo Clinic. This book supplements the advice of your personal physician, whom you should consult for individual medical problems.

For bulk sales to employers, member groups and health-related companies, contact Mayo Clinic Health Solutions, 200 First St. SW, Rochester, MN 55905, call 800-430-9699, or send an email to SpecialSalesMayoBooks@Mayo.edu.

Published by Mayo Clinic

© 2013 Mayo Foundation for Medical Education and Research (MFMER), revision 2018

Library of Congress Control Number: 2013935416

First Edition

4 5 6 7 8 9 10

## Image credits

NAME: 94988149.JPG/PAGE: COVER, 9, 61, 299, 339/CREDIT: © ISTOCKPHOTO/THINKSTOCK — NAME: CREAGAN_EDWARD_T_12MY/PAGE: IV/CREDIT © MFMER — NAME: 78486136.JPG/PAGE: 16/CREDIT: © COMSTOCK/THINKSTOCK — NAME: 101430348.JPG/PAGE: 17/CREDIT: © HEMERA/THINKSTOCK — NAME: I20906321.JPG/PAGE: 19/CREDIT: © ISTOCKPHOTO/THINKSTOCK — NAME: 71040508.JPG/PAGE: 20–23, 38–39, 44–45, 58–59, 102–103, 126–127, 148–149, 198–199, 230–231/CREDIT: © STOCKBYTE/THINKSTOCK — NAME: 78493223.JPG/PAGE: 30/CREDIT: © COMSTOCK/THINKSTOCK — NAME: 74226923.JPG/PAGE: 46/CREDIT: © MARIA TEIJEIRO/DIGITAL VISION/THINKSTOCK — NAME: 144875493.JPG/PAGE: 57/CREDIT: © ISTOCKPHOTO/THINKSTOCK — NAME: 86505611.JPG/PAGE: 64–65/CREDIT: © JUPITERIMAGES/BANANASTOCK/THINKSTOCK — NAME: 126106696.JPG/PAGE: 70/CREDIT: © ISTOCKPHOTO/THINKSTOCK — NAME: 57283712.JPG/PAGE: 80/CREDIT: © GEORGE DOYLE/STOCKBYTE/THINKSTOCK — NAME: 162571068.JPG/PAGE: 83/CREDIT: © ISTOCKPHOTO/THINKSTOCK — NAME: 89518199.JPG/PAGE: 87/CREDIT: © COMSTOCK/THINKSTOCK — NAME: 76812611.JPG/PAGE: 100/CREDIT: © CREATAS/THINKSTOCK — NAME: 100848080.JPG/PAGE: 110/CREDIT: © HEMERA/THINKSTOCK — NAME: AA051018.JPG/PAGE: 113/CREDIT: © RYAN MCVAY/DIGITAL VISION/THINKSTOCK — NAME: 87786691.JPG/PAGE: 121/CREDIT: © JUPITERIMAGES/PHOTOS.COM/THINKSTOCK — NAME: 155911815.JPG/PAGE: 125/CREDIT: © ISTOCKPHOTO/THINKSTOCK — NAME: 75547691.JPG/PAGE: 134/CREDIT: © STOCKBYTE/THINKSTOCK — NAME: 87568485.JPG/PAGE: 136–137/CREDIT: © HEMERA TECHNOLOGIES/ABLESTOCK.COM/THINKSTOCK — NAME: 78629214.JPG/PAGE: 154/CREDIT: © PIXLAND/THINKSTOCK — NAME: 200305422-001.JPG/PAGE: 157/CREDIT: © PHOTODISC/THINKSTOCK — NAME: 78287802.JPG/PAGE: 158/CREDIT: © GOODSHOOT/THINKSTOCK — NAME: 137059243.JPG/PAGE: 161/CREDIT: © ISTOCKPHOTO/THINKSTOCK — NAME: 157256088.JPG/PAGE: 164/CREDIT: © ISTOCKPHOTO/THINKSTOCK — NAME: 150640632.JPG/PAGE: 169/CREDIT: © F1ONLINE/THINKSTOCK — NAME: 73016781.JPG/PAGE: 170-171/CREDIT: © DORLING KINDERSLEY RF/THINKSTOCK — NAME: 7727686.jpg/PAGE: 182/CREDIT: © POLKA DOT/THINKSTOCK — NAME: FIG20-020-02.PSD/PAGE: 185/CREDIT: © MFMER — NAME: FIG21-021-02.PSD/PAGE: 185/CREDIT: © MFMER — NAME: FIG22-022-02.PSD/PAGE: 186/CREDIT: © MFMER — NAME: FIG23-023-02.PSD/PAGE: 186/CREDIT: © MFMER — NAME: FIG25-025-02.PSD/PAGE: 186/CREDIT: © MFMER — NAME: FIG26-026-02.PSD/PAGE: 186/CREDIT: © MFMER — NAME: FIG01-001-2.PSD/PAGE: 187/CREDIT: © MFMER — NAME: FIG02-002-02.PSD/PAGE: 188/CREDIT: © MFMER — NAME: FIG03-003-02.[SD/PAGE: 188/CREDIT: © MFMER — NAME: FIG05-005-02.PSD/PAGE: 188/CREDIT: © MFMER — NAME: FIG04-004-02.PSD/PAGE: 188/CREDIT: © MFMER — NAME: FIG10-010-02.PSD/PAGE: 189/CREDIT: © MFMER — NAME: FIG13a-013-02.PSD/PAGE: 189/CREDIT: © MFMER — NAME: FIG13b-013-02.PSD/PAGE: 189/CREDIT: © MFMER — NAME: FIG12-012-02.PSD/PAGE: 189/CREDIT: © MFMER — NAME: FIG11-011-02.PSD/PAGE: 190/CREDIT: © MFMER — NAME: FIG16-016-02.PSD/PAGE: 191/CREDIT: © MFMER — NAME: FIG14-014-02.PSD/PAGE: 191/CREDIT: © MFMER — NAME: FIG28-028-01.PSD/PAGE: 192/CREDIT: © MFMER — NAME: FIG15-015-02.PSD/PAGE: 192/CREDIT: © MFMER — NAME: 153720416.JPG/PAGE: 194/CREDIT: © ISTOCKPHOTO/THINKSTOCK — NAME: PYRAMIDIMAGE.PSD/PAGE: 202, 218/CREDIT: © MFMER — NAME: 97689694.JPG/PAGE: 203/CREDIT: © ISTOCKPHOTO/THINKSTOCK — NAME: 56359785.JPG/PAGE: 204/CREDIT: © PHOTODISC/THINKSTOCK — NAME: 98045007.JPG/PAGE: 208/CREDIT: © ISTOCKPHOTO/THINKSTOCK — NAME: 119505733.JPG/PAGE: 209/CREDIT: © ISTOCKPHOTO/THINKSTOCK — NAME: SKD259362SDC.JPG/PAGE: 210/CREDIT: © STOCKBYTE/THINKSTOCK — NAME: 77295209.JPG/PAGE: 212/CREDIT: © POLKA DOT/THINKSTOCK — NAME: 96924168.JPG/PAGE: 220/CREDIT: © ISTOCKPHOTO/THINKSTOCK — NAME: 100889745.JPG/PAGE: 220/CREDIT: © HEMERA/THINKSTOCK — NAME: 98001570.JPG/PAGE: 220/CREDIT: © ISTOCKPHOTO/THINKSTOCK — NAME: DES_001.JPG/PAGE: 220/CREDIT: © STOCKBYTE/THINKSTOCK — NAME: SKD186474SDC.JPG/PAGE: 221/CREDIT: © ISTOCKPHOTO/THINKSTOCK — NAME: 153893566.JPG/PAGE: 221/CREDIT: © ISTOCKPHOTO/THINKSTOCK — NAME: 166732724.JPG/PAGE: 222/CREDIT: © ISTOCKPHOTO/THINKSTOCK — NAME: 152539492.JPG/PAGE: 224/CREDIT: © ISTOCKPHOTO/THINKSTOCK — NAME: 140219493.JPG/PAGE: 225/CREDIT: © ISTOCKPHOTO/THINKSTOCK — NAME: 161947376.JPG/PAGE: 227/CREDIT: © ISTOCKPHOTO/THINKSTOCK — NAME: 78397101.JPG/PAGE: 232/CREDIT: © BRAND X PICTURES/THINKSTOCK — NAME: 100441955.JPG/PAGE: 238/CREDIT: © HEMERA/THINKSTOCK — NAME: 200413265-001.JPG/PAGE: 242/CREDIT: © STOCKBYTE/THINKSTOCK — NAME: 104113000.JPG/PAGE: 247/CREDIT: © ISTOCKPHOTO/THINKSTOCK — NAME: 111944267.JPG/PAGE: 249/CREDIT: © ISTOCKPHOTO/THINKSTOCK — NAME: 154197301.JPG/PAGE: 252/CREDIT: © ISTOCKPHOTO/THINKSTOCK — NAME: 100838175.JPG/PAGE: 257/CREDIT: © HEMERA/THINKSTOCK — NAME: dv1135098.JPG/PAGE: 262/CREDIT: © DIGITAL VISION/THINKSTOCK — NAME: 126840366.JPG/PAGE: 265/CREDIT: © ZOONAR/THINKSTOCK — NAME: 111957827.JPG/PAGE: 271/CREDIT: © ISTOCKPHOTO/THINKSTOCK — NAME: 135018438.JPG/PAGE: 280/CREDIT: © ISTOCKPHOTO/THINKSTOCK — NAME: 104451350.JPG/PAGE: 286/CREDIT: © ISTOCKPHOTO/THINKSTOCK — NAME: 78154471.JPG/PAGE: 290/CREDIT: © BANANASTOCK/THINKSTOCK — NAME: 78154749.JPG/PAGE: 297/CREDIT: © BANANASTOCK/THINKSTOCK — NAME: 75677151.JPG/PAGE: 302/CREDIT: © STOCKBYTE/THINKSTOCK — NAME: 80619183.JPG/PAGE: 311/CREDIT: © CREATAS/THINKSTOCK — NAME: STK323633RKN.JPG /PAGE: 314/CREDIT: © STOCKBYTE/THINKSTOCK — NAME: 161145408.JPG/PAGE: 320/CREDIT: © WAVEBREAK MEDIA/THINKSTOCK — NAME: 120416_MAYO_SLIDE7_SHOT20.PSD/PAGE: 327/CREDIT: © MFMER — NAME: 120416_MAYO_ SLIDE13_ SHOT28.TIF/PAGE: 327/CREDIT: © MFMER — NAME: Buttonhook_499.TIF/PAGE: 327/CREDIT: © MFMER — NAME: 120416_ MAYO_ SLIDE8_ SHOT21.TIF/PAGE: 327/CREDIT: © MFMER — NAME: DOORKNOBHANDLE_648.TIF/PAGE: 327/CREDIT: © MFMER — NAME: CANE.1.EPS/PAGE: 332/CREDIT: © MFMER — NAME: CANE.3.EPS/PAGE: 332/CREDIT: © MFMER — NAME: FIG60.JPG/PAGE: 332/CREDIT: © MFMER — NAME: FIG61.JPG/PAGE: 332/CREDIT: © MFMER — NAME: 86520278.JPG/PAGE: 334/CREDIT: © JUPITERIMAGES/COMSTOCK/THINKSTOCK — NAME: 157865736.JPG/PAGE: 352/CREDIT: © WAVEBREAK MEDIA/THINKSTOCK — NAME: 104832424.JPG/PAGE: 358/CREDIT: © ISTOCKPHOTO/THINKSTOCK — NAME: 105951730.JPG/PAGE: 381/CREDIT: © ISTOCKPHOTO/THINKSTOCK — NAME: 118838574.JPG/PAGE: 385/CREDIT: © ISTOCKPHOTO/THINKSTOCK

# Editorial staff

## Medical Editor
Edward T. Creagan, M.D., FAAHPM

## Managing Editor
Jennifer L. Duesterhoeft

## Product Manager
Christopher C. Frye

## Editorial Director
Paula M. Marlow Limbeck

## Creative Director
Daniel W. Brevick

## Art Director
Richard A. Resnick

## Illustrators
Joanna R. King, Michael A. King

## Editorial Research
Anthony J. Cook, Amanda K. Golden,
Deirdre A. Herman, Erika A. Riggin

## Proofreading
Miranda M. Attlesey, Donna L. Hanson,
Julie M. Maas

## Production
Downtown Bookworks, Inc., New York, NY
Sara N. DiSalvo, project manager
Laura J. Smyth, designer

## Contributing Editors and Reviewers
Julie A. Abbott, M.D.
Amindra S. Arora, M.B., B.Chir.
Ananda Basu, MBBS, M.D.
Brent A. Bauer, M.D.
J. Michael Bostwick, M.D.
Robert D. Brown, M.D.
Erik P. Castle, M.D.
April Chang-Miller, M.D.
Darryl S. Chutka, M.D.
Bart L. Clarke, M.D.
Stephanie S. Faubion, M.D.
Jean C. Fox, M.D.
Martha Grogan, M.D.
David S. Knopman, M.D.
Keith G. Kramlinger, M.D.
Edward R. Laskowski, M.D.
Mark Liebow, M.D.
Scott C. Litin, M.D.
Charles L. Loprinzi, M.D.
David E. Midthun, M.D.
Jennifer K. Nelson, R.D., L.D.
Paul D. Pettit, M.D.
Sheldon G. Sheps, M.D.
Lynne T. Shuster, M.D.
Paul Y. Takahashi, M.D.
John M. Wilkinson, M.D.

## Indexer
Steve Rath

## Administrative Assistant
Beverly J. Steele

# Preface

This book is one of the most important purchases you'll ever make. Why? Because it can help ensure that your later years are some of your best years.

Everybody knows the numbers; everybody reads the newspapers. We all know that individuals are living far longer now than in any time in history. We all know that modern medicine and technologies have pushed the envelope so that many people are still "finding themselves" well into their 80s and 90s. Does this happen by luck? Is this a roll of the dice? Absolutely not.

Living healthy isn't simply a reflection of personal genetics. It results from a combination of many factors including fitness, nutrition, preventive care, your personal outlook and your relationships — in addition to genetic influences. In other words, good health and well-being are generally the result of smart decisions and the right attitude.

*Mayo Clinic on Healthy Aging* is a compass. It's an instruction manual to help guide you and give you the tools you need to live life to its maximum — to do the things you've always wanted to do.

This book provides you the motivation, energy and knowledge to craft a future that's fulfilling and invigorating — no matter what that may be. The dedicated individuals who put this book together want you to fully enjoy what can be the most creative and meaningful years of your life.

The ball is in your court. Your hands are at the helm. The quality of your life now and in the future depends on the choices that you make today. Choose wisely!

Good luck and all the best as your personal journey unfolds.

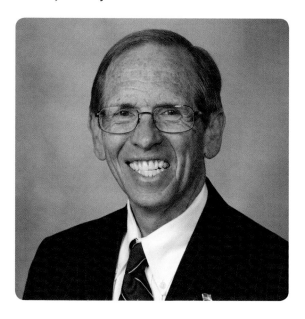

Edward T. Creagan, M.D., FAAHPM
*Medical Editor*

# Table of contents

# Part 1

# Taking charge of your future

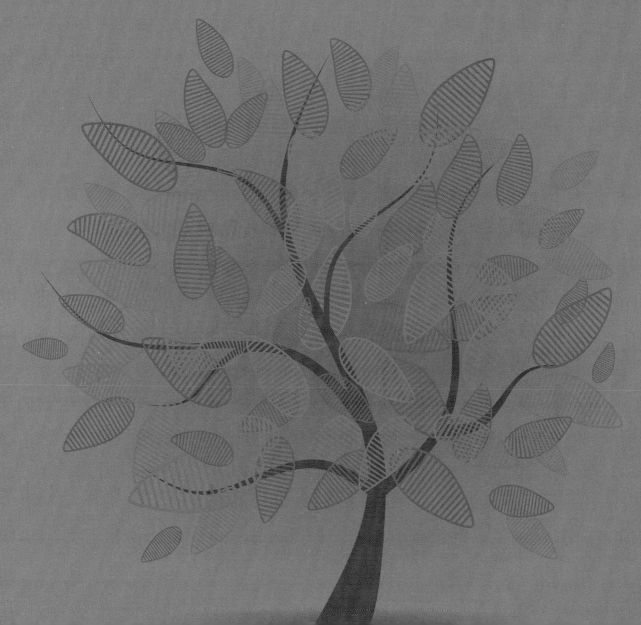

# Chapter 1

# It's all about attitude

You don't like the thought of growing older? Well, guess what? You don't have to. Sure, the calendar may remind you that another year has passed, but that doesn't mean that you have to act, feel or look like you're old.

Getting older is a choice, not a sentence. You can just as easily make up your mind — and tell your body — to remain at age 50 the rest of your life, as you can accept the physical and mental declines associated with passage into your 60s, your 70s, your 80s and beyond.

The truth is, aging isn't a roll of the dice. You don't have to get old, if you don't want to. That's because getting older doesn't inevitably lead to disease, decline and dependence, as so many people believe. No matter what your chronological age, you can continue to enjoy good health, happiness and an active lifestyle.

Think about it. The years ahead can truly be a time of growth, creativity and renewal. Now that your children are grown up and out of the house and with more time on your hands, you finally can take the time to do the things you always wanted to do. For many people, these years present an opportunity to explore and discover new things, pursue long-awaited goals, nurture relationships and live with a keener sense of purpose and meaning. The "golden years" can be rich, indeed.

If you haven't yet reached retirement, it'll come sooner than you think — and it's never too early to start thinking ahead. To truly enjoy the years that await you, it's important to make good choices now that will lead you down the right path.

This book explores many aspects of what you need to do and need to know to live stronger, longer and healthier at any age! The chapters that follow will provide you with tips, tools and strategies to help you feel young for years to come. Keep in mind, there's no single definition of "successful aging." The process unfolds continually and varies from one person to another. If you've got the right attitude, the choices you make will be the right ones.

To get the most out of what's often termed the best years of your life, your first challenge is to examine your ideas and attitudes about aging.

# A new perspective on age-old questions

Since the dawn of history, philosophers, poets, scientists and explorers have set out to understand the mysteries of aging. What does it mean to grow older? How can we live longer? What creates fulfilling later years? Though no one has discovered the Fountain of Youth yet, ideas about age have certainly changed.

## What's old?

Wearing tight jeans and a leather jacket, Mick Jagger can tear up the stage and work a crowd into a frenzy. Is this guy old? Most people would say no. But Jagger is turning 70. Some of his contemporaries in their 60s and early 70s: Robert De Niro, Paul McCartney, Cher, Harrison Ford, Martha Stewart, Bruce Springsteen and Sigourney Weaver. Little Richard, Jack Nicholson, Dustin Hoffman and Clint Eastwood are even older. They are the new faces of "old."

It's not just rock stars and celebrities who are redefining what it means to be old. Across America, millions of older people are using their later years to create new lives. They're trying new careers, volunteering, going back to school and pursuing passions.

Clearly, old isn't what it used to be. And as America's 76 million baby boomers approach retirement, the definition of old will continue to evolve.

## Age is what you make of it

Age isn't just a number. Reaching age 18 doesn't automatically make someone a grown-up. This same way, you're not suddenly "old" when you hit 65, become a grandparent or go through menopause. You're only old when you think you are and act like it. Age is an attitude. Once again, just in case you missed it — age is an attitude. Of course, aging is a physical process. But it also encompasses the mental, emotional and spiritual aspects of a person.

While your body ages to some degree, your mind, for the most part, will stay as young as you feel. If you expect to live a long life filled with physical vitality, humor and close relationships, that belief can become the internal map that guides your future. But if you're convinced that your later years will bring emptiness, depression and sickness, these negative beliefs can actually make you age faster.

In a study of women's attitudes as they move into their 50s, 60s and 70s, more than half define aging well as feeling great, no matter what their age. They don't see themselves as slowing down or stopping — they're just getting started. Four in 10 women older than age 65 said there's no age they'd define

as "old." Most people who live long, healthy lives aren't exceptional. They're just regular folks who don't equate "old" with illness and inactivity. They keep running companies, painting, playing the piano, skiing, swimming, helping in the community, and enjoying good times with friends and family.

## What's a long life?

"Anyone can get old," said Groucho Marx. "All you have to do is live long enough."

"Long enough" is a relative concept, especially when viewed through the lens of history. One way to define a long life is to measure it against the average life expectancy — the average number of years a person can expect to live. In 2009, the latest figures available, the average life expectancy at birth in the United States was 78.5 years. But some of us will live to be more than 100.

Life expectancy has risen steadily over the centuries. During the Roman Empire, the average person reached the ripe old age of 22 years. By the Middle Ages, a person in England could expect to live to 33. In the early 1900s, life expectancies in developed countries ranged from 35 to 55.

# Saving the best for last

Creativity and productivity are ageless. Here are some well-known people who achieved great things in their later years.

- Frank Lloyd Wright was working on the Guggenheim Museum when he died at age 91.
- Georgia O'Keeffe kept painting well into her 90s, even as her eyesight failed.
- At age 70, Dr. William W. Mayo founded Mayo Clinic.
- Homemaker Irma Rombauer wrote *Joy of Cooking* at age 60.
- Former President Ronald Reagan was elected to his second term at age 73.
- Laura Ingalls Wilder wrote the "Little House" books in her 50s and 60s.
- Astronaut John Glenn returned to space at age 77, more than three decades after his first mission.
- In his 60s, Tom Coughlin coached the New York Giants to two Super Bowl wins.
- Michelangelo finished his last frescoes in the Vatican at age 75.
- At age 68, Lillian Carter, mother of former President Jimmy Carter, joined the Peace Corps and served for two years in India.
- Benjamin Franklin invented bifocal glasses when he was 78, to help correct his own poor vision.
- When she was 71, Coco Chanel introduced the Chanel suit.
- Robert Penn Warren became the first official poet laureate of the United States at age 80.
- At age 89, Mary Fasano became the oldest person to earn a degree from Harvard University.
- At 95, dancer and choreographer Martha Graham premiered her work Maple Leaf Rag.

# How long can you expect to live?

This chart shows how many more years, on average, a person can expect to live, based on current age, sex and race. Of course, these are just general estimates. If you smoke or drive without a seat belt, you lower your odds. If you have a healthy lifestyle, you might beat the odds.

**Average number of years remaining**

| Current age | All races male | All races female | White male | White female | Black male | Black female |
|---|---|---|---|---|---|---|
| 50 | 29.0 | 32.7 | 29.2 | 32.7 | 25.2 | 30.2 |
| 55 | 24.9 | 28.2 | 25.0 | 28.3 | 21.5 | 26.1 |
| 60 | 20.9 | 23.9 | 21.0 | 24.0 | 18.2 | 22.2 |
| 65 | 17.2 | 19.9 | 17.2 | 19.8 | 15.1 | 18.5 |
| 70 | 13.7 | 16.0 | 13.7 | 16.0 | 12.3 | 15.1 |
| 75 | 10.6 | 12.5 | 10.6 | 12.4 | 9.8 | 12.0 |
| 80 | 7.9 | 9.4 | 7.9 | 9.3 | 7.7 | 9.3 |
| 85 | 5.8 | 6.8 | 5.7 | 6.8 | 6.0 | 7.1 |

Source: National Vital Statistics Reports, 2011

Life expectancy also varies according to where you live. Americans aren't the longest-lived people in the world. That distinction belongs to the Japanese, who live on average to almost age 83.

Other factors affect life expectancy, too. Women live longer than do men. In the United States, white individuals tend to outlive black individuals. For a white woman, life expectancy in 2007 was 80.8 years. For a black man, it was 70.0.

## Genes and long life

Many people assume that longevity depends to a great extent on inheriting good genes. No matter how much or little they exercise or how healthy or unhealthy their diet is, they figure their health in later years will be determined by genes. That's a myth.

Genes play only a minor role in longevity. Your gene pool is responsible for

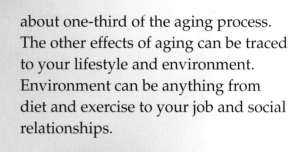

about one-third of the aging process. The other effects of aging can be traced to your lifestyle and environment. Environment can be anything from diet and exercise to your job and social relationships.

Genes may cause premature death from conditions such as Huntington's disease and cystic fibrosis. But once you've survived into later life, your own behavior plays a much more important role in future longevity.

If your father and grandfather both died young of a heart attack, you may be inclined to believe the same fate awaits you. But while you may have a genetic tendency for heart disease, factors such as diet, exercise, blood pressure, stress and tobacco use play significant roles in whether you actually develop a heart condition. You can outfox some of your genes.

## What's a better life?

Living well means more than just living longer. Longevity doesn't mean much if you're lonely, bored, depressed or in poor health. There's a difference between more years alive and more life. Some people live to a very old age but are miserable and bitter. Others find a

# Simple recipe for a good life

If you're the type that likes things short and sweet, here's one definition of a good life you may appreciate. A good life is having:

- **Someone to love.** People generally are healthier and happier when they have someone or something to love or care for, whether that's a spouse, children, grandchildren or a pet. Spending time with family and friends helps ward off depression and reinforces healthy behaviors.
- **Something to do.** When you're actively engaged in the world, you feel challenged and productive, which is key to satisfaction. Being involved — seeking opportunities to learn, build and love — gives you a sense of purpose and identity.
- **Something to look forward to.** For many people, later life is a time to explore new ventures, give back to others in the community, or share wisdom with family and friends. People like to know that they've challenged themselves or that they've made a difference — and to see the outcomes of their efforts.

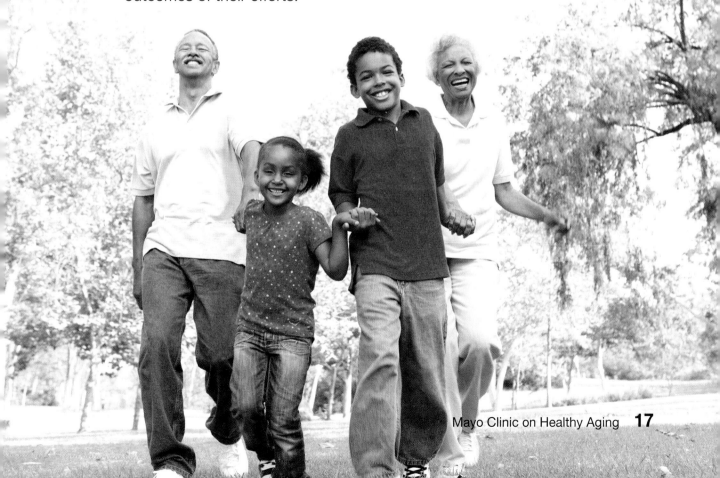

sense of purpose and zest for life even though they have a chronic illness or disability.

The top concern people express as they enter their later years isn't money worries or physical problems, but a sense of meaning and purpose in life. For many people, a fulfilling life — or a "better life" — is one in which they feel they've made a contribution, no matter how small or big that may be. Yes, optimal aging includes good health, but it also encompasses love, companionship, creativity, productivity, concern for others, learning and a hopeful outlook.

# How to live to your full potential

Good health and well-being don't happen by accident. They depend on the decisions you make and the habits you adopt. To fully enjoy the years ahead of you, you need to take steps to safeguard your health.

The American Cancer Society predicts that more than half of all cancer deaths could be prevented if Americans just took better care of themselves — stopped smoking, exercised more, ate

healthier and got recommended screening tests. And studies show that regardless of whether you're 50 or 70, exercising every day or nearly every day can reduce your risk of heart attack, stroke, high blood pressure, diabetes, osteoporosis and other health problems.

It's also important to remember that you're more than just your body. Good health means staying strong emotionally and mentally — having an optimistic attitude and maintaining connections with friends, family and community.

Not all diseases and conditions are avoidable. However, many of the most serious ones can be prevented by adopting habits and behaviors that promote good health. This book discusses key factors to not only good health, but also an enjoyable and meaningful life. They include:

- Having a purpose in life
- Enjoying a healthy diet
- Keeping physically active
- Maintaining a healthy weight
- Avoiding tobacco and excessive alcohol
- Preparing for retirement
- Challenging your brain
- Keeping socially and spiritually connected

- Cultivating a positive attitude
- Seeing your doctor regularly

By following these steps you'll feel good about yourself — and as a result, come across as young — no matter what your age.

This doesn't mean you have to focus on your health to the exclusion of all other things. Good health is simply about keeping your life balanced and making sure that the choices you make now will benefit you in the years to come.

And, remember, it's never too late to clean up your act. For instance, if you quit smoking, your risk of heart disease begins to fall almost immediately. And after five years have passed, your risk of a stroke is about the same as it is for someone who never smoked at all.

## What are your goals?

Most people fantasize about how they'll spend their later years — working on their golf game, travel-ing, painting, reading all

# A tale of two couples

Following are the stories of two couples and how their actions — or their inactions — have affected their retirement. Both couples had goals for their later years — visions of how they wanted to spend their retirement days.

One couple has been able to fully enjoy their time together. For the other couple, retirement hasn't gone quite as they had hoped.

Are you on the right path to getting the most out of your best years?

## Dealing with the hand they dealt

Mary and John seemingly had everything. In their middle 40s, they had a profitable business, their children were doing well in school, and any concerns about health and wellness were simply in the far-distant future. They felt no need to exercise, no need to watch what they ate, no need to ratchet down their stress level. They had "the world by the tail." Then the world started to come crashing down.

In his late 40s, John awoke on a Monday morning with crushing chest pain like an elephant was standing on his chest. John was rushed to the hospital and underwent a dye test showing severe blockage of multiple coronary arteries, which supply blood to the heart muscle. John underwent a quadruple vessel bypass, had a stormy recovery, but did recover. John was told that if he didn't exercise, change his diet and decrease his frantic lifestyle, he would be facing big trouble. Like many individuals, John thought he was "bulletproof" and made virtually no changes to his daily routine.

In her late 40s, Mary also was told that the quality and quantity of her life would be severely compromised unless she watched her weight, quit smoking and let go of some of her many civic and community responsibilities. Despite some emerging medical problems, Mary kept going. She didn't have time to worry about her health.

The realization of their actions — or inactions — came just a few years ago. A once in a lifetime opportunity arose when they received an invitation to tour some of the major capitals of Europe, an award John had won for his years of leadership. They were in a group of approximately 18 to 20 fellow travelers. The trip was not particularly arduous, but by midday John and Mary clearly "ran out of steam." Because of their weight, each developed back pain, hip pain and severe knee pain. Both were taking handfuls of pain medications, which in turn caused stomach upset and required the use of additional medications. They simply couldn't keep up with their fellow travelers, some who were 10 to 15 years older.

John and Mary are now nearing 60 and still headed down the same path, knowing they're on an unhealthy course. The two had looked forward to spending time with their grandchildren. However, neither has the energy nor the vitality to go to the park, the zoo or the circus.

The ultimate tragedy is that John and Mary's present circumstances were clearly predictable, avoidable and modifiable. By making a few changes in their lives, these golden years could have been wonderful.

Is it too late for John and Mary to set out in a new direction? Absolutely not.

## Looking forward to each tomorrow

Ken sums up the sweetness of his retirement years by quoting author Tom Robbins: "It's never too late to have a happy childhood."

Now 74, Ken retired 15 years ago after working steadily since age 12, when he got his first part-time job. Growing up, he was expected to contribute to the family income. He didn't have much time to just kick back and be a kid. So when he retired, Ken reacquainted himself with some of life's simpler pleasures.

"At first, while my wife, AJ, was still working, retirement meant I could read all day if I chose, and sometimes I did," Ken says. "I also bought a basketball, and I remember shooting a lot of baskets on my own that first year after I retired. I rode bicycle a lot, too. I played video games. I watched movies. I think I was enjoying some of the childhood I had missed."

The following year, AJ retired, at age 58. They were both in good health and were financially secure. "We had no outstanding debts, our house and car were paid for and our three children were 'launched,'" Ken says. "We lived sensibly and had been saving money for years." Starting with this solid foundation, the couple created a satisfying new life for themselves.

Ken and AJ hadn't necessarily planned to retire early, but both had experiences that spurred them into action. Ken's wake-up call came with the death of a good friend. "John was just a little older than me, and our interests were very similar," Ken explains. "He had a heart attack in his late 50s, and not long after that he chose to take early retirement. He moved to the south coast of England and was really enjoying life when he got an aggressive cancer and died a few months later.

"Looking back now, I know that John's death affected me profoundly. My father had died of cancer at age 47. I began to dread being deprived of my 'golden years.'" After his friend's death, Ken made the decision to retire.

AJ had a similar aha moment. One of her colleagues, who retired at age 65, became ill and died suddenly. "It made me realize that there were things I wanted to do before I died, so maybe I should take early retirement."

For AJ, one of the greatest rewards of retirement is being able to travel and do other things without the time constraints of a full-time job. The couple travels three or four times a year. Visits to their children and grandchildren take them to both coasts, and they visit England or other parts of Europe every year. The two find traveling broadening and educational. "We read about the countries we plan to visit so we know what we want to do and see," says AJ.

AJ and Ken have also pursued "a whole new bunch of interests and activities," as AJ puts it. She has taken college courses in French, music appreciation and piano. She and a friend regularly attend orchestra concerts. AJ has a long list of books to read, and every spring she can't wait to start working in her flower garden.

Ken got his first computer after retiring. Having a keen interest in England, he found an online group of like-minded enthusiasts who share observations and travel tips. Ken is also learning about woodcarving and enjoys cooking.

Both Ken and AJ try to follow a healthy lifestyle. They walk at least 30 minutes a day most days and eat a healthy diet. Both volunteer at a nearby hospital, and they share a love for their two cats.

Ken and AJ have noticed some challenges with age. Ken used to be a marathoner, but injuries curtailed his running days. Staying physically active isn't always easy.

AJ says she isn't as strong as she used to be. "I need to pace myself more than in the past. When we are having company, I start planning more ahead of time."

Still, both are thoroughly enjoying this stage of their lives. "I feel at peace," Ken says.

those books they never got around to, fixing up the house.

What are your dreams? What do you want to do each day? Remember, the possibilities are limitless. Jim, a former executive in the computer industry, turned his energy to curriculum development for a college. Rudy, who used to own a restaurant, now volunteers at an art museum, giving tours. Two sisters retired from their city jobs to run a small cafe in Wyoming. Bob and Joan are touring the country in a recreational vehicle, earning money along the way by working at state parks. It's common to hear older adults say they're busier now than when they were working. That's good!

Take a few minutes now to think about the years ahead of you. What are your goals? Do you have a plan — or an idea — for how you want to spend these years? Identify some things that you'd like to achieve in different areas of your life. Your goals can be as simple as meeting friends for coffee a couple of times a week or as complex as opening a bed-and-breakfast or going back to school.

Why do this? Because goals give you something to strive for, a reason to live, something to look forward to. Whether they're short-term or long-term, small or big, goals can make life happier and more meaningful. Let curiosity and passion be your guides. And aim for what's most important to you. Your goals might be things you've always wanted to do but have never tried, or something that you've never even considered.

As you read through this book, keep your goals in mind.

# Chapter 2

# Planning ahead

Today's baby boomers are redefining what it means to retire. They see retirement as a time to retool their lifestyles and revitalize their lives rather than sit back and watch the grass grow.

Retirement simply isn't what it used to be. Americans who retire today at ages 65 to 67 still have one-quarter to one-third of their lives left to live after retirement. In contrast, when Social Security was launched in 1935, life expectancy was about age 63, so most people lived just a few years past retirement, if they made it that far.

With so many years to spend in this next phase of life, you need activities to fill your day and money to live on. That's why the prospect of retirement is both exciting and scary for many people. Exciting because of the many opportunities it presents — to pursue interests, travel, start a new business or different type of career, spend time with family, learn, and explore. Scary in that along with freedom and new hobbies come worries. Will I have enough money to live comfortably? Where will the money come from? Will I be bored? Will I miss work and colleagues?

Retirement is a huge step and an important transition. Like any major life change, retirement can be stressful. It brings changes in your daily routine, income and financial status, family relationships and friendships, social roles, and identity. Some people handle the changes well and others don't.

Having a plan can help you manage the stresses and anxiety of retirement and will give you a much better chance of enjoying this exciting stage of your life. This chapter provides suggestions for what you should be thinking about now — before you're retired — to help make the transition a smooth one. If you're already retired, we provide some tips on ways to enjoy this new phase of your life.

# The importance of early planning

While it's impossible to predict exactly how your retirement will go, a realistic plan for the future can increase your odds of achieving your goals and dreams. Research suggests that people who plan ahead end up with more resources when they're ready to retire. When you establish your basic goals — including your retirement age, the lifestyle you want and the income you'll need — then you can plot how to achieve them.

Even if you love your job and plan to keep working as long as possible, it's still important to have a financial plan in case your work or health status changes. You'll want to have enough money saved so that work is an option rather than a necessity.

But retirement planning involves more than putting away money. You also need to think about what you'll do with your time when work and commuting no longer consume 40 to 60 hours a week. Planning ahead can ensure a retirement that's emotionally and physically satisfying as well as financially secure.

## Start sooner — not later

Many people put off planning for retirement. They may find the process daunting or downright scary. Or they think it's fine to wait until a year or so before retiring to start thinking about what's next. Others worry that investing for retirement is a dicey proposition, given the ups and downs in the stock market.

Retirement planning — both the financial and lifestyle aspects — should start early. Ideally, you should begin saving money early in your career and continue to do so steadily until you stop working. But no matter what your age, it's never too late to start saving money or to save more. For every 10 years that you put off setting aside money for retirement, you'll have to save three times as much to reach your nest egg goal.

It's equally important to think about what you're going to do during retirement well before you actually retire. Even people who have thoroughly charted the financial side of retirement often haven't given the same thought to how they'll spend their time during retirement or where they'll live. As one retiree noted, "Some people spend more time planning a two-week vacation than they do planning their retirement."

Start the planning process when you're in your late 40s and early 50s. If you wait until you're on the verge of retiring, you may find that you can't afford to do the things you want to. People who count on developing new interests or becoming involved in new activities after retirement often find these things don't happen. Midlife is the time to cultivate the habits of body, mind and heart.

# Questions to guide your planning

As you start planning for retirement, there are a number of issues to consider. Do you want to retire early, or will you continue to work at least part time past your full retirement age? Do you plan to travel extensively? How's your health? Do you hope to move when you retire? What other financial goals do you have besides retirement?

Once you've figured out your priorities, goals and hopes, you can take steps to reach them. The following questions will help you plan and dream.

## What am I going to do?

When you retire, you may find yourself with more free time on your hands than you've had since the summer vacations of your youth — maybe more than ever. This prospect triggers delight and anticipation in some people and dread and anxiety in others.

Many people look forward to the leisure time they'll have for gardening, traveling, painting, golfing and spending time with grandchildren. They intend to fully savor the freedom to sleep in or take a daily nap.

If you've worked all your life, it may indeed feel good to "do nothing" for a while. But after the first few months, the allure of endless free time begins to fade. Many retirees struggle to find activities that are meaningful. Even if you live in a warm climate and play golf every day, you still likely won't be able to fill every minute with leisure activities. Spending time with the grandkids is great, but how many hours a day can you do that?

For individuals who have been so centered on their careers, they can't imagine life without the structure, the routine and the rewards of work. They have trouble envisioning life after retirement and sometimes even refuse to acknowledge that their work patterns will change as they grow older. This is a particular risk for the high performer — failing to plan for retirement is the Achilles' heel of many corporate superstars.

Either approach to retirement — rosy fantasy or utter denial — lacks a sense of reality. A realistic plan should focus on specific activities you anticipate being involved in. The more specific you can be about how you want to spend your time, the more likely it is that you'll be able to turn that vision into reality.

Chapter 3 delves further into this topic and can help you explore and identify activities after retirement that not only are enjoyable but also provide satisfaction and meaning.

## Am I healthy?

Good health is an important component of quality of life in your retirement years. Even very old people can lead vigorous, active, involved and productive lives if they're reasonably healthy. If you're in poor health or have a disability, you'll be limited in what you can do with your free time.

In planning your retirement, consider how physically active your lifestyle will be. Do you see yourself golfing, playing tennis, walking, hiking or swimming? What about playing with your grandchildren or traveling? You need to be in good physical shape for these activities.

Before you retire, take a good look at your health. Are you in shape now, or do you need to take steps to improve your health so that you can enjoy an active retirement? If you haven't seen a doctor in a while, schedule a checkup.

If you have concerns about your health or have a chronic medical condition such as a heart condition or diabetes, talk to your doctor about things you can do now to ensure optimal fitness as you get older. For example, if you're overweight, talk to your doctor about a sensible plan for losing weight.

Establishing a habit of regular physical activity now not only will help keep you in shape so that you can enjoy a variety of activities later but also is an excellent way to ease the stress of the transition to retirement. It also gives you something to do on a daily basis and can serve as a base from which to explore new sports or hobbies.

## Am I financially stable?

Financial security is one of the major concerns — and stressors — among people approaching retirement age. Whatever your retirement plans, you'll need money to live comfortably and do many of the things you enjoy. Almost everyone wonders if they'll have enough money for retirement.

Unlike previous generations of retirees, who got by on Social Security, company pensions and small savings accounts, most people now are largely responsible for planning their own retirement. And today's retirees have to account for many more years of retirement than earlier generations did.

Living well in retirement requires skillful planning, saving and investing. Without good planning and discipline, there's no guarantee that your retire-ment income will cover your expenses, let alone allow you to travel or buy that lake cabin you dream of.

The sooner you start planning financially for retirement, the better. If your figures come up short, you may be able to take action to make up the difference.

### How much money will I need?

The first step in figuring how much you'll need is to establish your retirement goals, including the age at which you want to retire and the lifestyle you'd like to lead. On average, most people should plan to live 30 years past retirement.

The age at which you retire can have a big impact on how much money you'll need for retirement. By working longer, you'll have more time to put money into your retirement accounts. In addition, you won't be drawing money out of them as soon, allowing them to continue to grow. The earlier you want to retire, the longer your assets will need to last.

Your retirement age also affects your Social Security benefits. In 2013, for example, partial benefits begin at age 62, while full benefits are available between ages 65 and 67, depending on your year of birth. For each

## Financial security and your health

It's well known that money doesn't buy happiness — before or after retirement. But not having enough money can be a major source of stress. And the stress of not having adequate financial resources can affect your health.

Research indicates that people with sound finances generally cope better with illness than do people who don't have the funds they need. One likely reason is that they're not burdened by the stress and anxiety of the cost of their medical care.

Along with diet, exercise and social ties, adequate financial resources are a component of well-being. You don't have to be rich, but it helps to have a feeling of financial security.

year beyond that you wait to begin collecting Social Security, your benefit increases until age 70. Your benefit is reduced, however, if you begin collecting it as soon as you're eligible, at age 62.

Calculate your expenses. Once you've determined at what age you'll likely retire, the next step is to calculate how much money you think you'll need for retirement. Many financial planners use ballpark figures, such as 80 to 100 percent of your pre-retirement income, adjusted for inflation. But depending on your individual circumstances, you may need more or less than what you make before retiring.

If you plan to travel a lot or move to a more expensive area, you may need a higher yearly income than you had before retiring. But many retirees can live comfortably on less — especially if you've paid off your mortgage, you plan to downsize your home or you have fewer expenses, such as education for your children. Keep in mind, though, that your health care costs are likely to go up in retirement, and taxes will continue to take a portion of your money.

To estimate your retirement expenses, you have to know how much you're

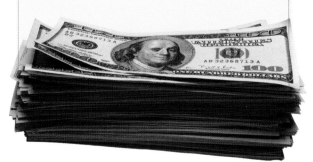

spending now. If you don't keep track of your expenses on a yearly basis, start now. Over the next year, record approximately how much money you spend on various items and activities.

A quick way to get a ballpark figure of your annual expenses is to take your after-tax income, and deduct from it the amount of money you contribute yearly to your retirement and savings accounts. If, for example, you earned $65,000 after taxes and you contributed $5,000 to your retirement account and deposited $5,000 into savings, you'd subtract $10,000 from $65,000. That leaves $55,000, a reasonable approximation of your current spending.

### Where will the money come from?
Most people fund their retirement through a combination of income sources and investments. Options for these may include:

**Pension plan.** About 20 percent of American workers at private companies, and many government workers, are covered by traditional pension plans. Defined-benefit plans offer regular payments throughout retirement.

**Social Security.** Social Security pays the average retiree about 40 percent of pre-retirement earnings. Although looming shortfalls in Social Security funds have made headlines and prompted political debate, for now the system is still running as promised. It's possible that future retirees will see their benefits trimmed or postponed. But if you're near retirement or already retired, it's probably safe to assume you'll get your currently scheduled benefits.

The higher your pre-retirement income, the smaller the role Social Security will play in your retirement income.

**Part-time work.** More than three-fourths of future retirees plan to work at least part time during retirement, according to AARP (formerly known as the American Association of Retired Persons). But it's important to be realistic about how much money this will bring in. Moving in and out of the workforce is more difficult after age 70, and many of the jobs people take in retirement pay less than did their previous employment. For example, if you move from a corporate job to part-time consulting or running a small business, you may make considerably less money. In general, earnings from work shouldn't form a core part of your retirement plan.

**Retirement savings and investments.** The difference between your projected retirement income and your retirement expenses can be made up by pre-retirement savings. Your investment portfolio may include a tax sheltered savings plan, such as a 401(k), 403(b) or profit-sharing plan offered by your employer, or an individual retirement account (IRA). When planning for retirement, assume a conservative rate of return on your investments — 4 to 8 percent.

To weather the ups and downs of the financial markets, experts recommend diversifying your investments in different industries and different forms, such as stocks, bonds, mutual funds and real estate. Diversification is more important than ever, given the stock market downturns of the past decade. If you happen to retire when the market is down, you could end up with much less income than you expected.

### Am I on track?

Compare how much money you think you'll need to retire with how much you're likely to have, based on your current savings and investment patterns. If you need help in doing this, you can seek the help of a financial planner. Otherwise, software tools are available that calculate retirement projections. And several websites offer online calculators that help you determine if you're saving enough for

retirement. To see if you can afford your retirement dreams, estimate the expenses involved in various lifestyle activities and compare the results with your projected income and savings.

If your calculations show that you're not on track for attaining your goals, re-evaluate your plans and consider what changes could be made, such as working longer or saving more. Conventional wisdom holds that most people should put away yearly at least 10 percent of their annual gross income toward retirement. But if you've procrastinated saving and are far short of your goal, you'll need to save significantly more than that.

**Account for inflation.** Remember to adjust your figures for inflation. Even modest inflation can rob your dollars of their value — your money will buy less when you retire than it will today. The average yearly inflation rate since 1953 has been between 3 and 4 percent. Therefore, a reasonable assumption for inflation is about 3 to 4 percent a year.

### What if I'm coming up short?

If you've put off saving for retirement, you're not alone. The majority of Americans never calculate how much they need to save for retirement, and many Americans age 55 and older have saved

# Is a financial planner in your future?

To understand the big picture when it comes to financial planning, you either need to inform yourself about retirement planning or work with a financial adviser you trust.

A professional financial planner can help you make retirement planning decisions that are right for you. A planner can assist with your retirement goals and will look at your net worth (assets minus liabilities), current and projected spending, and sources of income. With your goals in mind, a planner can determine how much money you'll need to live on each month, taking into account taxes and inflation. And he or she can identify how much additional money you need to save to get there.

There are many types of financial advisers, including insurance brokers and bankers, who offer financial planning and advice. A certified financial planner (CFP) has obtained certification in financial planning. The required course of study includes retirement, insurance, investments and estate planning.

Make sure to choose a competent and qualified financial planner. Here are some questions you may want to ask when selecting a planner:

- What experience do you have?
- What are your qualifications?
- What services do you offer?
- What is your approach to financial planning?
- Will you be the only person working with me?
- How are you paid for your services?
- How much do you charge?
- Have you ever been publicly disciplined for any unlawful or unethical actions in your professional career?

Make sure you understand the services that will be provided — and how you fit in. Set specific, measurable goals. For example, instead of saying you want to be "comfortable" in retirement, quantify what that means. Ask questions about the recommendations your planner gives you. And be sure to re-evaluate your retirement plan periodically to make sure you're meeting your long-term goals.

less than $100,000. About two-thirds of older adults rely on Social Security for half or more of their income.

There are many possible detours on the road to a comfortable retirement — job loss, divorce, illness, disability, falling interest rates on fixed-income investments and stock market dips. Thousands of people have lost benefits when traditional pension plans failed because of company bankruptcies. Even without a catastrophic event, many family budgets are so tight that saving for retirement is impossible.

If you're coming up short on the money you need to retire, you can take steps to catch up:

**Delay retirement.** Postponing your retirement, even by a few years, gives you more time to save money, reduces the time you're living off your retirement money and may increase your Social Security benefit. If your employer offers medical coverage, working longer can also reduce your health care costs.

**Reduce your projected spending.** Consider downsizing your home or relocating to a lower cost area. If the value of your home has increased significantly, you may be able to come away with

a handsome profit. Moving from an expensive area to a place with a lower cost of living can make your money go much further. You can also cut spending on clothing and big-ticket items such as cars.

**Pay off your mortgage.** Getting rid of your mortgage by the time you retire can shave off thousands of dollars in interest and considerably lower your expenses. Another option may be to take out a reverse mortgage, a loan that allows borrowers age 62 and older to convert their home equity into tax-free monthly income. When the homeowner (or surviving spouse) dies, the loan is repaid from the sale of the house. Talk with a financial advisor about the pros and cons of these steps.

**Boost your savings.** Workers age 50 and older are able to contribute more to their 401(k) and IRA plans each year than are younger people. But you should also be aware of the tax implications of your investments, so that your contributions now aren't surpassed by your tax bills in retirement.

**Continue working part time.** Even a lower paying job can make a difference.

**Sell a valuable asset.** If you have a vacation home or other valuable asset, you could consider selling it and investing the money you make from the sale.

**Investigate your investment withdrawal options.** In general, it's best not to take money out of an IRA or 401(k) for as long as possible, so that you can take full advantage of the tax-deferred growth. At age 70½, you're required to begin withdrawing a minimum amount of funds from these accounts. But you do have options about how much and when to withdraw, and it's worth exploring what your best option is to stretch your retirement dollars.

# Where am I going to live?

Another major decision that often comes with retirement is where to live. Many retirees sell their house and move to a warmer climate or a retirement community. Others prefer to stay in their homes.

The decision about whether and where to move is a complex one, with many factors to consider.

**Economics.** If you live in a large urban area where the cost of living is high, it makes financial sense for you to relocate to a less expensive place, such as a smaller community in a state with low

or no income taxes. On the other hand, if your retirement dream is to live in a coastal area, your housing and other costs might increase.

**Lifestyle preferences.** Consider the kind of community you want to live in. Are cultural events important to you? Are there other retirees to socialize with? What recreational activities do you want to pursue? If you live in a northern state and hope to do a lot of golfing, hiking or biking, moving to a warmer climate may be appealing. If you want to keep working in some capacity, look for an area with a robust economy.

**Resources.** It's important to learn about the resources and services available for older adults in a community. These might include transportation, medical care and safety issues. If you currently use a state service, you'll need to find out if it's available in another state and what the eligibility requirements are.

## Moving vs. staying put
You may have good reasons to relocate, but before pulling up stakes, take time to think through the implications. Moving may result in the loss of some important connections. Most retirement experts advise staying close to friends and family. Retirement is a major life change, and you'll want to have a

support system in place to help with the transition. In addition, if you have aging parents, it may be challenging moving far from them. Finally, if you plan to work part time or as a consultant in your field, you may not have the network of contacts you need to establish yourself in another city.

Before moving to a new place, give it a trial run first. Rent a condo, house or apartment for at least a month or two to get to know the area. If you feel uncomfortable in the new surroundings, ask yourself why. It takes time to adjust to any new place, but if you keep feeling unsure, this might not be the right move for you.

### Is my home suitable for retirement?

Many people prefer to remain in their homes after retiring. But it's worthwhile to think about whether your home will continue to meet your needs as you get older. For example, if you have a bad hip or knee and have trouble climbing stairs, a two-story house may not be practical. Can your home be adapted if your physical abilities change?

Another point to consider is whether your neighborhood has taken a turn for the worse over the years. Has your once-desirable neighborhood seen an increase in crime or a loss of community resources, such as grocery stores or pharmacies? Having access to public transportation or local services may become more important.

You should also think about the expense of keeping up your home. Even if you've paid off your mortgage, you may need a new roof or windows, or maybe your furnace and other utilities are older and in need of replacement.

Many housing options, including condominiums and retirement communities, are geared specifically to retirees. Condos offer the comforts of home without all the upkeep. A retirement community can provide a variety of activities and services, such as social events and transportation and security. Life in a retirement community isn't for everyone, though. Some communities have restrictions on guests and pets. And some retirees miss being around people of all ages.

# Are you ready to retire?

After all the planning and preparation comes the decision to actually retire.

Are you ready? In addition to being financially prepared, are you psychologically up for the change?

Many people think they're expected to retire when full Social Security benefits kick in, but that's an outdated notion. As people live longer, some are choosing to work more years. If you're in your 60s and happy with your career, there's no hurry to retire if you don't want to. Many people work well into their 70s and 80s, either full or part time.

But at some point you'll probably want or need to leave your job. If possible, set a clear retirement date. Uncertainty about when you'll retire produces anxiety. Another option is to "step down" or ease into retirement, taking it in stages (see page 42).

Here are some questions to ask yourself to determine your readiness to retire.

## Are my finances in order?

Financially, can you afford to retire? You'll probably never feel 100 percent certain that you've saved all the money you'll need. Even people who are very well off feel some anxiety when they stop receiving a regular paycheck. If you feel quite sure that you've planned effectively and can handle a few bumps along the way, allow that to give you peace of mind.

## Do I have health care coverage?

The most expensive medical bills you'll ever have may be yet to come. A key part of being ready to retire is having adequate health insurance coverage. Many people don't retire until age 65 because that's the year they become eligible for Medicare.

Even if you're covered by Medicare, you may need to purchase additional insurance. Take a close look at your insurance situation to determine whether you need a supplemental policy. A surprising number of middle-class people become impoverished when they reach their 70s and 80s because they had unexpected holes in their health insurance coverage. You also need to investigate your options if you decide to retire before you're eligible for Medicare coverage or if you unexpectedly lose your job.

For more information on Medicare and supplemental insurance policies, see Chapter 12.

# Enjoying the sweet life

Edward and Vivien (Vi) make it look easy. After carefully saving and planning, they retired early and have crafted a full, satisfying life. They take care of themselves by exercising, eating well and keeping mentally challenged. They give to their community by volunteering in a host of ventures. Their social life is hopping. In short, it's the good life.

And it's all the sweeter for having been created almost literally from nothing, since both of them came from humble beginnings.

Growing up in the segregated South, Vi says her career choices were limited. She earned a degree in elementary education. After college, she moved to New York City and was working in the business field when she was introduced to Edward through a mutual friend. Edward worked at IBM. He joined the company in 1956 after a six-year stint in the military.

The couple married in 1965. Edward worked his way up to staff engineer, while Vi earned a master's degree in early childhood education. In 1974, Edward was transferred to the Midwest. He stayed with IBM for 34 years, and Vi worked as a schoolteacher and eventually became a principal. Over the years, they became very involved in their community, forming a network of friends through their jobs, church and other activities. These relationships became a foundation for a successful retirement.

Long before Edward and Vi were anywhere close to retirement, they were setting aside money for it. "I started saving the day I started working as a kid," Edward says.

He learned a hard lesson early on, when an aunt who was keeping his U.S. savings bonds for him while he was in the military cashed the bonds. Still, that didn't deter him. As soon as he left the service, he started saving again. He also took advantage of his company's matching funds program for retirement savings. Vi dedicated her income to savings, vacations and extra things the couple might need.

In addition to saving money, the couple researched "what one could do, where one could live," as Vi puts it. They traveled a lot before retiring — including trips to Europe, South America and every state in the U.S. — and decided that they were happy to keep living in the Midwest.

Edward retired in 1991 at age 61, and Vi followed suit a few years later. Vi says the timing was good: "I had completed the challenges that I wanted to, both as a teacher and as a principal, and I was feeling good about where I had carried the schools."

Since retirement, the two have continued to travel. They also keep busy with volunteer work. Vi serves on the board of several community organizations, is a county human rights commissioner, delivers Meals on Wheels, is on her church's worship committee and mentors young people in the community.

Edward, who has a deep, resonant voice, volunteers as a reader for the visually impaired and as a lay reader at his own church and other churches in the area. In addition, he does on-call hospice visits and mans the reception desk of one hospital and the information booth of another one. "It's interesting," he says. "You meet all types of people from all over the world. I find the volunteering lots of fun."

Edward and Vi also make time for a variety of hobbies and interests. On Edward's list are cooking, the computer, classical music and current events. Vi enjoys investing in the stock market. She also cites exercise as a hobby.

The couple owned a large house on several acres, but they recently downsized to a co-op apartment in a 55-plus building.

Both Vi and Edward are grateful for the chance to savor their later years. "I look back and see I really moved a long way," Edward says. "My brother and I used to ride the subway and say, 'Maybe one day I could be a subway conductor.'"

## Am I psychologically ready?

Changing your routine after many years of working affects you emotionally and psychologically. A sudden large increase in free time takes some getting used to, and if your income changes, that can affect the way you live and your self-perception. Retirement also brings a change in your social role and status. You may lose some of the rewards that come with having a job, such as daily contact with people of similar interests, the feeling of being needed and the knowledge that you're contributing.

Just as you work to get your financial portfolio in order, it makes sense to develop your "psychological portfolio," as author Nancy Schlossberg calls it. This includes your identity, relationships and need for meaningful involvement. After retirement, it's important to maintain social ties and address your emotional needs. You'll need to find new ways to achieve a sense of accomplishment, structure and status.

Feelings of loss, restlessness and anxiety are common during the first months of retirement. The more central work is to your identity, the greater the sense of loss you're likely to feel when that role disappears. Health problems, marital conflict, previous bouts of depression, and an ongoing sense of hopelessness and pessimism can sometimes lead to depression after retirement.

To help prepare yourself psychologically for the transition, accept that even the best planned retirement will have some bumps. Go in with your eyes open and leave time to adjust. Most people don't move seamlessly and painlessly from one major life stage to another. You'll probably have periods of uncertainty and even fear. Acknowledge feelings of loss and anxiety as normal.

Having a plan for what you want to do after retirement can help you make the psychological transition. If you have something else to look forward to — another exciting chapter in your life waiting to be opened — leaving work is often easier.

Finally, part of being psychologically ready is understanding that you simply can't anticipate everything that will happen. Adjusting to retirement often involves trying many different paths until you find the one that feels right. One retiree sums it up this way: "You can read and talk and plan, but you still have to go through it. You have to adapt as you go. As with any major life transition, expect the unexpected."

# Early retirement

Many people dream of escaping the day-to-day grind of a full-time job years early. While millions of people choose to retire early, many others are forced out of their jobs before their intended retirement date. They may be laid off or offered an attractive early retirement package.

If you're thinking of retiring early — or you don't have much choice about it — here are some things to keep in mind.

- Make sure you have sufficient financial resources and health care insurance. If you retire at age 55, you may have to fund your retirement for 30 or 40 years. You'll also need some type of health care insurance to cover you until you qualify for Medicare.
- If your employer offers you an early retirement package, evaluate the offer carefully. Does it include health benefits? Good severance pay? A pension? You may want to discuss the offer with a financial planner before accepting it.
- Retiring at a younger age, when you're likelier to be in good health, can give you the chance to do more-vigorous activities.
- Early retirees have more time to test and try various activities and interests to find those that will be satisfying over the long term.
- If you retire early and most of your friends don't, you may find yourself with no one to socialize with. You'll have to adopt strategies for making new friends. Before deciding on a planner, make sure you understand the services that will be provided — and how you fit in. It's important that you play an active role in the decision-making. Set specific, measurable goals. For example, instead of saying you want to be "comfortable" in retirement, quantify what that means. Ask questions about the recommendations your planner gives you. And be sure to re-evaluate your retirement plan periodically to make sure you're meeting your long-term goals.

### Easing into retirement

If you're uncomfortable about jumping into retirement, consider a "step-down" process. This might mean working part time, working at your company in a different capacity or getting a part-time job in a different field before retiring. Many people find that retiring in stages or taking a trial run or two works best.

According AARP, approximately one-third to one-half of retirees work these so-called "bridge jobs" before they retire. An AARP survey also found that 7 out of 10 workers age 45 and older plan to work during their retirement. But they want greater flexibility and autonomy in their jobs than they may have had during their earlier years.

For many people, a combination of less work and more leisure time is preferable to full retirement, at least for a few years.

## Accepting the changes of retirement

Retired Mayo Clinic psychiatrist Robert Morse, M.D., reflects on the changes in identity that often come with retirement:

"If you had a positive career experience and enjoyed your work and colleagues, expect to feel some loss. If you don't experience some grief, you might wonder what's wrong. I missed relationships with my colleagues and many patients, and I missed the intellectual stimulation. Anticipate this as a normal part of change. If not, you may misinterpret it as, 'Oops, I made the wrong decision.'

"The loss of identity as a professional is very real. It's a blow to your self-esteem. You must have enough positive input from other sources, such as family, friends and grandchildren, to make up for the loss. However, there's another trap in retirement in thinking that your life no longer has meaning because all of your value was tied up in your work. There are many ways to define meaning and many roles in life that are meaningful."

# If you're having trouble with retirement

For some individuals, retirement is a real struggle. Retirement is uncharted territory for many people and often involves some tough emotional and psychological hurdles. You may need to give yourself 12 to 18 months to get a feel for what this phase of your life will be like.

It's natural to go through an adjustment period. If you're feeling depressed or overly anxious, however, or if you're not feeling better by the end of your first year of retirement, seek help.

Fortunately, a wide variety of resources are available to help people who are struggling with some aspect of retirement.

## Medical resources

A first step would be to talk to your family doctor. He or she may refer you to a psychologist or psychiatrist, who can help you deal with the issues you're facing. Psychologists often use various forms of psychotherapy, or "talk therapy," to help people with retirement issues. Psychiatrists, who are medical doctors, may prescribe medications in addition to psychotherapy, to deal with problems such as depression. Some psychologists and psychiatrists specialize in dealing with the concerns of older adults.

## Nonmedical resources

A host of local, state and national organizations and agencies offer services and help for older adults. Under the Older Americans Act, each year the federal government distributes tax dollars to states to provide services to seniors. If possible, make an appointment with a social worker who specializes in retirement issues.

The following agencies and organizations are good places to start when you're looking for information and help with retirement issues.

- **AARP.** AARP provides information on many aspects of retirement, including financial planning, retirement calculators and tax assistance.
- **SCORE.** The Service Corps of Retired Executives (SCORE), billed as "Counselors to America's Small Business," provides entrepreneurs

# Maintaining the 'people part'

Contrary to the advice typically given in books — including this one — Jerry didn't have a game plan for what he would do after retiring.

"I must admit I really didn't think much about what was in store," he says. "I thought, 'I'll make the decision to retire, and then we'll see what happens.'"

Jerry knew he wanted to step down from his position as a hospital administrator at about age 65. It was a busy job, and he was inundated with meetings. He looked forward to having more time to spend with his family and play golf. But there was one part of his job that he'd loved from the very beginning and he knew he would miss — the "people part of it."

And the people part was precisely what led Jerry to a fulfilling, active retirement. At the time Jerry retired, the president of the hospital's sponsorship board stepped down and Jerry was asked to fill the role. The sponsorship board was created to perpetuate the hospital's Franciscan Catholic identity and to reinforce the Franciscan values. Jerry became its first lay president.

It was a perfect fit: Jerry was able to use his skills and experience in a new capacity and contribute to a cause he believed in wholeheartedly. But the volunteer position wasn't as time intensive or demanding as his previous job, so he would still have time for his other activities.

"The good news is that I'm out of my wife's hair," he jokes. On a more serious note, he adds, "I hope I'm doing some good. What you get out of this personally is incredible. It's fun! I work with an outstanding group of men and women. It's a treat to come in and see them all."

Despite his ongoing commitments, Jerry still has plenty of time for the most important people in his life — his family and friends — and time to play golf.

Jerry and his wife, Patty, still live in the house they've owned for many years. "We've gone through the drill of thinking about whether to move or stay," Jerry says. "We're staying put." With so many years invested in their community, the couple has a wide social circle. They value their friends and social connections and don't want to give that up.

Fitness also is important to Jerry. He became serious about exercise after being diagnosed with diabetes several years ago. Now he walks or runs four or five times a week and tries to do some activity each day, whether it's stretching or helping his son on the family farm.

Jerry believes that good health — both physical and mental — is crucial to a happy, successful retirement. The other key, of course, is people: "First family, then friends. You need to stay connected and doing something meaningful. To be able to help others is priceless."

with free, confidential business counseling, either online or in person at nearly 400 chapter offices across the nation. This is a good resource for retirees who hope to start new businesses.

- **Place of worship.** Most churches, synagogues and other places of worship have fellowship or support groups, often geared toward specific age groups. Most clergy also provide counseling to members struggling with transitions.
- **YMCA or YWCA.** Many local organizations, including YMCA or YWCA centers, have services and activities for retired people.

- **Fraternal organizations.** Rotary Clubs, Lions Clubs, Elks Clubs, and other fraternal organizations provide a number of services and opportunities for older adults.
- **Senior citizen centers.** Most communities have senior citizen centers, which offer a variety of activities and services.

It's unlikely that all the pieces of a fulfilling retirement are going to magically fall into place all at once. If you're struggling now, take heart — with a little help and some planning, you can overcome barriers to a successful retirement and enjoy the years ahead of you.

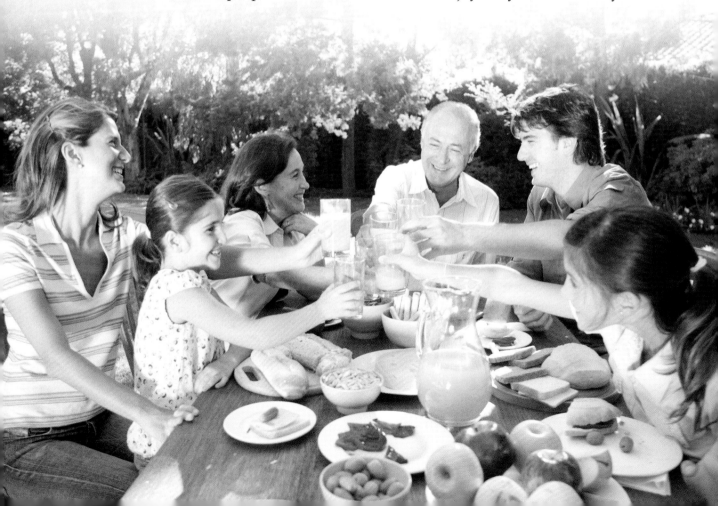

# Chapter 3

# Having a purpose in life

What role would you like to play in Act 2 of your life? What do you want to see, learn or understand? What kind of person will you be? What will make you feel like you still matter? What matters to you?

These questions deserve a thoughtful response. The second half of your life can be interesting, fulfilling and exciting — or it can be frustrating, boring and depressing. The difference is in the choices you make. These years offer an abundance of opportunities — traveling, learning, volunteering and deepening friendships and family relationships being just a few.

However, your goal should be not just to keep busy. Enjoying life at any age means taking part in activities that are meaningful to you — those that engage your body, mind and soul, that motivate you to get up every morning. This applies in retirement as well.

Leisure activities can occupy some of your day, but many people eventually get tired of too much recreation and begin to yearn for a sense of purpose. They want to feel appreciated and needed, absorbed and engaged. They want to make life better for others and feel connected to something larger than themselves.

To find satisfaction and fulfillment in your later years, you have to understand what's important to you. What makes you happy? What gives you comfort? The more you take part in activities that are personally meaningful to you, the more you'll enjoy this stage of your life.

# What's important to you?

Leaving a job that's played a major role in your life forces you to revisit the basic question of "Who am I?" If you've been a homemaker, your identity and roles may shift after your children leave home and again when your spouse or partner retires.

To make the most of your later years, you must understand who you are and what you need to thrive emotionally, physically, financially and spiritually. The more you know about what's important to you, the more successful you'll be in creating a new framework for the days, weeks, months and years after retirement.

These may be the sorts of questions you haven't thought about for a long time. During midlife, many are so busy with work or attending to the needs of families that they take little time for themselves. This can lead to physical, mental and emotional exhaustion. If you're feeling depleted, your effectiveness and enthusiasm for work and home responsibilities can be sapped. If this sounds like your life, it's even more important to take time to think about your needs and desires.

## Know thyself

To strategize and plan the activities with which you'll fill your upcoming years, take time to think about who you are. Below are two tools you can use to evaluate your needs, wishes, dreams and responsibilities.

## Information gathering

Answer the following questions honestly, based on who you are right now — not who you think you should be, who you think you will be or who you think others want you to be.

- What do I like to do?
- What makes me happy?
- What gives me pleasure, and what's fun?
- Were there things I wanted to do, see or experience but didn't have time for when I was working?
- What stimulates me and makes me think?
- When do I feel needed?
- What makes me feel valuable and important?
- When and where do I feel at peace?
- Am I meeting my self-care needs, such as getting exercise and rest?
- Am I spending time with other people and also alone?

- What's my definition of free time? How much do I want?
- When do I feel creative? What activities can I "get lost in" or find fascinating?
- What creates anxiety in my life? What makes me worried?
- Where is home to me? What makes that place feel like home? Where do I want to live that feels healthy and satisfying?
- Who do I like to spend time with?
- Who do I not particularly like to spend time with?
- What do I want to have done that will be remembered when I die?
- Am I helping others? What can I do to make a difference?

After you've answered these questions, write down what you think is the most valuable information you learned and what's most important to remember as you plan for the future. Pay attention to the questions that were difficult for you, and see if you can understand why they were.

## Life scripts

Another tool for better understanding yourself is your "life scripts" — the roles you play in life. To start, begin with a list of the personal and professional roles you play now, such as wife, husband, mother, father, grandparent, friend, household manager and traveler. Estimate how much energy you currently put into each of these roles and how much satisfaction you get in return. Use a scale of 1 to 10 to rate your satisfaction.

Next, consider new roles that you might want to pursue in your later years, such as a new hobby, as well as roles that might be inevitable, such as caring for aging parents. Take into account your responsibilities, needs and dreams.

Finally, work on easing out of roles that bring low satisfaction and invest more time in those you want to emphasize. For example, how much time do you want to spend with family and friends? How much of your identity and personal satisfaction stems from your job, compared with other roles you play in life?

# Determining your purpose in life

Meaningful activities support what you're trying to get out of life and help you feel connected to why you're here. They give you something to strive for,

a reason to live and something to feel excited about each day.

Having a sense of purpose can keep you from waking up one morning, looking back on your life and saying, "What happened?" As Mark Twain observed, you will have regrets and remorse for the things you did not do, rather than for what you did.

A sense of purpose can mean different things to different people. For many people, it includes a feeling that they matter — that others depend on them, are interested in them and are concerned about what happens to them.

Spending time on the things that are meaningful to you and that you enjoy can help you feel better about yourself and improve your mood and your attitude toward life.

Researchers believe that engagement with life — purposeful activities and close relationships — is one of the main components of a high quality of life. Without a sense of mission — a passion for something or someone — some people become vulnerable to depression, which can lead to poor self-care and health problems. The feeling that you matter and that others need you also is crucial for mental health.

## So, then, how do you find your purpose?

### Make a wish list

**Allow yourself to dream about all the things you'd like to do.** Pay attention to your inner voice, asking yourself, "How can I use my talents?" and "What is really important to me?" Your later years provide a chance to live unfulfilled dreams or develop underused talents.

**Write down the activities you see yourself doing, from part-time work to hobbies.** Try to include more than just solitary pursuits, such as reading, watching TV or walking. Keep in mind that a list heavy on material things, for example, buying a new "toy" or redecorating your house, won't likely be satisfying for long.

**Make your list as specific as possible.** Many people have a few general ideas, such as traveling or taking classes. But a more specific idea, such as creating a family website or starting a landscaping business, allows you to take steps before retiring that will help you later. If you plan to learn a new skill, such as watercolor painting, where and when will you do it?

Take into account the many different parts of your life — work, family, social relationships, health, intellectual development, values and beliefs. There are many avenues that might inspire you.

### Test and build on your ideas

Once you've come up with a list of things you think you'd like to do, test run your dreams and hone any skills and contacts you'll need to make them work.

It's a good idea to do a reality check of your ideas. Some people find themselves unexpectedly bored with their planned activities. Or their plans to start a new business or find an interesting part-time job are more difficult than they anticipated.

If you can, take the time in midlife to get some hands-on experience with the activities you imagine yourself doing in retirement. You may think you'll enjoy consulting or volunteering, but that's just a guess until you actually try. In addition, unless you have some experience, you may not be able to get the job or volunteer position you want.

One man loved art and imagined himself spending much of his free retirement time painting. But when he took art classes after retiring, he found he wasn't good enough at painting to really enjoy it.

If you're thinking of turning a hobby, such as gardening, into a business, you'll need small-business skills. You could start now by taking adult education classes that will prepare you to run a small business and by talking to others who have done similar things to see if you're up to the effort involved.

If you hope to keep working in some capacity — in your field, a new career or your own business — inventory your interests, talents and achievements, and brainstorm ways to build on them. It's also important to create and maintain a network of potentially helpful friends and colleagues who can assist you.

# Exploring new horizons

As work becomes a less consuming force in your life, your purpose will almost certainly change. Your daily routine won't be anchored by the schedule, pace and structure of work. If you've been a homemaker, you may still have many of the same chores and responsibilities, but your relationships and the time you spend with your children and your spouse or partner may change.

This is a great time to re-examine your priorities and develop hobbies and activities that provide a new sense of purpose. There's no right or wrong activity. What matters is whether it engages and motivates you.

As you plan for your later years, it can be helpful to find "retirement role models" — people who have retired successfully, who are energized and satisfied. Ultimately, each of us must forge our own path, but you can learn from people who have gone before you.

The pages that follow offer some suggestions on activities that can provide meaning and stimulation, allowing you to build a satisfying, full life.

## Pursue interests and hobbies

What intellectual or physical pursuits do you find fascinating, fun or pleasurable? The list might include researching your family history, cooking, gardening, reading, woodworking, rock climbing, listening to music, attending concerts or plays, watching football, playing bridge, tinkering in the garage, or scrapbooking — to name a few.

If you're in your 40s or 50s and don't participate in interesting activities, start exploring hobbies that intrigue you. Some retirees seem to forget how to be interested in new things — even though they have time for hobbies, they don't pursue them.

Here are a few tips for finding and pursuing interests:

- **Have fun.** If it feels more like a duty, consider something else. Look for activities that leave you feeling energized, not drained.
- **Consider joining a group to share your hobby with other enthusiasts.** Community centers, senior centers and civic groups often have clubs for people with common interests.
- **Be realistic about your expectations.** If you're just learning woodworking, start with a simple project. Keep initial costs low until you're sure you want to keep up the hobby.
- **Consider your space limitations.** If you're going to tinker in the small-engine-repair business or take up catering, do you have room for the activity and its equipment?

## Take a class

You're never too old to learn — and doing so provides the mental stimulation that helps keep your brain healthy (see Chapter 7). Studies on aging show that people with higher levels of education do better later in life than do people who fail to fully develop their intellectual capacities.

Classes can help you refresh old skills or develop new ones, especially as technologies rapidly change. Taking a class also gives you a chance to study for the sheer joy of learning. For most adults, the goal of schooling early in life was to acquire work-related skills. Many people had to interrupt their education in their younger years because of family or work responsibilities.

You can take classes at a local community college or university on any subject that interests you, without having to work toward a degree. Or you can go back to school to earn a college degree or advanced degree, if that's what you'd like to do.

## See the world

Whether you've dreamed of hitting the road in a recreational vehicle (RV), joining an environmental group for an eco-adventure in Costa Rica or taking a romantic trip to Paris, your later years finally give you the time to travel. Let your sense of adventure guide you.

Travel can be expensive, so consider your budget when planning a trip. Also watch for and take advantage of senior discounts, such as reduced airline fares for seniors.

Half the fun of traveling is planning. Begin by learning about the area you plan to visit and the importance of the sights you'll see. Figure out how you want to travel — airplane, car, RV, train — and how long you can afford to stay. And think about whether you want to travel alone, with a spouse or partner, with friends, or as part of a group.

Tours for older adults no longer involve just shuttling from one site to another on a bus. Group travel today includes educational, cultural, historical, environmental and adventure treks. You can join other like-minded retirees to learn a language, paint, cook, hike or volunteer. Tours offer fun, the chance to meet new people, and opportunities to learn and participate in a range of activities.

## Get a part-time job

Many people who enjoy the challenges and social interactions of the workplace want to keep working at least part time after reaching the traditional retirement age. Paid employment may be a good option if you need the income or to stretch your retirement fund. A job can also boost your self-esteem and add to your quality of life. In addition to providing regular contact with people, work gives you a feeling of being needed and of contributing — a sense of purpose.

You don't necessarily have to keep doing exactly what you've been doing. Options include working in the same field, but with a different company, getting a part-time job in the same field or a new one, starting a new career, or transforming a hobby or interest into a business.

Start by determining your goals, and then evaluate your skills and the job market. You probably have more skills than you realize — don't forget to include experience from volunteer work, hobbies, and home and social roles.

If you're thinking about changing careers or getting a part-time job in a new field, consider these steps:

- Assess your skills. Write them down.
- Network with friends and business colleagues to help you get leads on jobs that may be available.
- Find out if you'll need formal training for the job you want.

## The wisdom of age

Researchers who study the aging process point out that the old saying is often true: "Age brings wisdom." Wisdom can be defined in many ways. It includes the lessons learned over the course of a lifetime as well as personality characteristics such as kindness, compassion and fairness. Wise action, researchers suggest, is focused on long-term goals rather than immediate gain. It takes into account the community, not just the self.

With age, many people find that their sense of satisfaction depends less on external or material objects than on an inner sense of integrity and satisfaction.

Seeing the bright side, not taking yourself too seriously, being able to "Spin straw into gold" — these are some of the qualities of a wise old age.

---

- Consider volunteering in the field you're interested in to get some hands-on experience and make connections.

If you're hoping to market yourself as a consultant or expert in your field, or to start your own business:

- Arrange to work with (or at least have a conversation with) someone else who's already successfully running a small business.
- Create a contact list of people who can help you market yourself or your business.

- Determine how much money you'll need to start a business and keep it going.
- Develop a business plan. Don't be afraid to seek expert advice if you need to.

## Volunteer your time and talents

Many people say that one of the most fulfilling activities they do is community service and volunteer work. Many nonprofit organizations wouldn't survive if it weren't for dedicated volunteers.

Volunteers contribute not just their time and energy, but the skills and wisdom gained from a lifetime of experience.

By volunteering your time and talents, you're also helping yourself. For decades research has shown a link between quality of life and involvement with other people. Regular volunteering can improve your physical and psychological well-being and may even help you live longer. When you volunteer, you feel needed and valued, and you tend to feel better about yourself and the world around you. You're likely to be less isolated and less preoccupied with your own problems.

People who work to improve the world or help others tend to maintain a sense of vitality. They find that their contributions can make a positive difference. Other benefits include staying busy and productive, making new friends, and savoring the satisfaction that comes with doing something you believe in.

Volunteer work can also increase your sense of belonging within a community. Many people are grateful for the chance to give back to their community and country. As Theodore Roosevelt said, "What we do for ourselves dies with us. What we do for our community lives long after we are gone."

There are numerous volunteer options in your community. Places that often need help include hospitals, schools, libraries, food banks, scout troops, religious organizations, parks, environmental programs, historic sites, and organizations for children and youth.

Volunteer with an organization whose cause you support, and choose activities that fit your time and abilities. Some of the many organizations and agencies to consider include the United Way, Area Agencies on Aging, Service Corps of Retired Executives (SCORE), National Coalition for Literacy, Habitat for Humanity, Special Olympics, Red Cross, Peace Corps, AmeriCorps VISTA, and Retired and Senior Volunteer Program (RSVP), Senior Companion Program and Foster Grandparent Program, all part of Senior Corps.

A good way to learn about volunteer opportunities in your area is through your local newspaper or library. You can contact organizations directly or check their websites.

## Seek greater connections with family and friends

For most people, work is the steadiest source of structured companionship.

You see the same people day after day. When you retire, you may have to look for new ways to find social connections. As discussed in Chapter 6, maintaining social ties — spending time with family and friends — is critical for your emotional and physical health.

People who feel fulfilled in life generally have maintained friendships throughout their lives and continue to make new friends after retirement. Family commitments also may change over the years. As you get older, you may spend more time taking care of aging parents or an ailing spouse or friend. Or you may prioritize being with your grandchildren.

## Express your creativity

Expressing yourself in a creative way — drawing, painting, writing, sculpting, sewing, dancing, singing, taking photos, acting, making a film or video, playing an instrument, or writing music — enhances your enjoyment of life and gives it meaning. If you've ever had the urge to create, your later years are an excellent time to rediscover or further hone artistic impulses. Creativity isn't limited to a certain age range. Many artists experience a burst of sustained creativity after age 65.

Community centers often have classes in arts and crafts for people of all ages. There also are a variety of theater and music groups for older adults.

## Speak out

After retirement, you may have more freedom than ever to get involved in politics, government or community activism. Without the constraints of daily work, the demands of family life or the fear of losing a job, you can speak out and take action in support of policies or issues that you care about.

There are many ways to get involved, whether it's running for a board or office, working on someone else's campaign, keeping tabs on the latest legislation or initiating action to solve community problems.

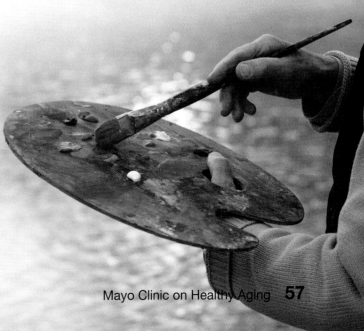

# A mission in life

When John, a plastic and reconstructive surgeon, retired, he didn't have to go looking for a renewed sense of purpose. As a child of missionaries, he grew up in Beijing. There he gained a deep commitment to caring for others, which continues to inspire his life and work. "I've been a person of faith most of my life," he says. "My faith teaches me that my function isn't just to love God but to love other people."

During his career, John specialized in, as he says, "the skin and its contents," including cleft lips and palates, congenital anomalies, head and neck tumors, and breast reconstruction. He was also involved in organ and tissue transplant surgery in its early years.

Before John retired in 1993, he made a list of things he might want to do in this next phase of his life. The list included some hobbies, such as regaining his skills on the flute, but his real interest was in doing something that would benefit the welfare of others.

John turned to his lifelong interest in overseas missions and began providing medical education and surgery in Asia, Africa and South America. Since then, he's traveled the world on dozens of medical missions with various faith-based and international organizations.

"Those little kids just melt your heart," John says. "You repair a cleft lip in 45 minutes to an hour, and you change that child's life."

He has also helped set up continuing medical education for doctors in Haiti and has provided treatment to people for everything from malnutrition to gallstones in Mexico, Ecuador, Indonesia and other countries.

John's "servant spirit" was cultivated from an early age. His father, who taught at the seminary of an interdenominational mission in Beijing, ministered to people in many countries.

"I was taught to look for something to do. If you saw something that needed doing, you just did it without being asked," he recalls.

He continues to be humbled by the people he meets in his travels. "They're so grateful for what's done for them," he says. "Sometimes you might feel a little sorry for yourself working under primitive conditions, and then you think about all the national physicians and how little they have to work with. You think, 'How was I so lucky to be born here and have everything I have?' These people have literally nothing at all."

Closer to home, John visits hospice patients at their homes a couple of times a week. He considers it a privilege to work with people who are near the end of life. "I took up hospice because I really missed the patients," he says. "Most of them I thought of as much as friends as patients." He also leads an interdenominational Bible study once a week.

To keep fit, John works out for 45 minutes to an hour every day except Sunday. "I'm still very busy, but I was overwhelmingly busy before I retired," he says. John does relax occasionally by reading, attending music concerts and visiting family. He and his wife, Janet, have five children and 10 grandchildren. The couple have been married for 56 years.

"Anything I've achieved I attribute to God first and my wife second," John says. "I admire and respect her tremendously. I don't just love her; I'm in love with her still."

# Maintaining your identity

Married individuals often face new challenges in their later years. You may be spending a lot more time with your spouse than you used to. This can lead to difficulties if you don't find a balance between shared interests and individual hobbies and pursuits. It's healthy for you as individuals and as a couple to pursue your own meaningful activities. Having your own hobbies and social activities separate from those of your spouse gives you established ties that you can rely on in the unfortunate event something should happen to your spouse.

Plus, your spouse just may not be interested in the same things you are. For example, perhaps you have been looking forward to doing a lot of traveling after retirement — but your spouse hates to fly and doesn't want to leave the house. One solution is for you to take some trips with friends or a group, such as your bridge club or your local veterans group.

Women often fare better than men do after retirement. That's because women usually have a wider array of social activities and friendships. In addition, women who have spent some of their lives staying at home with children already have found many ways to keep busy outside of the workplace. Household tasks, church or civic responsibilities, along with caring for children and grandchildren, give many women a strong sense of purpose.

In contrast, many retired men have far too little to do and not enough social contacts outside work. Men need to develop friendships, hobbies and interests outside of work before they retire. (Of course, it wouldn't hurt to learn to cook dinner, either!)

The more you can plan and prepare ahead of time, the less anxiety you're likely to experience when a big life transition such as retirement comes knocking at your door.

# Part 2

# Your action plan for a healthy life

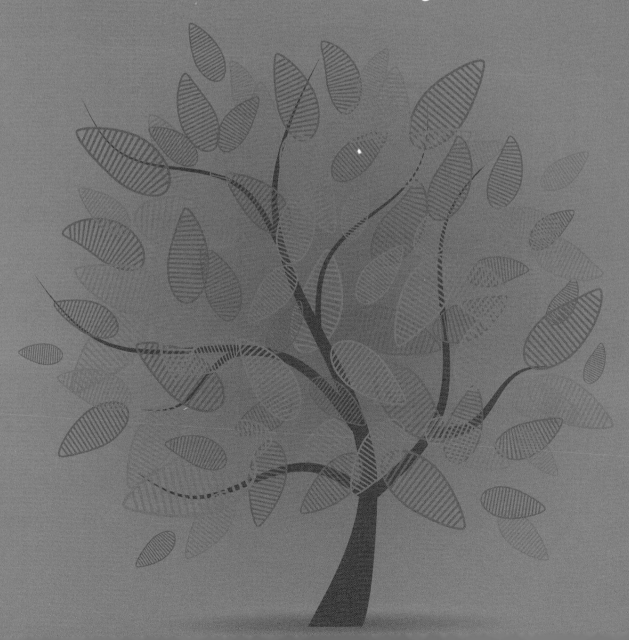

# Chapter 4

# Slow the flow

Until people begin to reach their fifth decade, aging rarely means much, even though it's a lifelong process that begins at birth. Young people typically feel immortal. It's only when certain physical changes begin to occur — the wrinkles on the face, the graying of the hair around the temples, the prescription for reading glasses — that you may truly start to realize you're getting older.

Physical changes associated with aging happen to everyone, but how and when your body changes is unique to you. Everyone ages at a different pace. Enormous variations exist between individuals at every age and in every part of the body. Genes, disease and lifestyle can all affect your rate of aging. So can your history of injuries and other physical or emotional trauma.

There are certain age-related changes that simply can't be prevented. If your hair starts turning gray at age 45, other than the help of some "chemical magic" from your hair stylist or the local drugstore, there's little you can do to prevent it.

For the most part, though, how quickly or slowly you age is influenced by how well you take care of yourself throughout life. Changes commonly attributed to aging are actually due to inactivity, smoking, an unhealthy diet and other lifestyle choices.

This chapter describes how your body systems change with age. More important, you'll find tips for slowing the aging process. By knowing what to expect and how to react, you can stay young regardless of your age.

# What causes aging?

It's a simple and unavoidable fact: Bodies — even healthy ones — grow old. What isn't so simple is explaining why this happens. The progressive wearing down of many bodily functions over time, a process known as senescence, is one of the least understood biological processes.

Scientists have proposed several theories to explain the aging process. One line of thinking holds that the damage done to cells and organs as they carry out their normal functions gradually causes things to go wrong. Another theory suggests that aging follows a biological timetable, a genetically programmed life span.

Researchers have discovered a variety of factors — genetic, biochemical and hormonal — that might contribute to the aging process. These include:

- **Cellular wear and tear.** Cells and tissues have vital parts that wear out.
- **Free radicals.** Accumulated damage caused by unstable oxygen molecules in the body (free radicals) causes cells to stop functioning.
- **Cross-linking.** In a process called glycation, blood sugar (glucose) molecules attach themselves to proteins, setting off a chemical chain reaction that ends in proteins binding together, or "cross-linking." This changes their structure and function and can disrupt cells' work.

- **DNA damage.** In the course of life, the body's basic building block, DNA, undergoes continual damage. The body has many ways to repair damaged DNA, but as the damage accumulates, genes, proteins and cells may malfunction, leading to disease and deterioration of tissues.
- **Programmed longevity.** Over time, certain genes switch on and off, causing physiological processes to shut down.
- **Hormonal changes.** A biological clock acts through hormones to control the pace of aging, similar to the way childhood growth and development is regulated.
- **Immune system changes.** A programmed decline in immune system functioning leads to increased vulnerability to infectious disease and diseases in which the body attacks its own cells (autoimmune disorders).

No single theory or phenomenon can completely explain why aging occurs — perhaps all of them play a role. Researchers generally view aging as many processes that interact and influence each other.

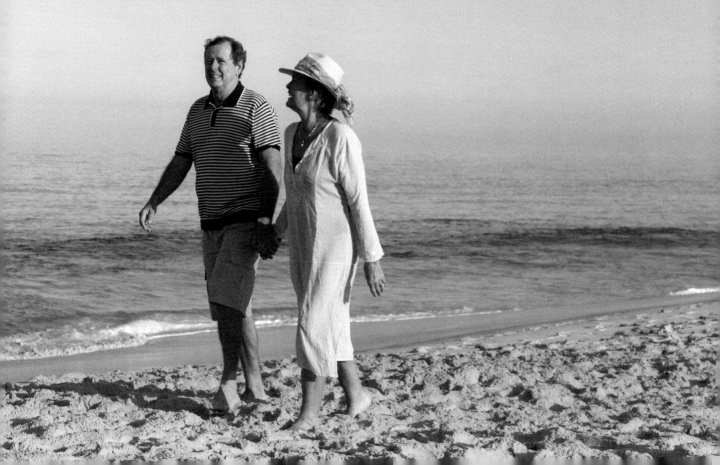

# Brain and nervous system changes

Over time, your brain loses some of the structures (axons) that connect nerve cells (neurons). Some of the brain's neurons are lost, but new connections are made in the remaining cells, and new nerve cells may form in some parts of the brain, even in older age. With billions of neurons and trillions of connections between them, the brain has more cells than it needs.

For most adults, mental performance stays about the same throughout life. However, as you get older, it may take you more time to do some mental tasks than it did when you were younger. For example, you might notice subtle changes in your ability to recall names or words and learn new materials. Occasional forgetfulness is a normal occurrence, and it doesn't mean you have dementia.

One of the most important age-related changes in the brain occurs in the arteries. The brain needs a constant supply of oxygen and nutrients from blood, delivered through several key arteries. Over time, fatty deposits can accumu-late in the artery walls, a condition called atherosclerosis. These deposits narrow the passageway through your vessels, putting you at risk of stroke.

The risk of brain diseases also increases with age. Sometimes the damage to cells in the brain and nervous system exceeds the ability of remaining cells to compensate for the loss. This can affect coordination, mental sharpness, muscular movement and muscle control.

## What you can do

The same things that keep your heart and blood vessels healthy — a diet low in fat, regular exercise and perhaps a daily aspirin — can help protect you against stroke. Other ways to minimize your risk of brain and nervous system disorders include:

- **Eating nutritious foods.** Nutrition is very important for healthy nerves. B vitamins help promote nerve transmission, and foods such as blueberries, strawberries and spinach are high in antioxidants, which also may help keep nerves healthy (see Chapter 9).
- **Limiting alcohol.** Consuming more than one or two drinks a day can raise your blood pressure and in-

crease your risk of stroke. Excessive alcohol can also injure nerve cells.
- **Quitting smoking.** Smokers have a 50 percent greater chance of having a stroke than do nonsmokers.
- **Challenging your brain.** Mental stimulation helps maintain brain function (see Chapter 7).

# Cardiovascular changes

Your cardiovascular system is made up of your heart, blood vessels (arteries and veins) and blood. This system sends fluids, nutrients, oxygen and other substances to body tissues and removes waste products such as carbon dioxide from them. A healthy cardiovascular system is key to the well-being of every organ in the body.

With age, changes naturally occur to your cardiovascular system. Your heart muscle becomes a less efficient pump, working harder to pump the same amount of blood through your body. The walls of the heart become stiffer, and the heart fills with blood more slowly. By about age 60, about 35 percent less blood circulates through the arteries of the heart (coronary arteries) than in earlier years.

In addition, your blood vessels gradually become less elastic. Arteries tend to thicken and become stiff, causing your heart to work harder to pump blood through them. This can lead to high blood pressure (hypertension), a condition that becomes increasingly common in older adults.

These normal changes that come with age generally don't affect the everyday functioning of your heart and blood vessels. In fact, at rest, the differences between younger and older hearts are relatively minor.

However, when an older heart has to work harder than normal, it has less reserve capacity to meet the sudden demands placed on it. In response to physical, mental or emotional stress — such as vigorous exercise, illness, worry or even excitement — the body needs more energy and oxygen than usual.

An older heart can't increase how fast it beats (heart rate) as quickly as a younger heart can. And it often takes longer for the heart rate and blood pressure in an older individual to return to normal after a stressful event. In other words, you might notice that your cardiovascular system can't roll with the punches quite as easily as you get older.

## Inactivity is riskier than age

The best measure of cardiovascular fitness is something called maximal oxygen consumption, abbreviated as VO2 max. It refers to the amount of oxygen consumed when exercising as hard as possible.

In men, VO2 max declines by about 10 percent with each decade of adult life. In women, it declines by about 7.5 percent a decade.

However, like other age-related events, changes in cardiovascular fitness can be modified by behavior. Studies have shown that VO2 max declines nearly twice as fast in sedentary older adults as in those who exercise. Being overweight and inactive leads to an even faster drop in aerobic capacity. In other words, lack of regular physical activity has as much — if not more — of an impact on cardiovascular fitness as does aging. An older person who is fit actually has a better VO2 max than does a younger person who's inactive and unfit.

The natural changes of aging alone generally don't cause cardiovascular disease. But when these changes are combined with certain lifestyle risk factors — including smoking, inactivity and obesity — the risk of serious disease increases.

This is why many cardiovascular diseases — including high blood pressure, coronary artery disease (the leading cause of heart attack) and congestive heart failure — are more common later in life.

## What you can do

Cardiovascular disease can be avoided by adopting good health behaviors. First of all, know your risk factors. In general, things that put stress and strain on the heart include:

- Eating foods high in fat and calories
- Obesity
- Smoking
- Lack of regular exercise
- Holding in emotions
- Stress

- Diabetes and other chronic conditions
- A family history of heart disease

Other healthy behaviors to maintain:

- **Stay physically active.** Regular aerobic exercise, such as swimming, cycling or walking, protects the cardiovascular system by increasing your heart's capacity to pump and keeping blood pressure in check. Exercise also helps control your cholesterol and weight (see Chapter 8).
- **Stop smoking.** Smoking raises your blood pressure and damages your blood vessels, increasing your risk of heart disease.
- **Maintain a healthy weight.** A healthy weight reduces your risk of high blood pressure, high cholesterol and heart attack (see Chapter 9).
- **Drink alcohol in moderation, if at all.** Light to moderate consumption of alcohol may help prevent heart disease, but heavy drinking can promote it. Experts recommend no more than one drink a day for women and individuals age 65 and older and no more than two drinks a day for men younger than 65.
- **Manage stress.** Relieving stress through relaxation can help prevent heart disease (see Chapter 5).

# Dental changes

How your teeth and gums respond to age depends on how well you've cared for them over the years. But even if you're meticulous about brushing and flossing, you may notice that your mouth feels drier and your gums have pulled back (receded). Your teeth may darken slightly and become more brittle and easier to break.

Older adults are generally at greater risk of gum disease, also known as periodontal disease. It's an infection that harms the gum and bone that hold teeth in place. When plaque stays on your teeth too long, it forms a hard covering called tartar. Plaque and tartar can damage your gums, causing them to become red and swollen and bleed easily. Over time, untreated gum disease can make your gums pull away from your teeth and form pockets that can become infected.

Dry mouth can make speaking, swallowing and tasting more difficult. Doctors once thought dry mouth was a normal part of aging, but they now know this isn't true. Dry mouth is, however, a common side effect of many medications. Hundreds of common medications, including painkillers, antihistamines, blood pressure drugs and

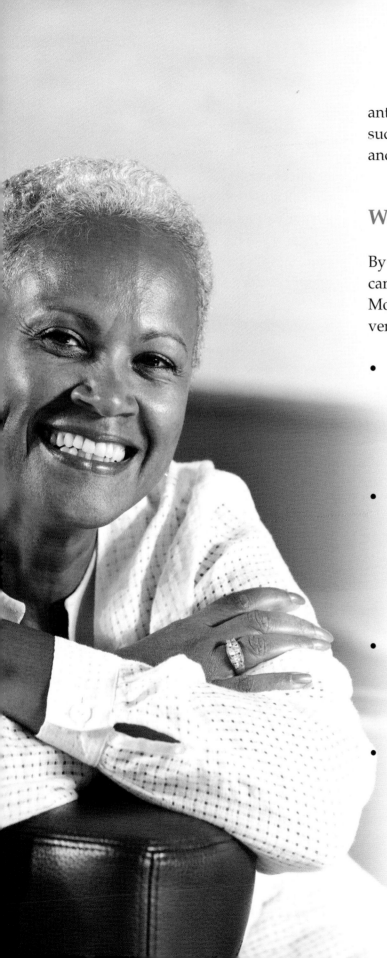

antidepressants, can cause side effects such as dry mouth, soft tissue changes and gum problems.

## What you can do

By taking good care of your teeth, you can protect them for years to come. Most dental and oral diseases are preventable and treatable at every age.

- **Brush your teeth at least twice a day.** Brush your teeth on all sides with a soft-bristled toothbrush and fluoride toothpaste. Be sure to clean both the outer and inner surfaces of your teeth and gums.
- **Floss once a day.** Careful flossing will keep your gums healthy by removing plaque and food that a toothbrush can't reach. Rinse after you floss. If you have trouble handling floss with your fingers, a floss holder or aid can help.
- **Visit your dentist regularly.** See a dentist at least once a year for a professional cleaning and checkup. Your dentist will check for cavities, gum disease and oral cancer.
- **Avoid tobacco products.** Tobacco used in any form, including cigars, pipes and chewing tobacco, increases the risk of gum disease and oral and throat cancers.

## Taste and smell

Most people enjoy a robust sense of taste throughout life. Over time your sense of taste may decrease a little bit, but the changes are generally so modest that most people don't notice. A loss of taste is more likely to be due to smoking, teeth and gum diseases, illness, or certain medications.

Beginning at about ages 40 to 50 in women and 50 to 60 in men, the number of taste buds on the tongue decreases. Sensitivity to the main taste sensations — sweet, salty, sour and bitter — doesn't change until after age 60, if at all. Foods may tend to taste bitter, and your tongue is less sensitive to salty and sweet tastes.

Much of what's thought of as taste actually involves smell. The two senses interact closely, and smells are needed to detect more subtle and complex flavors. The sense of smell declines slightly with age, but not enough to make a major difference for most people.

# Digestive changes

It's normal for the digestive process to slow as you become older. The stomach can't hold as much food because it's less elastic. Digested food moves more slowly through your intestines. The amount of surface area within your intestines diminishes slightly, and the small intestine may be less able to absorb certain nutrients.

The flow of secretions from your stomach, liver, pancreas and small intestine may decrease. The liver becomes smaller, and the enzymes it produces may work less effectively. As a result, it may take longer to rid the body of medications and other substances. This means the effects of drugs may last longer.

Digestive changes are often so subtle you may not notice them. But some problems can occur.

## Constipation

One of the most common digestive complaints among older adults is constipation. The passage of stools becomes less frequent and may be difficult and painful.

Although normal digestive changes contribute to constipation, many other factors can cause this problem. Lack of physical activity and not drinking enough fluids are generally the most common culprits. Other factors include a diet low in fiber, changes in diet, illness and a pattern of putting off bowel movements. Overuse of laxatives also can lead to chronic constipation.

## Heartburn

Heartburn — a burning pain in the chest that usually occurs after eating — is often more noticeable with age. It results when the valve located between the esophagus and the stomach (lower esophageal sphincter) opens, allowing stomach contents to come back (reflux) into the esophagus.

Occasional heartburn is common. Frequent heartburn is often associated with a common condition called gastroesophageal reflux disease (GERD).

## Lactose intolerance

In some older adults, the digestive tract produces less lactase, an enzyme needed to digest milk. This can result in problems digesting dairy products (lactose intolerance). People with lactose intolerance may feel bloated or have gas or diarrhea after consuming milk products.

## What you can do

Many digestive problems can be prevented or relieved with a healthy diet, exercise and other steps.

- **Eat a diet high in fiber and nutrients.** Eat plenty of fruits, vegetables and whole grains. Aim for 25 to 30 grams of fiber each day. Make sure you're getting the recommended amounts of vitamins and minerals.
- **Drink plenty of fluids.** Along with a high-fiber diet, fluids can help prevent digestive problems. Try to drink eight 8-ounce glasses of fluid daily. Water is the best.
- **Stay physically active.** Exercise helps keep your bowels moving and promotes regularity.
- **Try lactase products.** If digesting dairy foods is a problem, taking lactase tablets or drops (Lactaid, Dairy Ease) before eating dairy products

can help reduce bloating and abdominal pain.

- **Don't delay using the bathroom.** When you sense a pending bowel movement, go to the bathroom right away. Delaying bathroom use can contribute to constipation.
- **Avoid commercial laxatives.** Over time they can aggravate or cause constipation. Instead, consider a fiber supplement such as Metamucil or Citrucel.
- **To prevent heartburn, eat small, frequent meals.** Avoid foods and drinks that induce heartburn, such as fatty foods, alcohol, and caffeinated or carbonated beverages. It's also a good idea not to eat right before you lie down or go to bed. Over-the-counter antacids can help, but avoid using them for prolonged periods, because they can cause diarrhea or constipation. Taking acid-blocking medicines such as cimetidine (Tagamet) or ranitidine (Zantac) before meals also may help.

# Hearing changes

Structures in the ear that help with hearing and balance can gradually deteriorate. The most significant changes occur in the inner ear (cochlea).

## Hearing loss

Some people retain perfect hearing throughout their lives, but most lose some hearing sensitivity over time. About one-third of Americans older than age 60 have hearing problems.

Hearing loss may result from damage to parts of the inner ear, the nerves attached to it or hearing pathways in the ear. Excess or impacted earwax also can cause hearing trouble. Many other things can contribute to hearing loss, including damage from exposure to loud noises, certain medications, head injuries or illnesses. Men tend to have more severe hearing loss than do women of the same age.

Age-related hearing loss first affects your ability to hear higher frequencies. It might be harder to understand women and children and to hear conversations in large groups or when there's background noise. It might seem like other people are mumbling.

## Ringing in ears

Tinnitus also becomes more common with age. This is a persistent, abnormal ear noise — a ringing, hissing or roaring sound. It may be caused by exposure to loud noise, certain medications or a health problem such as high blood pressure or diabetes. It often accompanies hearing loss.

## Dizziness

As the structures in the inner ear wear down, some people experience dizziness or a feeling of unsteadiness on their feet. A spinning sensation, called vertigo, usually stems from a problem with the nerves and structures of your inner ear that sense movement and changes in your head position.

### What you can do

Medical treatment or surgery can help restore some hearing loss, especially if the problem is in the outer or middle ear. There's no known cure for age-related hearing loss, but hearing aids can help. With improved technology and new fitting options, hearing aids can produce dramatic improvements in hearing. Other products also can help you cope with hearing loss. They include TV-listening systems and telephone-amplifying devices.

You can prevent hearing loss from exposure to loud noise by using ear protection. If you know you'll be exposed to loud noise — loud enough to cause you to raise your voice to be heard by someone an arm's length away — wear earplugs that fit snugly or earmuff cushions that completely encircle the ear. Hearing protection is often recommended when using devices such as power tools, lawn mowers and snowblowers.

For persistent dizziness, see your doctor. It often can be treated with a simple procedure or balance retraining exercises. Medications may also help.

# Immune system changes

Your immune system defends your body against invaders such as bacteria, viruses, pollen and other foreign substances. This highly complex system is primarily made up of several different types of white blood cells. Your immune system also monitors your body for cells that have started malfunctioning, such as tumor cells.

With age, the immune system can become less effective. For the most part, these changes are so slight that they're hardly noticeable. But there are a few differences you may notice. With age, the body is less able to fight infections. It often takes older adults longer to recover from a cold or the flu than it does for younger individuals. Vaccines may not work as well in older adults. In addition, the immune system's ability to destroy malfunctioning cells, such as cancer cells, may slow down. This might be one reason why cancer rates increase with age.

## What you can do

The following strategies can help boost your immune system so that it's functioning at peak efficiency.

- **Eat well.** The immune system is sensitive to nutritional deficiencies, such as lack of zinc, vitamin E and vitamin B-6. In addition to eating a healthy diet, you might consider taking a daily multivitamin supplement (see Chapter 10).
- **Get regular exercise.** Regular exercise helps your immune system fight infection.
- **Manage stress.** Ongoing stress can weaken the immune system. Find healthy ways to deal with stress and relax, such as listening to soothing music, meditating or doing yoga.

# Metabolism, hormone and weight changes

One of the most common occurrences people comment on as they grow older is increased difficulty losing weight or maintaining a healthy weight. With age, your metabolism typically slows, meaning that your body functions by burning fewer calories than it once did. More calories are likely to be stored as fat. A major reason for this is that people tend to be less active as they get older. Changes in fat and lean body mass (including muscles) also cause shifts in body shape, which affect metabolism.

Metabolism is controlled by your body's endocrine system. This complex system is made up of organs and tissues that produce hormones, which regulate many body functions. With age, the hormones that regulate growth decrease, as do sex hormones. But not all hormones decrease in numbers. Some remain unchanged, while others increase.

## What you can do

Changes in metabolism, weight and hormone levels are inevitable, but exercise and a healthy diet can help minimize the negative effects.

- **Stay physically active.** Regular exercise helps boost metabolism and decrease body fat. It improves your cells' response to the hormone insulin, reducing your risk of diabetes. Exercise also increases the body's production of growth hormone and other "anti-aging" hormones.
- **Build strength to slow muscle loss.** Lifting weights (strength training) counters the loss of muscle mass that occurs with aging. Strength training can maintain or increase muscle mass.
- **Maintain a healthy weight.** Losing weight if you're overweight can help keep blood sugar levels in control, allowing the hormone insulin to work more effectively. This reduces your risk of diabetes.

# Respiratory changes

The muscles we use to breathe, such as the diaphragm, tend to weaken with time. The chest wall becomes stiffer, making it a little harder for the lungs to expand and contract. Maximum breathing capacity may decline by about 40 percent between the ages of 20 and 70. In addition, slightly less oxygen is absorbed from the air you breathe in.

Most people don't notice much change in the functioning of their lungs. However, vigorous exercise, such as running or biking up a hill, may be more difficult, especially for people who aren't physically fit.

With age, some people also become more vulnerable to respiratory infections such as pneumonia and the flu (influenza). The lungs may be less able to fight off infection, in part because the cells that clear debris from the airways are less effective. Adding to the problem, the immune system isn't as effective at fighting infection.

## What you can do

To protect your respiratory system:

- **Stop smoking and avoid second-hand smoke.** Eliminate smoke from your environment as much as possible. Many chemical compounds in tobacco smoke damage the lungs. Smoking also inhibits the ability of the lungs to clear bacteria from secretions in larger airways.

- **Exercise.** Aerobic exercise increases lung capacity and lessens the stiffening of the chest wall and lungs. Adequate exercise may also decrease your chance of getting a respiratory infection.
- **Avoid respiratory infections.** This means an annual influenza vaccination. If you're age 65 or older, get a pneumonia vaccination, as well.
- **Avoid environmental pollutants.** Stay away from chemical fumes and other irritants.
- **Eat a healthy diet.** Good nutrition is important for your lungs and immune system, boosting your ability to handle respiratory infections.

# Sexual changes

A healthy sexual relationship can positively affect all aspects of your life, including your physical health and self-esteem. Though movies and television might suggest that sex is only for younger adults, this isn't true. The need for intimacy is ageless.

Age does, however, bring physical changes that may affect your sexuality. One of the more common sexual changes is a gradual slowing of physical response time. It takes longer to become aroused, to complete the sexual act and to be ready to have sex again.

For women, most physical sexual changes are linked to menopause and reduced estrogen levels. It takes longer for the vagina to swell and lubricate when you're sexually aroused. The vagina's walls become thinner, drier and less elastic. These changes can make intercourse less comfortable. After menopause, some women also experience waning levels of sexual interest. This has more to do with a decrease in testosterone rather than in estrogen. Testosterone regulates your sex drive whether you're a man or a woman.

As men age, they may find it takes longer to achieve an erection. Erections may be less firm, and some men may not ejaculate with orgasm. You may also need more time between ejaculations. Aging doesn't cause erectile dysfunction (impotence), but older men are more likely to have it. Common causes are alcohol abuse, medications, smoking, and diseases such as diabetes and atherosclerosis.

These physical changes certainly don't mean that your sex life is coming to an end, but you may have to redefine some of your expectations and assumptions. Maintaining your ability to have sex as you age depends on your mind as much as your body. If you're embarrassed or ashamed of your changing sexual needs, your anxiety can affect your ability to become aroused. The stress of worrying too much about performance can trigger impotence in men or a lack of arousal in women.

## What you can do

There are ways to accommodate changing sexual needs, patterns and performance.

- **Take your time.** Longer foreplay can help men become aroused and may help stimulate natural lubrication in women. Taking things slowly can help you avoid anxiety about performance.
- **Use a lubricant.** If you're a woman experiencing vaginal dryness, try a vaginal moisturizer or lubricant, or talk to your doctor about vaginal estrogen therapy. Regular intercourse helps maintain lubrication and keep genital tissues more supple.
- **Talk with your partner.** Communication brings you and your partner closer. Discuss the changes you're going through and what your partner can do to accommodate you during sex.

- **Make changes to your routine.** Simple changes can improve your sex life. Change the time of day when you have sex to a time when you have the most energy. Because it may take longer to become aroused, take time to set the stage for romance, such as a romantic dinner or an evening of dancing. Try a new sexual position.
- **Manage your expectations.** If you didn't have sex very often as a younger adult, don't expect to have lots of sex as an older adult. Partners who enjoy frequent sex when they're younger are more likely to continue that as they age.
- **Take care of yourself.** A healthy diet, regular exercise and plenty of rest keep your body finely tuned. Avoid alcohol and illicit drugs, as excessive use decreases sexual function in both men and women. Find ways to relieve stress.
- **See your doctor if you're having problems.** Your doctor can discuss medications or other treatments that can help.
- **If you have a new partner, remember to practice safe sex.** All sexually active people — no matter what age — can contract sexually transmitted infections. Condoms are effective at preventing the transmission of most of these infections.

# Skeletal and muscular changes

Your bones reached their maximum mass in your mid- to late-20s. As you get older, they slowly shrink in size and density. In addition, the gel-like disks between the vertebrae of your spine become thinner. One consequence of these changes is that you might become shorter — the average person loses 1.5 to 3 inches in height over a lifetime.

Gradual loss of density weakens your bones and makes them more prone to fracture. Women lose bone mass more rapidly, especially in the years immediately after menopause. Not getting enough calcium and vitamin D in your diet can accelerate this process.

With age, muscle tissue (muscle mass) also tends to decrease. This loss starts at about age 30 and continues throughout life. Muscles, tendons and joints also lose some strength and flexibility. Most older adults experience some joint changes, ranging from minor stiffness to severe arthritis. The cartilage lining the joints may become thinner, and the joint surfaces may not slide over each other as well as they used to.

Research shows that loss of strength and muscle has as much to do with inactivity as it does age. If you continue to lead an active life, you can maintain much of the muscle strength that you enjoyed in your youth.

## What you can do

Taking care of your bones, muscles and joints throughout your life is key to maintaining an active lifestyle. There are several things you can do to lessen the impact of age-related skeletal and muscular changes.

- **Get regular exercise, including strength or resistance training.** Staying active is one of your best weapons. Even people who've never exercised before can build muscle mass and strength with regular exercise. Weight-bearing activities — things you do on your feet with your bones supporting your weight, such as walking and weightlifting — help strengthen and preserve your bones. Exercises such as swimming and water aerobics are easy on the joints for people with arthritis. See Chapter 8 for more information.
- **Consider practices such as tai chi, yoga or Pilates.** Tai chi helps im-

# Over-the-counter wrinkle creams

Many skin creams and lotions sold in department stores, in drugstores and on the Internet promise to reduce wrinkles and prevent or reverse damage caused by aging.

If you're looking for a face-lift in a bottle, you won't find it in a skin cream. But research suggests that wrinkle creams contain ingredients that may improve wrinkles slightly.

**Modestly effective**
- Vitamin A (retinol)
- Hydroxy acids

**Possibly effective**
- Alpha-lipoic acid
- Coenzyme Q10
- Copper peptides
- Growth factors
- Soy isoflavones
- Tea extracts
- Vitamin C
- Vitamin E

**Likely ineffective**
- Collagen

Combining the right skin cream with a proven treatment for wrinkles may help you achieve a younger looking face. The best approach is to avoid long periods in the sun without covering up or wearing sunscreen.

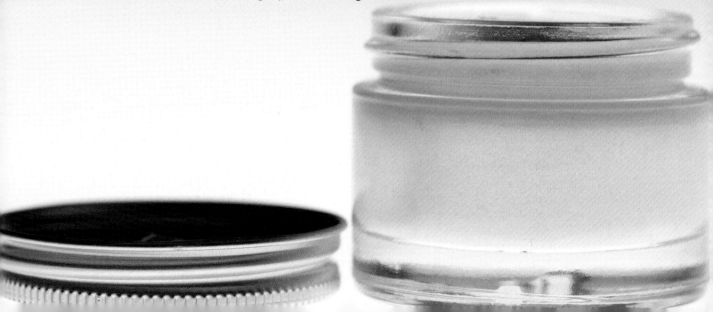

prove balance, while yoga increases muscle flexibility and strength as well as overall flexibility. Pilates is designed to strengthen the body's core muscles.

- **Eat a healthy diet.** Protein helps slow the muscle loss that occurs with aging, while calcium and vitamin D are essential nutrients for building and sustaining bone mass. Consider supplements if you can't get enough from your diet.
- **Maintain a healthy weight.** Excess weight puts stress and strain on your muscles and joints.
- **Don't smoke.** Smoking interferes with calcium absorption and can speed the loss of bone.
- **Limit alcohol.** Excessive consumption of alcohol can hasten bone loss.
- **Practice relaxation techniques.** Programs that teach you how to relax your muscles can help ease pain in your shoulders, back and neck.

# Skin and hair changes

Skin changes are among the most visible signs of aging. Everyone is affected, but how fast your skin ages is influenced by many factors, including heredity, nutrition, smoking, exposure to sunlight and other environmental conditions. Asian-Americans, African-Americans, American Indians and Hispanics tend to have fewer wrinkles and smoother skin as they grow older. Blue-eyed, fair-skinned people show more age-related skin changes.

With time, your skin becomes thinner, drier and less elastic. This can cause it to wrinkle and sag. Years of exposure to sunlight contribute to wrinkles and rough, blotchy skin. People who haven't spent much time in the sun often look much younger than their actual age. Smoking also causes wrinkles, yellowing and a leathery appearance.

Age spots, also known as liver spots, may begin to appear. These small, flat patches look like freckles. Growths such as skin tags, warts and other blemishes are more common with age. Though age spots and most growths are harmless, if their appearance changes, see your doctor to rule out skin cancer. Production of natural skin oils also slows with age. The loss of oils can cause red, scaly and itchy skin on your back, legs, arms or elsewhere.

Changes in hair follicles lead to graying and hair loss. Half the people older than age 50 have gray hair. Graying usually begins at the temples and works its way up the scalp. Gray hair often has a different texture.

Some thinning of hair also typically occurs in both women and men. Age, changing hormone levels, heredity and your sex cause some people to lose more hair than do others.

Men are more likely to lose hair as they age. By age 60, 80 percent of men are at least partly bald. Male-pattern baldness typically involves a receding hairline and hair loss on top of the head. A smaller number of women develop female-pattern baldness. A woman's part may widen, or her hair may look and feel thinner. Hormone changes after menopause sometimes cause facial hairs to coarsen and grow.

## What you can do

You can't undo years of exposure to the sun. But you can protect your skin from further damage.

- **Limit sun exposure.** Prevent sunburn by using sunscreen when outdoors, even in winter. Wear protective clothing and hats.
- **Eat well.** Protein is essential for healing and building new tissue, and without enough protein, skin becomes more fragile. Vitamins A, B and C are all important for skin health. Drinking plenty of fluids helps prevent skin injury.
- **Don't smoke.** Nicotine in cigarettes constricts the blood vessels that nourish your skin.
- **Keep your skin moist.** Moisturizers can't prevent wrinkles, but they can temporarily mask tiny lines and creases. To relieve dryness and itching, take fewer baths and showers, avoid antibacterial soaps, increase the humidity in your home during the winter and apply oils to your skin.
- **Learn more about wrinkle treatments.** If you're concerned about wrinkles, talk to a dermatologist. Retin-A, a prescription cream containing a synthetic derivative of vitamin A, has been shown to improve sun-damaged skin and make skin smoother. Botulinum toxin (Botox) injections, face-lifts, chemical peels and laser treatments also can help smooth wrinkles.
- **Learn more about hair-loss treatments.** If your thinning hair bothers you, consider your options. Medications can stimulate hair growth, or hair follicles can be surgically transplanted from other parts of your head. Toupees and weaves are op-

tions, too. If facial hair is a problem, you can bleach the hair or remove it by plucking, waxing or electrolysis or with hair remover. Removal doesn't stimulate further growth.

# Sleep changes

It's a myth that you need less sleep as you get older. Your need for sleep remains fairly constant throughout your life. But over time, sleep patterns tend to change. You may have a harder time falling asleep or staying asleep, and you may also find that you sleep less soundly. You may spend less time in "deep sleep," which helps your

body recover from the day's activities. As a result, you may feel less well rested and alert than you used to after a night's sleep.

In addition to altered sleep patterns, physical and psychological problems can interfere with sleep. Chronic pain, digestive problems, depression, anxiety and stress can contribute to insomnia. Medical conditions such as an enlarged prostate and diabetes cause a need to urinate several times during the night. Medications, including some antidepressants, bronchodilators, high blood pressure medicines and steroids, can disturb sleep. A snoring bed partner also can make it hard to get a good night's sleep.

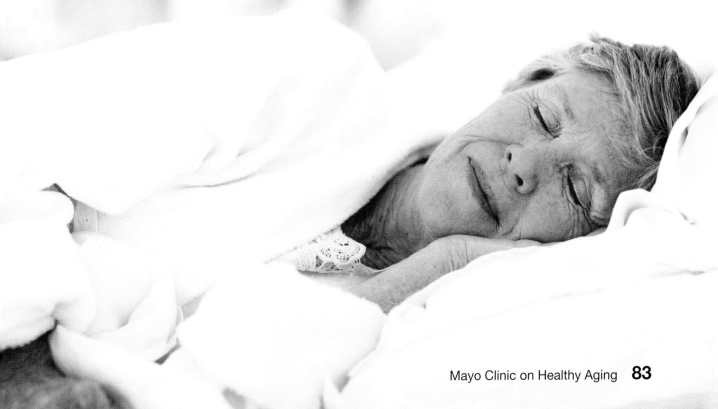

## What you can do

Good sleep habits can help minimize or prevent sleep problems.

- **Limit naps during the day.** Don't take a nap if doing so makes it more difficult for you to fall asleep at night. If you do nap during the day, keep it short, 15 to 30 minutes.
- **Minimize interruptions.** Close your door or create a subtle background noise, such as that from a fan, to drown out other noises. Drink less before bed so that you won't need to use the bathroom as often. Encourage a restless or snoring bed partner to see a doctor. Be cautious of a pet that sleeps with you. It can interrupt your sleep, and you may not be aware of it.
- **Create a restful environment.** Keep the bedroom at a comfortable temperature. Choose comfortable sheets, blankets and pillows, and a mattress that's neither too firm nor too soft. Use the bedroom only for relaxing activities.
- **Stick to a regular sleep schedule.** Go to bed at the same time every night and wake at the same time every morning.
- **Avoid substances that disrupt sleep.** During the late afternoon and evening, avoid stimulants such as caffeine, nicotine and decongestants that can keep you awake. Alcohol may make you sleepy at bedtime, but it increases awakenings later in the night.
- **Exercise daily.** Complete your activity at least five to six hours before you go to sleep.
- **Wind down gradually.** Take a warm shower or bath. Read a book or watch television until you become drowsy. Don't watch the news if it generally distresses you.
- **Be careful with medications.** Talk to your doctor before taking any sleeping pills, especially if you're taking other prescription medications. Ask whether your current medications may be contributing to insomnia.

# Urinary changes

The urinary system includes your kidneys, ureters and bladder. Kidney function gradually declines with age.

At about age 40, you begin to lose important filtering units within the kidneys, called nephrons. By the time you're 80, your kidneys are 20 to 30 percent smaller than when you were 20. As kidney function declines, you're more likely either to become dehydrated or to retain fluid.

Despite these changes, the kidneys have a built-in reserve capacity, and they continue to work normally as you get older. Only if you have a chronic illness, such as high blood pressure or diabetes, might these changes pose a problem.

The bladder also changes with age. Its walls become less elastic, so you can hold less urine. As a result, you may have to go to the bathroom more often. At the same time, bladder muscles may weaken, and the bladder may not empty completely when you go to the bathroom. This increases the risk of urinary tract infections.

Urinary incontinence is more common with age. In men, incontinence can result from noncancerous enlargement of the prostate gland, prostate cancer or prostate surgery. In older women, the lining of the tube through which urine passes (urethra) thins, and the tube itself shortens. The muscle that controls the passage of urine is less able to close tightly, and the pelvic muscles weaken, reducing bladder support.

Other factors that can contribute to incontinence include infections, excess weight, frequent constipation and a chronic cough. Several medications, including some used for depression, high blood pressure and heart disease, also can cause the problem.

## What you can do

To preserve your kidneys and bladder and prevent or manage incontinence:

- **Drink plenty of fluids.** However, excess fluids can result in having to go to the bathroom often. If you have problems with frequent urination at night, stop drinking liquids after about 7 p.m.
- **Limit or avoid alcohol and caffeine.** These beverages cause more frequent urination.
- **Be careful with medications.** Ask your doctor about safe use of over-the-counter pain relievers and other medications, including herbal and dietary supplements. Over-the-counter decongestants can tighten the muscles that control urine flow, making urination more difficult.
- **Follow a fixed bathroom schedule.** This may be more effective in preventing problems than is waiting for the need to go. Try to urinate all that you can during this time to empty your bladder completely.

- **Do pelvic floor exercises.** In both men and women, pelvic floor exercises (Kegels) can often help with mild to moderate incontinence. To do the exercises, imagine that you're trying to stop the flow of urine. Squeeze the muscles you would use and hold for a count of 10. Repeat this exercise four times a day. It may be two to three months before you begin to notice results. To maintain the benefits, keep doing them.
- **Keep active.** Inactivity causes you to retain urine.

# Vision changes

A change in vision is often one of the first signs of aging. By the time you're in your 40s, the lenses of your eyes become stiffer and less elastic, so you're less able to focus on nearby objects or small print. You start holding your reading material at arm's length. This change in vision is known as presbyopia. It can also cause headaches and eye fatigue from reading or other close work.

The sharpness of your vision — your eyes' ability to distinguish fine details — also gradually declines with age. Almost everyone older than age 55 needs glasses at least part of the time.

Other age-related eye changes can affect your sight. By the time you're 60, your pupils shrink to about one-third the size they were when you were 20. The pupils may also react more slowly to darkness or bright light. You might feel blinded in bright light or unable to see in a dark room. Glare from sunlight or reflected light becomes more of a problem. Some people have difficulty driving at night because of problems with glare, brightness and darkness.

With age, you become more at risk of common eye disorders.

## Cataracts

A cataract is a gradual clouding of the normally clear lens of your eye. Cataracts keep light from easily passing through the lens, resulting in blurred vision, double vision or seeing halos around lights. Cataracts can cause problems with vision at night and especially with night driving.

## Glaucoma

Glaucoma is the buildup of fluid within the eyeball to an abnormally high pressure. This condition narrows your field of vision and can damage the optic nerve. Glaucoma can lead to blindness if not diagnosed and treated.

## Age-related macular degeneration

This disease is the leading cause of severe vision loss in people over age 60. Age-related macular degeneration affects the macula, the part of the retina that provides sharp central vision. Signs and symptoms include hazy, gray vision and a central blind spot.

## What you can do

Because good vision is important to fully enjoying your later years, you want to take care of your eyes.

- **Have a regular eye exam.** Early detection is the best defense against serious eye diseases such as glaucoma and macular degeneration. See an eye specialist regularly, especially as you experience changes in your vision (see page 291). Seek prompt medical attention if you

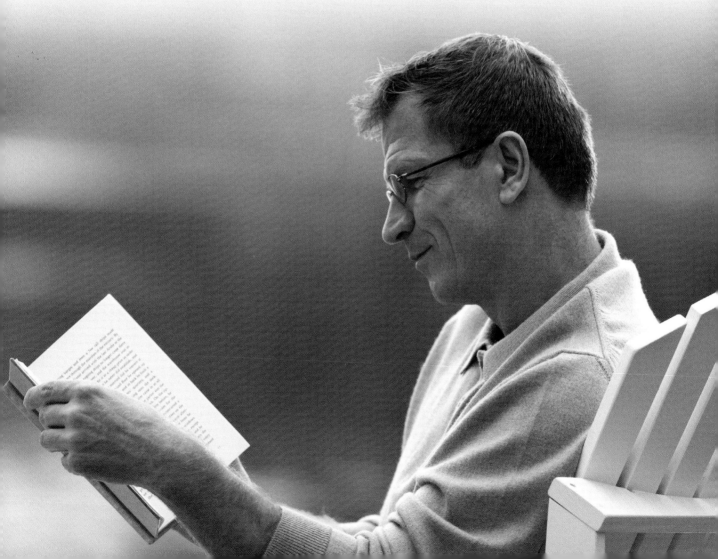

lose some or all vision in an eye or experience flashes of light in your visual field.

- **When outside, wear sunglasses and a hat or visor with a brim.** This can help reduce glare. Too much sunlight also increases your chance of getting cataracts.
- **Don't smoke.** Smoking increases your risk of cataracts.
- **Have adequate light indoors.** Even if you don't have vision problems, you'll need more light to see. It's more effective to increase the light on your work or reading material than to turn on an overhead light.
- **Use artificial tears solutions or eyedrops.** These products reduce symptoms of dry eyes. Aging eyes produce less tears.

all of these changes in one fell swoop or in their most extreme manifestations. And for some aspects of aging, there are things that you can do to help slow the natural timeline.

It's also possible to embrace these changes by cultivating a positive attitude. As Mark Twain said, "Wrinkles should merely indicate where smiles have been."

# An individual process

The list of physical changes that occur with age may seem long. Fortunately, most of these bodily "insults" occur gradually and often they aren't very — if at all — noticeable.

Remember that aging is an individual process. You're not likely to experience

# Chapter 5

# Respond to your risks

If you think that your genes rule when it comes to your health, you're missing half the picture. Yes, genetics are an important factor, setting the stage for health throughout our lifetimes. But the truth is that your health depends just as much on your lifestyle choices — especially in your later years. Research confirms that your weight, activity and stress levels, and health habits play a very large role in determining your overall well-being.

What does this mean? If some of your habits and behaviors are unhealthy, the sooner you change them and adopt healthier ones, the greater your chances of living to a ripe old age and enjoying those years.

So what are risky habits and behaviors? They're those activities or lifestyle choices that increase your likelihood of developing disease. For some people, a risk to their health may be inactivity or excess weight. For others, it might be a lifestyle filled with too much stress. For yet others, it may be smoking or drinking too much alcohol.

Whatever your risks are, it's never too late to change them. If you don't address certain behaviors now, your efforts to ensure that your years ahead are plentiful and enjoyable may be for naught.

Following is a brief overview of common health risk factors, and why these habits and behaviors can put your well-being in jeopardy. If you feel like the time is right to make a healthy change in one of these areas, we've included tips to help you get started.

# Inactive lifestyle

If you aren't physically active, it's time to get moving. Studies show that only about one-quarter to one-third of older adults participate in moderate physical activity three or more days a week.

Maybe you think it's too late to get anything out of exercise. In fact, the opposite is true. Compared with teens and younger adults, older adults actually have more to gain from becoming more physically active. That's because the older you become, the greater your risk of illness and disease. Exercise can help reduce that risk.

## Health risks

Lack of physical activity contributes to many chronic diseases and conditions. Here's a brief overview.

- **High blood pressure.** Too little physical activity increases your risk of high blood pressure by increasing your risk of being overweight. Inactive people, regardless of their weight, also tend to have higher heart rates. Their heart muscles have to work harder with each contraction — and that results in a stronger force on the arteries.

- **High blood cholesterol.** Lack of exercise can increase your level of low-density lipoprotein (LDL) cholesterol, the "bad" cholesterol. It can also lower your level of high-density lipoprotein (HDL) cholesterol, the "good" cholesterol.
- **Diabetes.** The less active you are, the greater your risk of diabetes.
- **Obesity.** Sedentary people are more likely to gain weight because they don't burn calories through activity.
- **Heart attack.** An inactive lifestyle contributes to high blood cholesterol levels and obesity, increasing your risk of heart attack.
- **Colon cancer.** If you're inactive, you're more likely to develop colon cancer. This may be because when you're inactive, waste stays in your colon longer.
- **Osteoporosis.** Weight-bearing activities, such as walking or lifting weights, help keep your bones strong. If you're inactive, your bones become less dense and more brittle, leading to osteoporosis and an increased risk of fractures.

## Why change?

Regular physical activity can improve your quality of life. With increased strength and endurance from daily exercise, routine tasks such as doing yard-work, washing the car, washing clothes or cleaning the house are easier to do.

Exercise will also give you more energy and vitality so that you can enjoy spending time with friends and family, traveling, doing hobbies, or whatever it is that you look forward to.

Equally important, regular exercise can reduce your risk of dying prematurely. Exercise helps prevent, delay or control a number of diseases and conditions that can cause injury or disability and shorten your life.

## Where to start

If you're inactive and you haven't had a physical examination within the past two years or you have a chronic medical condition, it's generally a good idea to see your doctor for a checkup before beginning an exercise program.

Once you've gotten your doctor's OK, ease your way into exercise. Then you can start working your way up to some healthy fitness goals. For more information on how to get started with an exercise program or how to include more physical activity in your day, see Chapter 8.

# Being overweight

As you know only too well, over time it can be more difficult to keep the pounds off. As you get older, you gradually lose muscle mass, which decreases your metabolism. If you don't also decrease the number of calories you eat or increase your activity level, you gain weight.

Having excess body fat is a serious threat to your health and future happiness. If you're overweight or obese, you're more likely to develop a number of potentially serious health problems.

Losing weight isn't easy, but it can be done — regardless of your age or weight. And doing so will greatly improve your quality of life during the years ahead.

## Health risks

Here's an overview of conditions commonly associated with obesity.

- **High blood pressure.** As fat cells accumulate, your body produces more blood to keep the new tissue supplied with oxygen and nutrients. More blood traveling through your arteries means added pressure on

# Is obesity an overrated health risk?

In recent years, obesity has been touted as a leading cause of preventable death in the United States, second only to smoking. In 2004, the Centers for Disease Control and Prevention (CDC) attributed 365,000 deaths annually to obesity. That number was later dropped considerably — to 112,000 obesity-related deaths a year.

Why such a great discrepancy? First, the second estimate uses newer data. Second, somewhat different statistical methods were used. Earlier estimates only reflected obesity-related health risks that people experienced in the 1970s. The newer data, some with follow-up through the year 2000, appear to reflect a real decline in the risk of dying from obesity-related diseases, such as heart disease.

Big improvements in controlling risk factors for heart disease may have resulted in far fewer people dying today from obesity. The new data may also reflect advances in lifesaving interventions for obesity-related diseases.

So, does this mean being overweight is less important than once thought? Not at all. This estimate only relates to deaths. Just as important are the diseases or conditions associated with obesity, including serious chronic diseases such as diabetes, heart disease, arthritis and some cancers. These are typically accompanied by pain and suffering, reduced quality of life, and medical costs for treatment.

It should be noted that obesity-related deaths don't adequately represent overall deaths related to poor nutrition and physical inactivity. People who are a normal weight can also die of heart disease caused — at least in part — by poor diet and lack of physical activity.

your artery walls. Weight gain also typically increases insulin, a hormone that helps control blood sugar. Increased insulin is associated with sodium and water retention, another contributor to increased blood volume. In addition, excess weight is often associated with increased heart rate and reduced transport capacity of your blood vessels. These two factors can increase your blood pressure and may lead to a burst blood vessel.

- **Diabetes.** Excess fat makes your body resistant to insulin, the hormone that helps transport sugar (glucose) from your blood into individual cells. When your body is resistant to insulin, your cells can't get the sugar they need for energy, resulting in diabetes. In fact, obesity is a leading cause of type 2 diabetes. If you're at risk of developing diabetes, you may be able to avoid the disease by losing weight.

- **Unhealthy cholesterol levels.** The same dietary choices that lead to obesity often result in elevated levels of low-density lipoprotein (LDL, or "bad") cholesterol and reduced levels of high-density lipoprotein (HDL, or "good") cholesterol. Obesity is also associated with high levels of triglycerides, another type of blood fat. Abnormal blood-fat levels can cause buildup of fatty

deposits (plaques) in your arteries, putting you at risk of heart attack and stroke.

- **Osteoarthritis.** Excess weight puts extra pressure on your joints and wears away the cartilage that protects them, resulting in joint pain and stiffness.

- **Sleep apnea.** Most people with sleep apnea are overweight, which contributes to a large neck and narrowed airways. In sleep apnea, your upper airway becomes intermittently blocked, resulting in frequent awakening at night and subsequent drowsiness during the day. Left untreated, the condition can lead to a heart attack.

- **Cancer.** Several types of cancer are associated with being overweight. In women, these include cancers of the breast, uterus, colon and gallbladder. Overweight men have a higher risk of colon and prostate cancers.

## Why change?

Losing weight will help you feel better. You'll feel better physically and have more energy for the things you've looked forward to doing, such as travel, hobbies and spending time with your grandchildren. And you'll feel better about yourself. If you've been frustrated because of your weight, the boost in self-esteem that comes from losing a few pounds can be a very welcome change.

Reaching and maintaining a healthy weight will also improve your health over the long term. And remember, you don't have to lose a lot of weight to enjoy health benefits. Modest losses of just 10 to 20 percent of your body weight can bring significant benefits including lowering your blood pressure and reducing your risk of cardiovascular disease, stroke and diabetes. If you weigh 200 pounds, that's losing as few as 20 pounds.

### Where to start

Slow and steady weight loss of 1 or 2 pounds a week is considered the safest way to lose weight and the best way to keep it off.

Begin by eating more healthy foods and fewer unhealthy foods and by getting some exercise every day. If you're worried that you can't lose weight on your own, talk with your doctor or a dietitian. And tell yourself that you can do it.

Having the right attitude is very important. To lose weight — and to keep it off — you need to examine and address

habits, emotions and behaviors that may have caused you to gain weight.

For more information on healthy weight loss, see Chapter 9.

# Excess stress

One of the biggest culprits in unhealthy aging is one you may not expect — stress. Increasingly, researchers are viewing stress — how much we face and how well we deal with it — as a critical factor in how well we age. Studies consistently show that people who do best at managing stress also tend to stay the healthiest in older age.

### Health risks

Stress occurs when the demands in your life exceed your ability to cope with them. Many things can cause stress — from simple things such as having to stand in line at the checkout counter to more-serious challenges such as caring for an ailing family member or adjusting to retirement.

Whatever the cause of your stress, if it's overwhelming you, you need to address it. Stress is a serious health risk.

When you experience stress, your heart beats faster, your blood pressure rises and your breathing may quicken. These responses are intended to help you flee from a dangerous situation or fight for your life. After the stressful moment (threat) passes, your body relaxes again.

The problem is, situations that aren't life-threatening — worrying about finances or an argument with a family member — can trigger this same response. If stressful situations pile up one after another, your body has no chance to recover, making you more vulnerable to long-term health problems.

Stress may contribute to the development of an illness, it may aggravate an existing health problem or it may trigger an illness if you're already at risk. Here's a brief overview.

- **Immune system.** Chronic stress tends to dampen your immune system, making you more susceptible to colds, the flu and other infections. In some cases, stress can have the opposite effect, making your immune system overactive. The result is an increased risk of autoimmune diseases, in which your immune system attacks your body's own cells.

- **Cardiovascular disease.** If you exhibit extreme increases in heart rate and blood pressure in response to daily stress, this may add to your risk of a heart attack. Such surges may gradually injure your coronary arteries and heart. Increased blood clotting from persistent stress also can put you at risk of a heart attack or stroke.

- **Gastrointestinal problems.** It's common to have a stomachache or diarrhea when you're under stress. Stress may also trigger or worsen symptoms associated with conditions such as irritable bowel syndrome or nonulcer dyspepsia.

- **Depression and anxiety.** Stressful life events — such as the death of a loved one — may trigger depression. So can chronic stress if you're prone to the disorder. Stress may also worsen the signs and symptoms of other mental health disorders, such as anxiety.

- **Other illnesses.** Stress worsens many skin conditions — including psoriasis, eczema, hives and acne — and can be a trigger for asthma attacks. Stress can also heighten your body's pain response. This may make the chronic pain associated with conditions such as arthritis, fibromyalgia or a back injury more difficult to manage.

# Exercises to help you relax

Following are some techniques you can use to calm your mind and body. Pick one or two and practice them so that they become natural, and you can apply them when you need them.

## Relaxed breathing

This form of relaxation focuses on deep, relaxed breathing as a way to relieve tension and stress. Before you begin, find a comfortable position. Lie on a bed or couch or sit on a chair. Then do the following:

- Inhale. With your mouth closed and your shoulders relaxed, inhale slowly and deeply through your nose to the count of six. Allow the air to fill your diaphragm — the muscle between your abdomen and chest — pushing your abdomen out.
- Pause for a second.
- Exhale. Slowly release air through your mouth as you count to six.
- Pause for a second.
- Repeat. Complete this breathing cycle several times.

## Progressive muscle relaxation

Progressive muscle relaxation is a technique that involves relaxing a series of muscles one at a time. Begin by sitting or lying in a comfortable position. Loosen tight clothing and close your eyes. Tense each muscle group for five seconds then relax for at least 30 seconds. Repeat once before moving to the next muscle group.

- **Upper face.** Lift your eyebrows toward the ceiling, feeling the tension in your forehead.
- **Central face.** Squint your eyes and wrinkle your nose and mouth, feeling the tension in the center of your face.
- **Lower face.** Clench your teeth and pull back the corners of your mouth toward your ears.
- **Neck.** Gently touch your chin to your chest, feeling the stretch in the back of your neck.

- **Shoulders.** Pull your shoulders up toward your ears, feeling the tension in your shoulders, head, neck and upper back.
- **Upper arms.** Pull your arms back and press your elbows toward the sides of your body. Try not to tense your lower arms. Feel the tension in your arms, shoulders and back.
- **Hands and lower arms.** Make a tight fist and pull up your wrists. Feel the tension in your hands and lower arms.
- **Chest, shoulders and upper back.** Pull your shoulders back as if you're trying to make your shoulder blades touch.
- **Stomach.** Pull your stomach toward your spine, tightening your abdominal muscles.
- **Upper legs.** Squeeze your knees together. Feel the tension in your thighs.
- **Lower legs.** Flex your ankles so that your toes point toward your face. Feel the tension in your calves.
- **Feet.** Turn your feet inward and curl your toes outward.

### Visualization

Also known as guided imagery, visualization involves lying quietly and picturing yourself in a pleasant and peaceful setting.

- Allow thoughts to flow through your mind. But don't focus on any of them. Tell yourself that you're relaxed and calm, that your hands are heavy and warm — or cool if you're hot — and that your heart is beating calmly.
- Breathe slowly, regularly and deeply.
- Think of a calming setting. Once you're relaxed, imagine yourself in a favorite place or in a spot of beauty and stillness.
- Let go. After five or 10 minutes, rouse yourself gradually.

Brain studies of people undergoing guided imagery sessions show that visualizing (imagining) something stimulates the same parts of the brain that are stimulated during the actual experience. If sitting by the ocean relaxes you, you may achieve the same level of relaxation through visualization as you would if you were actually there.

# Why change?

Reducing stress can help you to become a more productive and happy person. As you learn how to relax and manage stress, you may even find yourself enjoying things that once seemed burdensome. Just as important, letting go of stress can often improve your physical health.

# Where to start

There are many ways to deal with stress. Experiment with the following strategies to see if they can help you better manage stress.

- **Learn to relax.** Learning how to relax is an important first step in managing stress. Seek out activities that give you pleasure, be it exercise, art, music or some other hobby, and devote at least 30 minutes to these activities every day. You may also want to experiment with other relaxation techniques, such as deep-breathing and muscle relaxation exercises (see pages 96 and 97), yoga, or meditation.
- **Simplify and organize your day.** If your busy lifestyle seems to be a source of stress, ask yourself if it's because you try to squeeze too many things into your day or because you aren't organized. If you're overextended, cut out some activities or delegate some tasks to others. If your home or work environment is so cluttered that it's causing you stress, take the time to organize it.
- **Practice tolerance.** Try to become more tolerant of yourself and of situations over which you may have little control. Change is constant and certain changes — losses, disappointments and events that you can't control — will continue to occur, like it or not.
- **Learn to manage anger.** Anger can significantly increase and prolong stress if you remain angry for an extended period. Anger can even trigger a heart attack. Identify your anger triggers and find release valves — ways to release the energy produced by your anger. Exercise, writing in a journal or listening to soothing music are some ways to let go of anger.
- **Think positive.** In many cases, simply choosing to look at situations in a more positive way can reduce the stress in your life. Throughout the day, stop and evaluate what you're thinking and find a way to put a positive spin on any negative thoughts.

- **Seek professional help.** If these simple measures aren't helpful, don't be afraid to seek guidance from your doctor, a counselor, psychiatrist, psychologist or clergyperson. These people can provide you with additional and more-personalized tools for recognizing and managing stress. Many people mistakenly believe that seeking outside help is a sign of weakness. To the contrary, it takes strength to realize that you need help and good judgment to seek it.

# Excessive alcohol use

Alcoholism and alcohol abuse are less prevalent among older adults than among the general population, but that doesn't mean older adults are immune from this problem. Among adults who abuse alcohol, one-third develop the problem later in life, perhaps in reaction to retirement, failing health or the death of a spouse. Your body also seems to become more sensitive to alcohol as you become older. If your drinking habits don't change to compensate for that, you may find that you have a problem on your hands.

## Health risks

Drinking too much alcohol produces several harmful effects:

- **Sleep.** Alcohol causes sleeplessness and shallow sleep. Alcohol may help you fall asleep, but it frequently wakes you up in the middle of the night. Even moderate amounts of alcohol can disrupt normal sleeping patterns.
- **Brain and nervous system problems.** Excessive drinking can cause short-term memory loss and extreme fatigue. If you abuse alcohol and are deficient in nutrients, particularly thiamin, you may develop weakness and paralysis of your eye muscles, severe amnesia, and hallucinations.
- **Liver disorders.** Drinking heavily can cause you to develop an inflammation of the liver (alcoholic hepatitis). Hepatitis may lead to the irreversible and progressive destruction of liver tissue (cirrhosis).
- **Gastrointestinal disorders.** Excessive alcohol can cause inflammation of the lining of the stomach (gastritis), as well as stomach and esophageal ulcers. It can also interfere with the absorption of nutrients, and it can lead to inflammation of your pancreas (pancreatitis).

## How much is too much?

The National Institute on Alcohol Abuse and Alcoholism recommends that men who are age 65 and younger should have no more than two drinks a day. Women and anyone older than age 65 should have no more than one drink a day. The stricter amounts for people age 65 and older reflect the fact that, with age, your body processes alcohol more slowly.

Each of the following is the equivalent of one drink:
- 4 to 5 ounces of wine
- 12 ounces of beer
- 1 to 1½ ounces of 80-proof distilled spirits

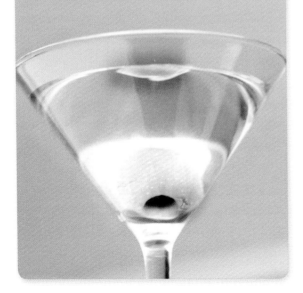

- **Cardiovascular system disorders.** Too much alcohol can lead to high blood pressure and damage your heart muscle. These conditions can put you at increased risk of heart failure or stroke.
- **Sexual disorders.** Alcohol abuse can cause erectile dysfunction in men. In women, it alcohol abuse can interrupt menstruation.
- **Cancer.** People who abuse alcohol have a rate of cancer that's higher than that of the general population. This is especially true of cancers of the mouth, larynx, esophagus, stomach and pancreas.
- **Drug interactions.** Alcohol can have dangerous effects when it interacts with numerous medications.

## Why change?

You may be reluctant to seek treatment for alcohol abuse or alcoholism. But by confronting your problem, you'll be taking the first step toward a healthier, more positive future. In addition to reducing your risk of serious health problems, seeking treatment likely will improve your relationships with family and friends. You'll also be able to think more clearly. Studies show that older adults benefit from alcohol treatment just as much as do younger adults.

## Where to start

If you feel guilty about your drinking, talk with your doctor. Even if you don't think you have a problem, but if your friends and family are worried about your drinking, take their concerns seriously.

If you're dependent on alcohol, cutting back isn't an option. Abstaining from alcohol must be a part of your treatment goal. There are many options to help people with alcohol problems. Treatment is typically tailored to your individual needs and may include counseling or a brief intervention — drafting of a specific treatment plan, which may include behavior modification techniques, participation in Alcoholics Anonymous (AA) or follow-up care at a treatment center.

# Smoking

If you're like many adults who smoke, you probably picked up the habit before its harmful health effects were widely known. Now that the facts are available, you may be so dependent on nicotine that quitting smoking seems impossible. Whatever your reason for continuing to smoke, it's never too late to stop. Even if you don't quit until later in life, doing so has proven health benefits.

## Health risks

When you inhale tobacco smoke, you're ingesting a toxic combination of more than 4,000 chemicals. This includes 63 cancer-causing agents (carcinogens) and trace amounts of such poisons as cyanide, arsenic and formaldehyde. The negative health effects throughout your body are numerous:

- **Cancer.** Smoking is a major risk factor for cancers of the mouth, larynx, pharynx, esophagus, lung, stomach, pancreas, kidney, bladder and cervix. It's the cause of almost 90 percent of all lung cancer — the most deadly form of cancer in the United States.
- **Chronic obstructive pulmonary disease (COPD).** Tobacco smoke damages or destroys tiny air sacs in your lungs called alveoli. The majority of deaths from COPD are related to cigarette smoking. The more years you smoke and the more packs you smoke, the greater your risk.
- **Cardiovascular disease.** The nicotine in tobacco smoke triggers your adrenal glands to produce hormones

# A second chance at life

Like many young men of his generation, Ed started smoking while he was in college. He started slowly, having an occasional cigarette in the fraternity house where he lived. But before long, the addictive power of nicotine took hold. Within the first year of starting to smoke, Ed was up to a pack a day — or more.

Ed continued smoking into his 50s, going through a pack and a half of cigarettes every day. He'd smoke when he was driving, talking on the phone or watching a particularly exciting sporting event on TV. "I suppose I smoked to relieve stress, but it was mostly an addiction," he says. "I got to the point where my brain just needed it three or four times an hour."

Ed tried to quit smoking cold turkey a couple of times. After one attempt, he remained smoke-free for three or four weeks. But the real turning point came when he had a heart attack at age 52. "After that, I made the decision to stop smoking," he says. "Plus, it was something my wife, Jerelyn, really wanted."

Because he was scheduled to undergo triple bypass surgery, Ed was advised not to use nicotine replacement therapy to treat his withdrawal symptoms. Instead, his doctors recommended the antidepressant bupropion (Zyban). Bupropion raises the level of a chemical in your brain called dopamine, the same chemical released by nicotine. Thus, it helps replicate the feel-good response you get from smoking. "I found bupropion very effective," Ed says.

After his surgery, Ed also participated in a weeklong, inpatient smoking cessation program. "That program taught me how to cope with the urge to smoke in other ways, such as with exercise and other distractions," he says. "The urge to smoke can be very short-lived, if you can distract yourself."

Ed hasn't had a cigarette since he made the decision to stop smoking. "Once I quit, I quit," he says. But that's not to say that the process was easy. "Smoking is a pretty powerful addiction. It's not impossible to quit, but it requires a lot of hard work. Nobody has it easy."

For Ed, one of the greatest allies in his quest to stay smoke-free is the passage of time. During the first year after he stopped smoking, he continued to experience frequent urges to smoke, especially when he was driving or talking on the phone. "For me, it took a year before I could really throw off my reliance on cigarettes," he says.

Since then, things have been easier, but Ed knows he's only a cigarette away from trouble. "The threat is still there. If I lit up today, I'd be back to a pack and a half a day in no time. But the passage of time helps break the habit. The further away you get, the easier it is to cope."

Now approaching age 60, Ed has been smoke-free for almost seven years — and has noticed dramatic changes in his life as a result.

"I certainly do feel better and healthier since quitting smoking and undergoing bypass surgery," he says. "Like a lot of my contemporaries, I tended to let my physical condition decline through inattention, and consequently, I paid a stiff price. But I got a second chance. Now I'm committed to lifestyle choices that I feel will prolong my life and make me feel better at the same time. For me, that means a regular exercise program. And, of course, no smoking."

Ed is also using the confidence he's gained and the skills he's acquired to help others make it down the same path. Ed works part time in the nicotine dependence unit at a local medical center. He spends evenings and nights with individuals who are attempting to quit smoking, simply keeping them company and helping them through rough points in the process.

He wants others to know that if he did it, they can quit, too.

that stress your heart by increasing your blood pressure and heart rate. At the same time, the carbon monoxide in tobacco smoke binds to hemoglobin in your blood, taking the place of valuable oxygen and reducing the amount of oxygen available to your heart and other vital organs. Smoking also contributes to the buildup of fatty deposits in your arteries (atherosclerosis). These changes all increase your risk of heart attack and stroke.

- **Other conditions.** Smoking increases your risk of respiratory infections, gum disease, cataracts and peptic ulcers. In men, it increases the risk of erectile dysfunction. In postmenopausal women, it increases the risk of osteoporosis and hip fracture.

## Why change?

When you stop smoking, your health will improve almost immediately. Within 24 hours, the levels of harmful carbon monoxide and nicotine in your system will decrease significantly.

Within a few days, your senses of smell and taste should improve. You may breathe easier, and your smoker's cough will begin to disappear.

Within 20 minutes of smoking that last cigarette, your heart rate drops. Within a year, your risk of heart attack is cut in half. Within two to three years, your risk is the same as that of a nonsmoker.

You'll also rid yourself of the unpleasantness associated with smoking — bad breath, yellow teeth, and smelly clothing and hair. And you'll set the right example for your children, grandchildren and friends.

## Where to start

Stopping smoking can be very difficult, especially if you've been smoking for many years. However, with today's medications and other smoking cessation strategies, your chances of success have never been greater. Talk with your doctor, and the two of you can work on a plan tailored to your needs and lifestyle to help you quit.

Generally, quit plans combine several different strategies, such as using a nicotine replacement product, attending a smoking cessation support group, or seeking individual counseling with a doctor, psychologist, nurse or counselor. Studies show that using more than one strategy increases your chances of becoming smoke-free.

## Resources for quitting smoking

Toll-free tobacco quit lines are available in every state in the United States and many countries throughout the world. Call the national quit line at 877-448-7848 to find the best fit for you. These online resources also can help you:

**American Cancer Society**
*www.cancer.org*

**American Heart Association**
*www.heart.org*

**American Lung Association**
*www.lungusa.org*

**Ex**
*www.becomeanex.org*

**Mayo Clinic Nicotine Dependence Center**
*www.mayoclinic.org/ndc-rst*

**National Cancer Institute**
Free Help to Quit Smoking
*www.cancer.org*

**Nicotine Anonymous**
*www.nicotine-anonymous.org*

**QuitNet**
*www.quitnet.com*

**Smokefree.gov**
*www.smokefree.gov*

Many smokers try to quit cold turkey — making a sudden, decisive break from smoking with little or no reduction beforehand. If this strategy appeals to you, make sure you're both emotionally and physically prepared to withstand the strong desire to smoke. Quit-smoking medication is usually recommended when using this method, to ease the withdrawal symptoms of nicotine addiction.

Other medications include nicotine patches, gum and lozenges, as well as prescription nasal sprays, inhalers and pills. These medications help control nicotine cravings and reduce the pleasurable effects of smoking.

If you don't succeed in quitting the first — or any — time, it's worth trying again. Your doctor may be able to help by adjusting the dose of your medication, recommending a different medication, or simply by providing advice and support.

# Family genes

The genes you inherit from your parents can increase your risk of developing certain diseases or disorders. Are there diseases that run in your family for which you may be at risk?

Key features that suggest an illness may be passed from one generation to the next (genetic) include:

- Early onset of symptoms
- The same disease in more than one close relative
- Certain combinations of diseases, such as breast and ovarian cancers within the same person or family

You can't change your family history; however, genes aren't destiny. In many cases, whether you'll actually develop a condition to which you may be genetically predestined depends to a great extent on your health habits.

## Health risks

Here's an overview of diseases and disorders that can run in families, resulting from one or more flawed genes passed from one generation to the next.

- **Alzheimer's disease.** Your risk increases if you have a parent, brother or sister with the disease, but usually there isn't a clear hereditary pattern.
- **Breast cancer.** If you have a first-degree relative (mother, sister or daughter) or other close relative (grandmother or aunt) with breast cancer, you may be at increased risk, especially if your relative was diagnosed before age 50.
- **Colorectal cancer.** Risk increases if you have a parent, sibling or child with colon or rectal cancer. If two or more first-degree relatives have it, the risk is even greater. Two hereditary conditions — familial adenomatous polyposis (FAP) and hereditary nonpolyposis colorectal cancer (HNPCC) — also may predispose you to colon cancer.
- **Depression.** You're at increased risk if a parent, sibling or child has depression. But other factors, such as stressful life events or a serious medical condition, also play a role for many people.

- **Diabetes.** You have a greater chance of developing type 1 or type 2 diabetes if a parent, brother or sister has the one of the conditions.
- **Eye disease.** A family history of macular degeneration, cataracts or glaucoma can increase your risk of developing these conditions.
- **Heart disease.** Your risk of heart disease is greater if you have a parent, grandparent or sibling with the condition. This is especially true if it developed at an early age.
- **High blood pressure.** If one of your parents has high blood pressure, you're at increased risk of developing the condition. If it affects both of your parents, your risk increases substantially.
- **Ovarian cancer.** Your risk increases if you have a mother, sister or daughter with ovarian cancer. If two or more first-degree relatives are diagnosed, the risk is even greater. A family history of breast or colon cancer also may increase your risk of ovarian cancer.
- **Parkinson's disease.** Studies show that people who have a parent or sibling with Parkinson's are at greater risk of developing the condition.
- **Prostate cancer.** Your risk is substantially increased if your father or brother has prostate cancer. Your risk is even greater if your relative's cancer was diagnosed at a younger age.
- **Stroke.** Your risk of stroke may increase if you have a parent or sibling who with a history of stroke. In some types of hemorrhagic strokes, you may inherit artery abnormalities that put you at risk of an aneurysm, which could rupture and cause bleeding into the brain.

## Why change?

True, you can't change your genes. But you can change your attitude toward diseases and disorders that may run in your family. Instead of simply waiting for a disease to develop for which you may be at risk, you can take steps to prevent it, slow its onset or reduce its severity. Being proactive, instead of reactive, may result in a better quality of life — and could even save your life.

## Where to start

If you don't know your family health history, contact your relatives and inquire about their health. In addition to your parents, brothers, sisters and children, be aware of diseases affecting your aunts, uncles, cousins, grandparents and grandchildren.

# Lapses and relapses

A lapse occurs when you revert to old behaviors once or twice. It's temporary, common and a sign that you need to get back in control.

A relapse is more serious. After several lapses have occurred in a short span of time, you're at risk of completely reverting back to your old behavior. You panic, afraid that you'll undo all your good efforts. You may give up and say, "I guess I just can't do it."

When lapses and relapses happens, calm down. Take a deep breath. Consider these tips for getting back on track when you have a lapse:

- Don't let negative thoughts take over. Remember that mistakes happen and that each day is a chance to start anew.
- Clearly identify the problem, then create a list of possible solutions. Pick a solution to try. If it works, then you've got a plan for preventing another lapse. If it doesn't work, try the next solution and go through the same process until you find one that works.
- Get support. Talk to family, friends or a professional counselor.
- Work out your guilt and frustration with exercise. Take a walk or go for a swim. Keep the exercise upbeat.
- Recommit to your goals. Review them and make sure they're still realistic.

What if you do relapse? Although relapses are disappointing, they can help you learn that your goals may be unrealistic, that certain situations create challenges for your plan or that certain strategies don't work.

Above all, realize that reverting to old behaviors doesn't mean that all hope is lost. It just means that you need to recharge your motivation, recommit to your plan and return to healthy behaviors.

For each family member, record his or her relationship to you, sex, year of birth, any illnesses, and the age at diagnosis. If anyone in your family has died, note the age at death and cause of death.

Also try to include information about lifestyle factors, such as smoking, alcohol use or obesity, that may have affected a family member's health.

Use this information to construct your pedigree. A pedigree is a chart that shows your family tree and indicates illnesses each family member developed and at what age. Begin with yourself, then move on to your parents and branch out from there.

Once your family health history is complete, take it with you to your next doctor's appointment. Together, you and your doctor can look for and analyze disease patterns throughout your family and discuss your particular risks. Your doctor can also make informed recommendations about screening tests you should have — and when. Earlier screening for a particular disease may result in early detection, when the odds for successful treatment are greatest.

Creating a pedigree can also help your children, grandchildren and other relatives track their own health.

# How to change behaviors

Making the decision to adopt a healthier lifestyle isn't easy. But the real challenge comes in putting your words into action. According to psychologists who study behavior change, quitting an unhealthy behavior can take anywhere from three to 30 tries. And there's no magic bullet for adopting healthier habits. Different techniques work for different people.

But there is good news. By planning your behavior change carefully and taking small steps, you increase your chance for success. Consider the following strategies.

- **Be specific.** State exactly what you want to do, how you're going to do it and when you want to achieve it. Start with goals you can achieve within a week or a month. If you have a big goal, such as stopping smoking, break it down into a series of smaller weekly or daily goals you can measure. "I want to look better" isn't a good goal because it's not specific and it's hard to measure. "I want to lose 5 pounds this month" is a better goal because it's specific and measurable.

- **Make it reasonable.** You may be setting yourself up to fail if you resolve never to eat chocolate again or to follow a two-hour-a-day fitness regimen. The test: Can you do this regularly over the long haul? If not, ratchet your goal down a notch.
- **Share it.** Going public can give you the peer support — or pressure — you need to succeed. So let friends and family know what you want to accomplish, from managing stress to avoiding alcohol. Tell them how they can support you.
- **Schedule it.** You have a better chance of accomplishing your goal — whether it's attending a yoga class or running two miles — if you make time for it on your calendar.
- **Find a partner.** You're more likely to show up for that smoking cessation class or AA meeting if a friend is there waiting for you.
- **Record your progress in a journal or activity log.** People who write down their accomplishments are more likely to keep moving toward their goals.
- **Reward yourself when you reach your goal.** A night out at the movies, a massage or a new tool for your garage can encourage you to keep up the good work.

Keep in mind that it takes about three months to develop a healthy habit. If you continue faithfully for that long, you'll be more likely to stay with it for the long haul.

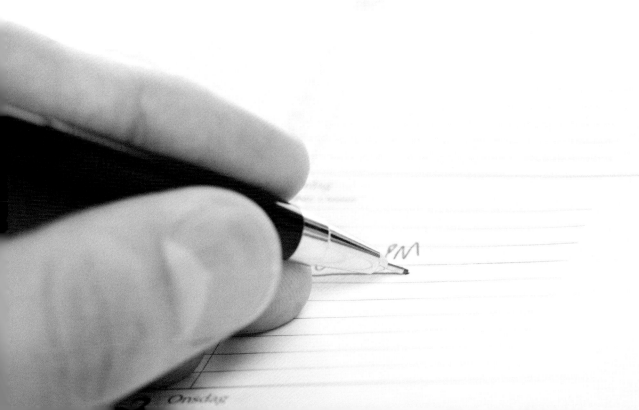

# Chapter 6

# Think positive and stay connected

Life is full of change. Some changes are anticipated and happy, such as finding a loving life companion or a fulfilling job. Others are more difficult — losing a loved one or going through a divorce. Later adult years, in particular, can present many changes. Children grow up and leave home. Parents need more help with daily activities. Partners and friends go through midlife crises or face serious illnesses. Daily routines and patterns change with retirement. Changes in your health begin to feel more apparent.

Coping with all of these changes can be overwhelming, especially when multiple changes occur at the same time or overlap, as they tend to do in later years. Some changes are so great that they may shift the course of your life in an entirely new direction.

Regardless of how changes come about, the way you handle them is perhaps the most influential factor in defining their impact on your health and happiness. Your attitude and your social and spiritual ties are tools you can use to more successfully adjust to change, no matter where life's path may take you.

## Changes and transitions

Changes occur throughout life. They're often little things. Your office is moved to a different building, or you develop a fondness for autobiographies rather than fiction. Whether voluntary or involuntary, or a little bit of both, most of us are equipped to handle small changes in our schedule or routine with little or no difficulty.

Transitions, on the other hand, are changes that alter your way of life in a profound manner, so much so that you may need to develop new dimensions to your identity to accommodate the transition. Marriage is a classic example. You go from being single and responsible for only your welfare to being a partner in a relationship in which you generally share goals, interests, responsibilities and living quarters. To establish a successful and loving relationship with another person requires compromise, and compromise almost always requires change in individual habits. Though many of these changes are small, together they may seem significant.

Other examples of life transitions include becoming a parent, changing careers, relocating, retiring from the work force, developing a chronic illness, or losing a family member or friend. In all of these, the changes involved become part of a transformative process, a move from one phase of life to another.

Author William Bridges, who has explored the concept of transition in his books, describes the transitional process as beginning with an ending, followed by a middle, or "neutral zone," and finally succeeded by a new beginning. So, although it may seem paradoxical, a transition typically starts with an end.

It should be noted that there is a difference between anticipated endings — those endings that are planned and often less traumatic — and unanticipated endings. Unanticipated endings can be much more difficult to accept and manage and may require different transitional skills.

## Ending

Every ending, even if it's viewed in a positive light, involves some form of loss. Retirement, for example, may be something you've been looking forward to, a well-deserved reward for all those years of hard work. Yet when the day arrives and you don't have to get up in the morning and get ready for work, you may find that you don't quite know what to do with yourself. What are you now, if you're no longer an architect, secretary or business owner? What should your morning routine be? What will you do during the day?

Or, perhaps, you're a homemaker and your spouse has recently retired. He or she is now around the house all day, depriving you of your autonomy and privacy and interfering with your normal routine. These losses may seem relatively small, but they often catch people off guard because they weren't considered beforehand.

Losses that accompany the death of a spouse are much more pronounced and can seem overwhelming. Again, there's loss of the familiar and loss of future plans and dreams.

When you experience the ending of a chapter in your life, it's important to acknowledge the losses that accompany it, no matter how great or small.

## Middle

The middle period, the passage between the ending and the beginning, can be particularly difficult. During this time, it's impossible to go back into the past but you can't quite move forward yet either. It's not uncommon at this point to feel anxious, uneasy and vulnerable. You may even feel a certain amount of panic about what to do next. Unfortunately, there are no shortcuts. The only way to reach the next phase is through the passage of time.

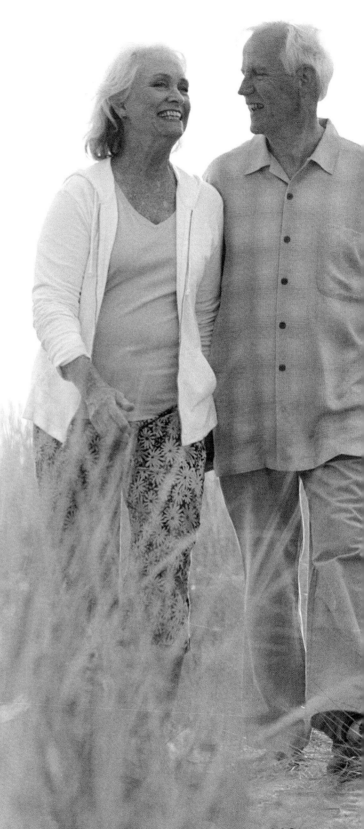

But you can make use of this time. While it's OK to begin formulating a plan for your next steps, it's also OK not to make any plans — to be still for a while. This middle passage is an opportunity to pause and rediscover what's meaningful to you. Is the direction of your life aligning with your priorities and interests? This time to step back and reflect may make it easier to make the right changes when you're ready.

As you move through this period, remember to take care of your basic necessities. Eat well, stay active, get adequate rest and keep involved with important relationships. Doing these things will go a long way toward easing your transition.

## Beginning

After a while, you'll begin to notice that you're gaining more confidence, more familiarity with your new way of life and perhaps more hope about the days ahead. You may even begin to feel excited about the possibilities that lie before you. This is a wonderful time of new awakenings, new thoughts and new experiences.

Don't be afraid to take pleasure in this new phase. You won't be discrediting what you've lost. Rather, you'll be affirming the power of your past experiences to make you the healthy, strong and vibrant person you've become.

It may help to return to the analogy of your life as a musical composition. There may be many transitions in your composition, and you may only hear certain notes at a time. But if you step back every once in a while, you may catch strains of the entire symphony.

# Optimism and your health

As you make your way through life and the various transitions it brings, you'll find that an optimistic attitude can make your days more enjoyable and less stressful. But did you know that your attitude also plays a role not only in how well you'll live but also in how long you may live? Your mind and your body are closely intertwined.

## Optimists live longer

Increasing evidence suggests that being an optimist or a pessimist has an effect on your health. One par-

# How to tackle transitional stress

Going through a major life change can be stressful. Chronic stress can be harmful to your emotional and physical health. Here are some practical suggestions for keeping stress under control during this time:

- **Reach out to friends and family.** If they live far away, stay in touch by phone or email. Conversations don't have to be long, and emails can be brief. The important thing is to stay connected.
- **Keep your strength up.** That means eating right, exercising regularly, and avoiding drugs and alcohol. Make sleep a priority. Lack of sleep is cumulative, and constant fatigue can be a trigger for depression. Too much sleep, however, can be counterproductive as well.
- **Protect your time.** If you feel overwhelmed, eliminate activities that aren't absolutely necessary.
- **Get back to the basics.** It may be more difficult to cope with everyday demands while you're adjusting to a life change. Keep things simple by working on one task at a time.
- **Practice forgiveness.** Try to be more forgiving of yourself and of situations over which you have no control. Be realistic with your expectations of how you should feel or not feel. It's normal to feel uncomfortable or disoriented during a transition period. Some days will always be better than others.
- **Avoid negative people.** Cultivate relationships with people who will boost you up rather than bring you down.
- **Accept change as a constant.** People who can roll with the punches generally come out of transitions more successfully than do those who refuse to be flexible.
- **Maintain a sense of humor.** Not everything has to be deep and dark. Laughter relieves tension and relaxes your muscles as well as your mind. Lighten up with a funny movie or a friend who makes you laugh.
- **Focus on things that give life meaning.** This may include a spiritual journey or greater involvement in your faith community.

## Can you become an optimist?

People generally don't choose to be optimists or pessimists. The attitude you take toward life events is likely a combination of genetics, early environment and life experiences.

But that doesn't mean you're stuck with your attitude. Pessimism may be changeable to some degree. By being mindful of the ways in which your viewpoint brings you down or influences how you think, you may be able to view some events in a different manner. Here are some suggestions:

- **Be aware of negative thoughts.** Pay attention to the messages you give yourself. When you catch yourself thinking that life is terrible, stop the thought in its tracks.
- **Put things in perspective.** Some people are so negative that even when small things go wrong, they feel as if they're cursed. Remember, everyone has ups and downs and nobody's life is perfect.
- **Try reframing.** Reframing can help you find the good in a bad situation. If you've lost your job, for example, look at it as an opportunity. A job change can allow you to learn new skills and meet new people.

ticular Dutch study found that older adults with an optimistic disposition — people who generally expected good things rather than bad things to happen — lived longer than did those who tended to expect doom and gloom.

At the beginning of the study, more than 900 participants filled out surveys that assessed their well-being, including their sense of optimism. The survey asked participants to respond to statements such as "I often feel that life is full of promises" and "I do not make any future plans." After accounting for factors such as age, sex, smoking, alcohol consumption, physical activity, socio-economic status and marital status, those who scored high on the optimism scale had a 29 percent lower risk of early death than did participants who scored low on the scale.

- **Count your blessings.** Gratitude can help you focus on what's right in your life. Look around you and make a mental list of all the things you take for granted but for which you are truly grateful.
- **Forgive and let go.** Learn from your mistakes, forgive yourself and move on. Also try to forgive others. Hanging on to a hurt or a wrong done to you by someone else only gives that hurt more power over you.
- **Savor the good times.** Good memories can get you through the bad times, so savor the moments when all is well with the world and store them up for future reference.
- **Pursue simple pleasures.** If you find satisfaction in the small things in life — a sunny room, a relaxing cup of coffee, time spent with friends or family — you won't need spectacular events or extravagant purchases to make you happy.
- **Be kind.** Turning toward others can make you forget about yourself. Being kind to friends and strangers can relieve some of the tension in their lives and make you feel better about your own.
- **Focus on things that give life meaning**. This may include a spiritual journey or greater involvement in your faith community.

In this study, a positive outlook appeared to be particularly protective against death from cardiovascular problems. Highly optimistic participants were 77 percent less likely to die of a heart attack, stroke or other cardiovascular event than were highly pessimistic participants. These results held true regardless of whether the participants had a history of cardiovascular disease or high blood pressure.

A study conducted at Mayo Clinic reported similar results. Researchers examined the relationship between explanatory styles — how individuals explained the causes of life's events — of more than 800 participants and the group's mortality rate during a 30-year period. The researchers found that individuals who had a more pessimistic explanatory style died younger than did those who were more optimistic.

Participants who were classified as optimists tended to believe that the causes of bad events were temporary, not their own fault and limited to the present circumstances. Pessimists, on the other hand, tended to blame things on themselves, feel that the current situation was going to last forever and feel that the bad event would undermine everything.

## Optimists live better

Using the same group of people for a different study, Mayo researchers examined the association between explanatory style and self-reported health status. Thirty years after filling out the original questionnaire that determined whether they were optimists, pessimists or a mix, a group of the participants answered a series of questions relating to their physical and mental health. Those who had an optimistic explanatory style reported fewer health limitations, fewer problems with work or other daily routines, less pain, more energy and greater ease with social activities. In addition, they reported feeling more peaceful, happier and calmer most of the time.

Other studies have shown that optimists have fewer incidences of coronary artery disease, and if they do undergo heart surgery, they have a better recovery and better health afterward.

To the contrary, studies during the past few decades suggest that people who have pessimistic views of life events are prone to depression, have a weakened immune system, and use medical and mental health care services more frequently.

## Finding the link

Scientists aren't sure exactly how optimism provides the health benefits that it does or how pessimism can translate into poorer health and earlier death. In the Dutch study, optimism was associated with higher levels of physical activity, moderate alcohol use, less smoking, a higher educational level and living with a spouse. But even after adjusting for these factors, optimism still had an independent effect on mortality.

Part of the explanation may be that optimists, by their very nature, tend to report better health. However, in the Dutch study, optimists lived longer than pessimists, even if they had chronic illnesses or physical disabilities.

It's possible that optimists cope more effectively with life events than pessimists do and have habits that are more likely to promote health and recovery, such as taking medications as prescribed or following a treatment regimen. There also may be biological differences involving factors such as the immune system, genetics and hormones.

# Social companionship and your health

Your relationships also play a vital role in your health and sense of well-being.

In a survey done by the National Council on Aging, titled "American Perceptions of Aging in the 21st Century," nearly 90 percent of respondents thought that having close relationships with family and friends was very important to having a vital and meaningful life, ranking above a number of other factors, including health.

Throughout life, strong family ties and good friendships contribute to mental and emotional well-being. But studies also show that people who enjoy "social support" — strong relationships with family, friends and partners —

tend to not only have better health but also live longer.

## The health benefits of friendship

Increasing evidence suggests that physical factors such as blood cholesterol levels, heart rate, blood pressure and your immune system are affected by psychosocial factors, such as your attitude and your relationships. Whereas social isolation can contribute to illness and poor health, having strong connections with the outside world appears to reap many rewards.

### Extends life
More than a dozen studies link social support with a lower risk of early death. In one study, for example, researchers monitored the health of nearly 7,000 Californians for more than 17 years. They found that those lacking social connections were two to three times as likely to die younger as were their more socially connected counterparts.

### Boosts recovery
After reviewing more than 50 studies examining the link between social support and cardiovascular disease, researchers concluded that individuals

without social support have worse recovery rates after a heart attack. People with social support may be more motivated to recover and adhere better to treatment regimens. Lack of social support appears to carry the same weight as other cardiovascular risk factors, such as high cholesterol, smoking and high blood pressure.

### Bolsters immunity

It's clear that stress can suppress immunity. Love and friendship help to reduce stress. Interestingly, one study found that people with more diverse social networks were less susceptible to the common cold.

### Improves mental health

Having people to talk with when difficult times come along provides a psychological buffer against stress, anxiety and depression. Even when you don't have a crisis in your life, social networks increase your sense of belonging and self-worth, promoting positive mental health.

### Reduces anxiety

Studies have found that people hospitalized for heart disease who have strong social and religious ties are generally less anxious about upcoming medical events and procedures.

Individuals with higher support levels are less prone to anxiety in general, which, in the case of cardiovascular disease, is associated with increased risk of death and sudden cardiac death.

### Protects against mental decline

One mind can sharpen another. A study involving a group of older adults living in Spain found that having multiple social ties ranging from intimate to extended, maintaining frequent contact with these individuals and playing an important role in their lives help to preserve mental ability.

Another study examining the link between social networks and mental sharpness found that study participants who frequently interacted with larger networks, such as civic and church groups, better maintained their mental sharpness (acuity) over time.

## Finding the link

Knowing that social support has a positive impact on health raises the questions of how or why.

Researchers suspect that being connected with others protects your physical health in a number of ways:

## Your pet: A lifesaver?

You may already know that the companionship and unconditional love a pet provides is priceless. But did you also know that caring for a pet can bring you health benefits?

Various studies have shown that living with and caring for a cherished animal may:

- Help you cope with stress
- Lower your heart rate and blood pressure
- Help you live longer after a heart attack
- Improve your mood and sense of well-being
- Reduce loneliness, if you live alone
- Help you become more active

One study found that one-year survival after a heart attack was higher among people owning dogs than it was among those who didn't have a dog. Another study demonstrated that pets can buffer how people react to stress. People with animal companions had lower heart rates and blood pressure levels. They also had smaller increases in those levels when put under stress, and faster recovery from elevated levels after stress. Yet another study found that older adults who owned pets were less likely to become depressed, were better able to tolerate social interaction and were more active than were their counterparts who didn't have pets.

- Reduces stress
- Motivates you to engage in healthy behaviors, such as walking regularly or quitting smoking
- Allows you to receive direct expressions of affection, esteem and respect (socio-emotional support), which in turn might increase your biological resistance to disease
- Enables you to get better or more-prompt medical care, or actually providing you with medical care if needed
- Provides you with practical help when needed — for example, assistance with household chores and transportation

## How to build a support network

Casual friendships may come and go. But most people at any age have an inner circle — a group of friends and family to whom they can turn when they need support. Although the members of this inner circle may change over time, the size usually remains fairly stable during the course of a lifetime.

To build and maintain a strong network of family and friends, invest in some key relationship strategies:

- **Make relationships a priority.** One of the best support sources is a healthy, fulfilling long-term relationship. Don't take your spouse or partner for granted. Take time to be there for each other. In addition, make time to regularly do something with your friends.
- **Recognize the importance of give-and-take.** Sometimes you're the one giving support, and other times you're on the receiving end. Letting family and friends know you love and appreciate them will help ensure that their support remains strong when times are rough.
- **Respect boundaries.** Although you want to be there for friends and family, you don't want to overwhelm them either. Respect their ways of communicating. Find out how late or early you can call or how often they like to get together.
- **Don't compete with others.** This will turn potential rivals into potential friends.
- **Avoid relentless complaining.** Nonstop complaining is tiresome and can be draining on others.
- **Adopt a positive outlook.** Try to find the humor in things.
- **Listen up.** Make a point to remember what's going on in others' lives. Relate any interests or experiences you have in common.

- **Resolve to improve yourself.** Cultivating your own honesty, generosity and humility will enhance your self-esteem and make you a more compassionate and appealing friend.

## Break away from unhealthy connections

As you seek to expand your social network, beware of support systems that are unhealthy, oppressive or rigid. These can be just as damaging as having no connections at all.

If people in your social support system are continually stressed or ill, for instance, you may suffer along with them. If your friends place heavy demands on your time, or if you're unable to meet their needs, you may find yourself increasingly anxious or depressed. You may also pay a psychological toll if you feel obligated to conform to your friends' beliefs or ideas.

# Spiritual ties and your health

In addition to an optimistic attitude and a strong support network, scientific studies suggest that religious beliefs and practices and spiritual well-being can have a positive influence on the quality of your life and your ability to cope with stress and adversity. Like optimism and social support, a strong sense of spirituality can improve your physical and mental health.

## Defining spirituality

People often use the word *spirituality* interchangeably with *religion*. Although there's considerable overlap between the two concepts, the terms aren't necessarily synonymous. While religion typically refers to a formal system of beliefs, attitudes or practices held by a group of believers, spirituality is more individualistic and self-determined. There may be as many definitions of spirituality as there are people in the world — one common definition is "a personal search for meaning and purpose in life."

Many people consider themselves to be both spiritual and religious. Spirituality and religion both push you to turn inward and reflect on your own life and its purpose. Your spiritual beliefs can help you prioritize your life and develop interests that have the potential to be most fulfilling.

At the same time, spiritual beliefs and practices help you to connect to something larger than yourself. This may include the divine, the people around you, humanity in general, art or music, the natural world, or all of the above.

## What the research shows

The relationship among religion, spirituality, and mental and physical health is garnering increasing medical attention.

More studies are suggesting that when you believe in something larger than yourself, you strengthen your ability to cope with whatever life hands you.

People who attend religious services tend to enjoy better health, live longer and recover from illness faster and with fewer complications than do those who don't attend such services. They also tend to cope better with illness and experience less depression.

## Finding the link

Researchers aren't quite sure of the mechanisms through which religion and spirituality appear to promote mental and physical health. Here are some factors likely thought to play a role.

### Social support

Whether you attend a church, synagogue or mosque, these religious settings usually have a built-in social support structure that's readily available to its members. And as you just read, social support has many positive effects on health.

Most religious congregations offer assistance ranging from emotional support and spiritual guidance to practical support such as meals and housing. In addition, religious communities offer a variety of friendship opportunities.

Religious social ties may be especially helpful in easing transitions such as children leaving home, retirement or the death of a spouse. In addition, as people age, they may depend on fellow members to help them with household tasks, shopping or transportation.

### Coping resources

Your religious beliefs may help you make sense of the world around you — especially during times of crises or when tragedies arise.

Turning to God or another higher power for comfort and strength may provide relief from stressors in life that can have a negative impact on your health.

## Health benefits of religion and spirituality

### Physical health
- Longer life
- Less cardiovascular disease and less mortality from cardiovascular disease
- Lower blood pressure
- Better immune function
- Healthy behaviors: more exercise, better nutrition, better sleep, less smoking, and increased use of seat belts and preventive health services
- Better functioning among disabled people
- Fewer hospitalizations, shorter hospital stays

### Mental health
- Less risk of depression and better recovery from depression
- Less anxiety and more rapid recovery from anxiety disorders
- Less substance abuse
- Decreased risk of suicide
- Greater well-being, hope and optimism
- More purpose and meaning in life
- Greater marital satisfaction and stability
- Higher social support

Adapted from Koenig H.G. Religion, spirituality, and medicine: Research findings and implications for clinical practice. *Southern Medical Journal.* 2004;97:1194 and Mueller P.S. et al. Religious involvement, spirituality, and medicine: Implications for clinical practice. *Mayo Clinic Proceedings.* 2001;76:1225.

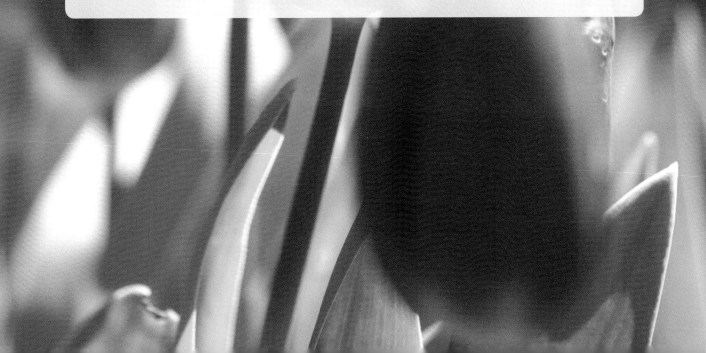

# Armed with optimism

To say that Margaret lived with breast cancer most of her life is true. She was first diagnosed with the disease in 1957 at the age of 39. And she managed cancer for nearly 50 years.

Margaret's cancer was first diagnosed when she discovered a lump in her left breast and brought it to the attention of her doctor. She quickly underwent surgery to remove the breast.

Since that initial diagnosis, Margaret underwent numerous major and minor surgical procedures and radiation therapy. Over the years, she had more than 25 separate surgical procedures, which have removed more than 65 tumor nodules. In between surgeries — to keep new tumors from developing or at least slow their growth — she took multiple anti-cancer hormone therapies. She did this on and off for more than 20 years. When the effects of one medication wore off, she switched to another.

So why are we telling you about Margaret? Because, despite battling breast cancer day in and day out for more than half her life, Margaret lived well.

Armed with a positive attitude, deep religious faith and strong commitment to help others, she never let her cancer interfere with her goals and ambitions. In telling about her cancer recurrences, Margaret stated, "I took them one at a time, and was glad to get rid of them. And then I went on living each time. I think you make use of each day."

After Margaret's first operation, she and her husband, Walter, traveled to Tanzania, East Africa, to teach at a college there, an experience they found extremely enlightening. Margaret continued to teach English for many years after returning to the United States.

Since childhood, Margaret always enjoyed writing. After she was diagnosed with cancer, she found that her daily journal helped her face and then let go of her worries and fears — writing became her therapy. Following her retirement, with more time on her hands, Margaret's writing took on a broader scope. She wrote a book about the lives of several generations of a Norwegian immigrant family, based, in part, on her own family's experiences.

Additional books and collections of poetry followed, including a book about her personal battle with cancer.

Throughout her life, in addition to traveling with her husband and raising a son, Margaret kept busy with volunteer work: helping at the local nursing home, reading to children in the Head Start program, teaching community education classes and participating in various civic organizations.

For Margaret, volunteer work was another coping tool — her way of coping and carrying on. "I think taking an interest in other people makes a lot of difference. If you just go around thinking about yourself, it can cause you problems."

Margaret continued to live a full life until she fell on some ice while out walking and broke her hip. After that incident, her breast cancer seemed to become more aggressive. Almost 50 years after her breast cancer was diagnosed, Margaret died at the age of 88.

So why did Margaret do so well despite her breast cancer that kept recurring? The specialist who cared for Margaret the last two decades of her life readily admits that he doesn't know. Under the microscope, Margaret's cancer looked like a routine type of breast cancer. Why it acted so differently from virtually all of other such cancers is a real mystery. Hopefully, it's a mystery that can one day be solved.

But it is safe to say that Margaret's optimism and her strong social and spiritual connections were part of the reason why Margaret enjoyed a fulfilling 50 years. During times when it would have been easy to become depressed, overly anxious or frustrated, and just throw in the towel, Margaret never did.

Margaret's story is a great reminder that despite challenging circumstances, it's possible to enjoy a meaningful and long life.

## Be aware of the negatives

Not all encounters with religion and spirituality are positive. If you become part of a religious organization with the expectation of receiving emotional support and spiritual guidance and instead you become enmeshed in gossiping, fighting and complaining among members, the resulting experience may do more damage to your health than good. In such cases, it may be helpful to seek out a more stable and positive organization that better meets your needs.

Other instances in which religion or spirituality may have a negative impact on health include refusing medical treatment or preventive health measures for religious reasons.

Belief in something larger than yourself also may help you to accept and cope with events that are beyond your control. By learning to accept those things that can't be changed, you're able to devote more energy to events in your life that you can control.

In addition, the feeling of hope, prominent in many faiths, may boost your immune system.

### Social regulation

Research suggests that people who belong to religious communities are less likely to smoke or abuse alcohol or drugs, more inclined to view physical activity as a priority, and less likely to carry or use weapons, get into fights and engage in risky sexual behavior than are those who are less religious.

### Forgiveness

The practice of forgiveness is prominent in religion. There's evidence that forgiving others promotes mental and physical well-being, possibly by:

- Relieving the forgiver of the burden of pent-up anger and resentment
- Re-establishing social ties that may have been a major source of support
- Promoting positive emotions, which can reduce anxiety and reduce blood pressure

### Prayer

A survey of Americans on prayer reported that around 90 percent of Americans pray, including a large number who pray at least once a day.

Engaging in ritual activities, such as prayer or meditation, promotes relaxation, which is characterized by lowered blood pressure, heart rate, breathing rate and metabolic rate. This may have a protective effect, particularly against high blood pressure.

## Developing your spirituality

Spirituality is an evolving process. It's shaped by your upbringing, personality and experiences, and it matures as you age.

Going through life transitions can affect your awareness of spiritual matters and highlight your spiritual needs. At a basic level, spirituality is linked to self-discovery and the development of your inner self.

Attending religious services, joining a charitable organization and volunteering in your community are a few ways to express and expand the spiritual side of your life. Many people find that these activities bring an added sense of purpose to their lives as they see their time and talents put to positive use.

Many people use prayer or meditation to reflect on their inner lives. Sometimes, just shutting off the television and sitting quietly can help you get in touch with inner thoughts and feelings. Writing down your thoughts can help you sort them out and allow you to examine them later.

Still other people find inner spirituality — what they often term *inner peace* — through music, dance, art or exploration of nature.

To help you gain a better understanding of yourself and become more acquainted with your spiritual side, ask yourself the following questions:

- What gives my life meaning and purpose?
- What gives me hope?
- How do I get through tough times? In what circumstances do I generally find comfort?
- How do I connect to my place of worship? (If you belong to a religious community.)
- What are my three most memorable experiences in my life so far?
- How have I survived previous losses and transitions in my life?

- What helps get me through the daily grind?
- When — a particular time or instance — did I feel that all was right with the world? What caused me to feel that way?
- When — a particular time or instance — did I feel my life was particularly meaningful? What caused me to feel that way?
- Was there a time when I was filled with a sense of awe?

# A final example

Imagine a person admitted to the hospital with advanced cancer. Aggressive chemotherapy and radiation are ordered to give this person a fighting chance — but what are the odds? How will this person tolerate the treatments and how will he or she handle this ordeal?

Clinical experience and overwhelming evidence show that attitude, social support and spiritual factors will all have some bearing on how this person will fare.

That's not to say that simply thinking happy thoughts or meditating will make the cancer go away — biology is a fact of life. However, when faced with this problem, the individual who will do well, whether that's being cured or having a peaceful end-of-life transition, typically has a number of characteristics:

- A partner or advocate that connects with the person and can speak on his or her behalf.
- A sense of community — whether it's faith based, socially based, or simply a camaraderie of friends — for support and encouragement.
- An acknowledgment that life isn't always fair and that the good guys don't always win. But with an equal acknowledgment that we each have gifts to share.
- Some element of spirituality — a belief in a power or an energy above him- or herself that can be a source of comfort and strength.

It may not be a quick recipe for survival, but it certainly helps.

# Chapter 7

# Challenge your brain

William Safire said it best. "Never retire." This was the advice the longtime *New York Times* columnist gave as he penned his last editorial for the newspaper. That, and to keep on changing. At the age of 75, Safire left his newspaper career to work with the Dana Foundation, a philanthropic organization dedicated to advancing and sharing with the public its interests in science, health and education.

According to Safire, one of his main reasons for switching careers at 75 was to extend the life of his brain, to keep his "synapses snapping." As he aptly put it, "We can quit a job, but we quit fresh involvement at our mental peril."

His example may be worth copying. As he himself would point out, increasing evidence suggests that the phrase "Use it or lose it" may indeed apply to the body's most powerful organ — the brain.

So what can you do to prevent memory loss and Alzheimer's disease? Unfortunately, the answer isn't simple. Although the popular press has extolled the brain-boosting powers of many different things — from wild salmon to coconut milk — there's no proven way to reduce the risk of developing abnormal plaques and tangles in your brain, which are the hallmarks of Alzheimer's disease.

What we know today is this: If you haven't been diagnosed with a memory problem, you can take simple action steps to cultivate good memory habits and maximize your everyday memory. Healthy lifestyle habits can also enhance your brain function and prevent memory problems.

Some of these steps may also increase your resilience to Alzheimer's disease. Research shows that two people with the same amount of plaques and tangles, measured by brain imaging, may experience very different symptoms. For one person, the plaques and tangles are debilitating; for the other, they cause no noticeable change in everyday life.

How is this possible? One explanation is that some people are simply more resilient to the physical damages happening in the brain, maybe because their brain cells and connections are stronger. This resilience — also known as a "cognitive reserve" — may be something you're born with (such as intelligence), or it may be something you can influence through lifelong mental stimulation and other lifestyle choices. More research is underway to better understand this and other risk factors for Alzheimer's disease.

In the meantime, you can make the most of your memory. In this chapter, you'll find practical strategies to improve your ability to remember important information, activities to exercise your brain and lifestyle habits that can also make a difference.

# Common changes over time

Will your mental abilities change as you age? Research indicates the answer is yes, they probably will. Just as you may notice changes in your vision, hearing or balance, you may experience the following common changes in brain function:

- It may take a little longer to learn new things. You either learn less in the same amount of time or need more time to learn the same amount, compared with when you were younger.
- It may be harder to recall some names, faces, dates, places and other pieces of factual information.
- It may be more difficult to handle multiple tasks at the same time. You may need to focus on only one task and accomplish it well before turning your attention to the next task.
- You may experience memory lapses, such as forgetting where you parked the car in a crowded lot or where you put your keys. This is a common complaint of people age 50 and older.

All of these changes can be scary, so it's worth noting that there are many regions of the brain that generally aren't touched by age. This includes the areas that store language and word meanings, creativity, wisdom, and procedural memory — which are the skills and procedures for doing activities, such as brushing your teeth or riding a bicycle. Using these unchanged areas to your advantage can actually help you overcome some of the age-related changes in other areas.

It's also important to remember that no two people age in the same way. There are older adults who live into their ninth decade with their golf swing and memory intact. But that's probably not a realistic or likely goal. Most people experience at least some subtle changes in memory as they age. Your mental strengths and weaknesses as a young adult are likely to continue as you get older. If you've always been good at remembering people's names, you're likely to maintain this skill. But if you've always had trouble remembering names, you're likely not to get much better at it with age. In fact, this type of problem may even get worse.

Happily, most experts believe that you can improve your memory, if you're motivated to change your everyday habits. This is great news, but it isn't always easy. Despite good intentions, many

people don't find the time or motivation to work on their memory, until they're faced with an early-stage dementia diagnosis that spurs them into action. By reading this book, you're already taking a big step toward proactively protecting your memory. Now, it's time to roll up your sleeves and get started on changing your everyday habits.

# Strategies for staying mentally sharp

It's never too early to start developing habits that can help offset age-related memory changes. Here are six practical strategies that can improve your everyday memory and ability to process information. These strategies may also help you keep your brain in shape:

## 1. Keep a calendar

In today's world, you may find yourself bombarded with lots of details from all directions — names, numbers, passwords, to-do lists. If you feel like your brain wasn't particularly well-designed to lug around this type of information,

# Memory training at Mayo Clinic

Many of the strategies described in this chapter are part of an innovative memory training program called Healthy Action to Benefit Independence and Thinking (HABIT), which was developed by Mayo Clinic experts. HABIT is a 10-day intensive, outpatient program in Rochester, Minn., for people who have been diagnosed with mild cognitive impairment (MCI) — an intermediate stage between the expected cognitive decline of aging and the more serious decline of dementia — or early-stage dementia, as well as their caregivers.

In this setting, Mayo Clinic specialists work together to help participants learn new habits that compensate for changes in their mental functioning, so they can maintain their independence. Key features include:

- Training with a memory-tracking calendar and organization tools
- Supportive group therapy
- Brain fitness
- Meditation and yoga practice
- Information about brain-healthy diets, sleep hygiene and other wellness topics

This program was designed for adults with known memory problems, but many of its strategies are ideal for healthy adults of all ages who are ready to improve their memory.

you're right. When you're trying to track too many tedious details, you're actually more prone to memory lapses.

An effective calendar and organization system can help you get over information overload. If you start developing this habit at a young age, you'll cope better as you get older — but it's never too late to start.

In fact, this type of system is the foundation of the Mayo Clinic HABIT program (see page 134). Participants in the Mayo Clinic program learn to use a highly structured calendar and note-taking system during 12 one-hour counseling sessions over six weeks. The goal is to make this system an established habit that is stored in the procedural memory, because this type of long-term "habit" memory is preserved in the aging process. Then the system can become a substitute (prosthesis) for memory.

It works the same way as a physical prosthesis — such as a walker. Rather than trying to fix or change the functioning in the brain, the organization system provides a way to compensate for loss of memory, just as the walker compensates for loss of balance.

The success of this system hinges on its counseling program. But you can apply some of the key concepts to a calendar system of your own. There is a wide variety of tools that can help you organize and remember appointments and tasks — from paper calendars to smartphones and tablet computers with many applications (apps) designed for this very purpose. Whatever you choose, follow these key ideas:

## Choose one tool

Rather than relying on multiple sticky notes and papers throughout your home, purse and pockets, pick one comprehensive tool that you can (and will) take with you at all times. Look for something that's small enough to fit into a man's breast pocket or a woman's purse. It can be a paper datebook or a smartphone with multiple apps — whatever suits your style.

## Develop a method to track different categories of information

Most of the information you need to remember on your daily to-do list will probably fall into one of three categories:

- Events that happen at a particular time (such as appointments and meetings)
- Tasks that need to get done, though not at a scheduled time (including work tasks, home chores and medications that need to be taken)

# Forgetting: What's normal and what's not

The following information, based on information from the Alzheimer's Association, gives examples of the differences between ordinary mental glitches and disease-related decline. Remember that occasional forgetfulness is normal, whereas forgetfulness caused by disease is ongoing and becomes progressively worse.

**What's often normal**

- Occasional forgetfulness — forgetting an assignment, a deadline or a co-worker's name, but typically remembering them later
- Occasional difficulty with familiar procedures — balancing a checkbook
- Difficulty with tasks that aren't readily familiar — setting up to record a television show or using the settings on a microwave
- Occasional disorientation — forgetting the day of the week or what you need from the store
- Visual changes related to aging — poor visual clarity, difficulties with night driving
- Occasional trouble finding the right word to use
- Occasionally misplacing things — forgetting where you put your wallet or keys
- Poor judgment from time to time — choosing not to wear a sweater or a coat on a chilly night

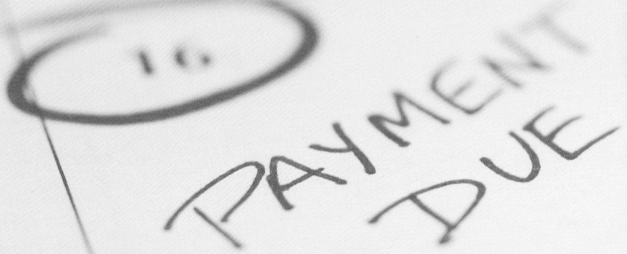

- Occasional loss of initiative — tiring of housework, business activities or social obligations
- Developing very specific ways of doing things — becoming irritable when a routine is disrupted

**What may be a sign of a more serious medical condition**

- Memory loss that disrupts daily life — forgetting important dates or events or asking for the same information over and over
- Challenges in planning or solving problems — trouble following a familiar recipe or keeping track of monthly bills
- Difficulty completing familiar tasks — trouble driving to a familiar location or remembering the rules of a favorite game
- Confusion with time and place — getting lost on your own street or forgetting where you are, how you got there or how to get home
- Trouble understanding visual images and spatial relationships — difficulty reading, judging distance, and determining color or contrast
- New problems with words in speaking or writing — forgetting simple words or substituting inappropriate words or having trouble following or joining a conversation
- Misplacing things and losing the ability to retrace steps — placing things in unusual places, losing things and being unable to go back over the steps, accusing others of stealing
- Poor or decreased judgment — using poor judgement when dealing with money, paying less attention to grooming
- Withdrawal from work or social activities — removing self from hobbies, avoiding being social
- Changes in personality — becoming confused, suspicious, depressed, fearful or anxious, easily upset outside of a comfort zone

Adapted from "Know the 10 Signs," Alzheimer's Association, 2012

- Addresses, phone numbers and other contact information for the key people in your life

Designate a separate section in your datebook or phone to track each type of information. It's easier to remember and process information when it's separated according to category, rather than being jumbled together in one big list of dates and details. You can also benefit from a short journal or note-taking area, where you can record important events that happen throughout the day, such as news from an important phone call.

### Use the system at least three times a day

Frequent, regular use is the only way to turn your calendar system into a routine habit. Set a regular schedule for reviewing your calendar system during routine times, such as upon waking or during meals. Of course, younger adults are likely to use a calendar system much more frequently — ideally, every time you schedule or complete a new meeting, appointment or task.

### Mark tasks when they are complete

Use an X or some other notation. This makes it easier to track unfinished items and leaves no question about whether routine tasks, such as taking medications, were done on a particular day. If you think your memory is still sharp enough to skip this step, think again. It's wise to establish this habit early. And you'll likely benefit from a motivating sense of accomplishment as you mark off tasks.

Over time, you'll surely develop your own strategies, shortcuts and abbreviations that make your calendar system work best for you. That's great! Experts agree that there isn't one right way to keep a calendar. The best calendar system is just the one that suits your individual needs and takes the least amount of time and energy to maintain.

## 2. Clear the clutter

Nowadays, there are whole stores devoted to selling bins, baskets, cases, containers, hooks and hangers. So there's no shortage of organization options and inspiration for your home. You don't have to alphabetize every drawer and shelf. But keeping your environment clutter-free can help minimize distractions and improve your memory.

### Create a system for belongings, just as you do for information

Store frequently used items in the same place, whether at work or at home. Carry your car keys or house keys in the same location every time you use them — always in the same pocket or handbag — and always return them to a designated spot when you're finished with them. Keep the kitchen utensils that you use for certain tasks together in convenient locations, for example, bowls with measuring cups or knives with cutting boards.

Use a toolbox to store tools that you may need every once in a while, such as a hammer, pliers and wrench. Always put the tools back when you're done using them so that you know where they are for next time.

### Put your paperwork in order

It's not easy to wrangle in the endless stream of junk mail, bills, bank statements, meeting notices and special announcements that you receive each week. Instead of letting paper accumulate in miscellaneous piles, sort mail and other documents as soon as you get them. As you sort, ask yourself: "Will I ever need this document again?" If the answer is yes, keep it. If the answer is no, throw it away right away.

Next, separate the items in the "yes" pile into designated folders, files or baskets for the following categories of paperwork:

- Items that require a response or action. This category includes bills that need to be paid and invitations that need an RSVP. Corral these to-do items into a basket or file as they come into the house. Then set aside time to address these tasks at least every week.
- Important information that you'll need to consult only occasionally. Examples are tax records; statements for your checking, savings and investment accounts; insurance policies and other key contracts; and owner's manuals for appliances, cars and other possessions. Create special files for safekeeping of these items. At least once year, review these files and purge anything that's irrelevant.
- Items to read at your leisure. Gather magazines, newsletters and brochures into a "to-read" file that can be read at any time. Keep these items together and save them for bedtime reading or weekend relaxation or even your next plane trip.

## 3. Stand at attention

Attention happens when you focus on a task, interaction or event. This skill is an important part of memory processing. It takes attention and concentration to input information into your brain at the beginning of the memory process, so it can be stored properly and retrieved when you need it. However, it can be difficult to sustain your attention as you age.

Slowing down and focusing on the present can help. Before you start a conversation or task, take a few deep breaths. Then look closely at the person or task in front of you. You can also use your senses (sight, hearing, taste, touch and smell) to help you focus on the present. Thinking about smells or sounds around you can bring awareness of your surroundings and help you concentrate and remember. Here are some other tips for improving your attention:

### Minimize distractions
Turn off the radio or TV while you're reading instructions or having a conversation. Pull the earbuds out of your ears. Control your work environment to reduce interruptions, such as shutting the office door when you need to concentrate on a report. And, what about the chimes, rings and alerts coming from your phone or other technology devices? Consider silencing your phone and computer for a couple hours each day — or at least while you're working on a project.

### Do one task or activity at a time
Whenever possible, do one thing at a time. Choose to focus for a set period of time and then take a break.

### Use selective attention
You rely on this type of attention anytime you have a conversation in a crowded restaurant. You tune out background noise and other conversations to focus on a select task — in this case, whatever your dinner companion is saying.

You can use this same technique to be selective about what you're trying to remember. Remind yourself of what's truly important and what's of less priority. When meeting many new people at the same time, for example, try to focus on retaining just a handful of key names — better to remember a few than to be confused about everyone. When reading a news article, give it a skim to consider what facts or ideas may be the most important to remember, then return for the full details.

## 4. Use memory tricks

Studies on memory suggest a number of memory techniques may be useful aids. Experiment with the following time-honored tips to see which ones work best for you. Most prompt you to encode information more efficiently — that is, to mentally focus on information when you first encounter it and to manipulate it in such a way that it helps you remember. Approach these memory techniques as if you're playing a game — have fun with them. Being creative (or even outlandish) with these techniques can make them more effective.

## Make associations

One way to remember something new is to associate it with something that you already know. Making intentional connections gives information meaning and makes it more likely that you will remember it. You did this as a child when you learned to recognize Italy on a world map by remembering that the country is shaped like a boot, or that the state of Michigan resembles a mitten.

Association can also work for learning definitions and people's names. For example, to remember that the port side of a boat is the left side (and not the right), you can connect the fact that that the words port and left both have four letters — whereas as right has five letters. This helps associate port and left in your memory.

Try these tips to make associations as you learn new names:

- Think of other people you know well with the same name, such as a favorite uncle or a close neighbor.
- Associate the new name with an image, if one comes to mind. (For example, link the name Robin with a bird. Or picture Robert Green covered in green paint.)
- Associate the new name with a noticeable feature of that person or some information about how you know each other. (For example, Tall Timothy or Concert Catherine.)

You can also use association to retrieve memories. Say that you're trying to remember the name of a person you worked with 10 years ago and haven't seen since. If that name doesn't pop immediately into your mind, try to think of something associated with that person that you do remember. Visualize the building you both worked in, the location of your offices or the name of your supervisor. Prompting your memory with related details helps you retrace your mental path to look for information, just as you might retrace your physical path to look for your keys. And it often yields the information you want.

## Repeat, rehash and revisit

Repeating new information helps you pay attention to it and encode it properly. It helps to repeat factual information — such as names and numbers — several times when you first try to learn it. For example, when you meet new people, try to use their names in conversation right away to help you remember them. The same technique works for directions. Repeat directions out loud a few times to properly process the information and order of steps.

Similarly, when you want to remember key concepts or ideas, talk about them with others. If you want to remember the main ideas of a book you've just finished, summarize them in a conversation with family and friends. Turning your thoughts into words will help you pinpoint the most important information and formulate your opinions.

You may also want to review relevant information in advance of a special event — such as paging through your high school yearbook before attending a class reunion in order to remember names and faces.

### Other memory techniques

Here are more tricks of the trade that may help you remember new information:

- **Break it down.** Divide large amounts of information into meaningful, manageable chunks. You do this already when you break down a 10-digit phone number, such as 8005551212, into the area code, three-digit local phone exchange and four-digit personal number: 800-555-1212. Apply the same technique to remember your driver's license ID, computer password or other long numbers. You can also chunk a long list of items or directions into smaller groups. For example, rather than trying to remember a grocery list of seven random items, think of the list as four vegetables and three fruits.

- **Picture it.** Create a vivid mental image of the information you want to remember. Creativity works particularly well with this technique. For example, if you store your Thanksgiving roasting pan in the basement closet between holidays, you might remember its location by picturing a turkey running around that closet.

- **Write it down.** Making notes or lists can help you remember information. In addition, the act of writing involves mental actions that often stay with you. So writing down the name of a restaurant you want to try may help you remember the restaurant even if you misplace the note. Recording a sequence of events and your feelings about them in a journal may help you remember the experience, even if you never reread the passage.

- **Use a cue.** A cue is anything that signals you to do something, be it an object or a sound or even a smell. Many people like to place objects in uncommon locations in order to help them remember. For example, place letters to mail in your pathway to the front door so that you don't forget them as you leave the house. Or stick reminder notes on the bathroom mirror or the refrigerator at night to make sure you do something the next morning. You can also use auditory cues, for example, setting your watch alarm a few minutes before appointments.

## 5. Cross-train your brain

One way to keep your mind sharp may simply be by exercising it. Just as regular physical activity improves your heart and lung capacity, regular brain training may improve your brain function.

Early research on science-based brain-training programs — which include a structured set of exercises, designed to train specific areas of the brain — is positive. These brain-training programs may increase your ability to focus and your speed of processing — and may even help build that cognitive reserve described at the beginning of this chapter.

The Mayo Clinic memory-training program dedicates 10 hours of time to a scientific, computerized brain-fitness program, which consists of listening exercises that get progressively trickier. Participants wear headphones and are asked to distinguish between high- and low-pitched sounds, for example. To start, the sounds are slow and distinct. Then, sounds go faster and faster, until they ends up sounding almost like a click. Another exercise asks participants to distinguish between similar syllables such as "doe" and "toe." The goal of all these exercises is to improve speed and accuracy of sound (auditory) processing in the brain. Revving up this type of processing may improve overall brain functioning in older adults.

You'll find a range of available online brain-training programs, computer software programs and smartphone apps, with varying price points and scientific merits. Do your homework before you purchase any program. Or start with brain-exercise books and free online games that are designed to stretch and strengthen your brain. Crossword puzzles, number games and everyday activities also provide opportunities for mental aerobics.

Just keep in mind the following general guidelines for brain training — which happen to be very similar to those for fitness training.

### Be regular

It takes regular physical activity to get your body in shape and reduce your risk of heart disease. The same is likely true of brain training. To make a noticeable change in your brain functioning, you need regular workouts, not just occasional card games. In fact, in one successful study of cognitive training, participants trained for one hour each day, five days a week, for a total of eight weeks.

### Vary your routine

A good fitness program includes a mix of different exercises designed to work the whole body. The same cross-training concept applies to brain training. So, if you're about to start your 100th crossword puzzle, it's time to put down your pencil and shake up your workout. Aim for a combination of exercises and activities to stimulate the whole brain, including the areas that control visual processing, sound processing, sequencing, spatial relationships, language and more.

Look for a brain-training program that targets a range of skills. Or seek out everyday activities that work different areas of the brain. For example, try jigsaw puzzles to sharpen your spatial relationship skills. And attend classical music concerts or lectures to test your sound processing.

### Challenge yourself

The brain fitness software used in the Mayo Clinic memory-training program automatically adjusts in difficulty, based on the users' responses, so that everyone always gets about 85 percent of answers correct. As a result, the program is challenging — but not straining. Follow the same principle in your own efforts. Choose a level where you can't get everything right. Move from beginning exercises to intermediate or advanced exercises, as needed.

### Focus on speed

Dedicate some time to improving your speed of processing, since speed is an important part of memory that typically slows with age. Think Slapjack instead of Solitaire. The former is an easy childhood card game, but you can't win without quickly slapping the Jacks as they're placed on the pile. Test your Slapjack speed against one of your favorite five-year-olds, or seek out other fast-paced brain games, such as Memory (Concen-

## Resources for brain training

If you're interested in brain training, you'll find hundreds of options, including books, websites, smartphone applications and computer software programs. Here's a small sample of the available options:

Paid online programs and computer software
- BrainHQ, *www.positscience.com*
- MindFit, *www.mindfit.com*
- Happy Neuron, *www.happy-neuron.com*
- Lumosity, *www.lumosity.com*

Free online games and puzzles
- AARP games, *http://games.aarp.org*
- Enchanted Mind, *www.enchantedmind.com*
- Maze Works, *www.mazeworks.com*
- Ravensburger Web Puzzles, *www.ravensburger-webpuzzles.com*
- Your Amazing Brain, *www.youramazingbrain.org/testyourself/default.htm*

tration) or Minesweeper. Or try your usual crossword puzzles and number games against a timer, rather than allowing yourself an endless amount of time to complete them.

## 6. Try new things

Lifelong learning and mental stimulation are sure to make life more interesting and enriching. And it's possible that these activities may also lower your risk of memory decline and Alzheimer's disease. Although you may not be able to do some things as well as you did them before, age shouldn't stop you from pursuing new frontiers. Studies show that older adults learn new skills as well as younger adults do. While younger adults may be able to mentally process faster, older adults can apply more wisdom and experience.

Don't be afraid to test your limits. Excitement is an important part of learning. Former president George H. W. Bush celebrated his 75th birthday by sky diving. The first time he made a parachute jump was when his plane was shot down over the Pacific Ocean during World War II. After that experience, he promised himself he would one day jump out of a plane for fun.

If you're not one for skydiving, creative work may be more your style. Artist Georgia O'Keefe, after discontinuing her work for years, returned to painting and sculpting at the age of 86 and went on to receive the Medal of the Arts. When he was in his seventies, film director Clint Eastwood was nominated for three Academy Awards over a four-year period. He won for "Million Dollar Baby" — a film that earned 68 year-old Morgan Freeman his own Oscar for best supporting actor. More recently, at the age of 88, actress Betty White became the oldest person to guest host "Saturday Night Live," and she won a Primetime Emmy Award for her efforts. Architect Philip Johnson also worked into his nineties and continued to exert influence on the design and aesthetics of buildings. Quite simply, it's never too late to turn out some of your best work.

On the other hand, it doesn't take celebrity status to expand your horizons. Here are a few ways to get you started:

- Stay curious. Take adult or continuing education classes — learn yoga or Pilates, or try your hand at painting or creative writing.
- Volunteer your skills or knowledge to the local school system or to a civic or charitable organization.
- Stay up to date on new technology, such as computers, cameras and telecommunications — you can do it cheaply by reading trade journals and visiting specialty stores.
- Use the Internet to access a wealth of information on a topic that's interesting to you. Research new recipes, gardening or golf trends, travel prospects, biographies, or historical stories.
- Travel to new places, be it a far-flung destination or a new ethnic restaurant in your hometown.
- Stay in touch with family and friends and look to expand your circle of acquaintances with new, stimulating friendships.
- Join a book club or other discussion group.
- Attend local concerts, lectures and plays to explore the cultural life of your community.
- Research family history and publish your account.

The experience of age provides a rich backdrop for developing skills, embracing change and integrating new knowledge into your life.

## 7. Take care of yourself

Caring for your body also will help your mind. Staying physically active, getting enough sleep, limiting your alcohol intake and managing your stress levels all contribute to keeping your brain at its optimum functioning level.

### Stay physically active

Keep active, even if that's just going for a walk. Physical activity improves blood flow, which brings increased oxygen to the brain and reduces your risk of heart disease and stroke, which may ultimately reduce your risk of mental decline and illness. It's also possible that physical activity helps the brain by decreasing the harmful effects of stress hormones. Some research even suggests that physical activity may promote regeneration of brain cells or the birth of new ones.

One study, based on data from nearly 19,000 women between the ages of 70 and 81, showed that long-term regular physical activity was associated with higher levels of mental functioning and less mental decline, an effect similar to being three years younger. In addition,

the activity didn't have to be strenuous to have an effect: Walking at least an hour and a half a week at a leisurely pace provided mental benefits.

The same appears to be true for men. Another study showed that older men who walked regularly were less likely to develop dementia. A study of Dutch, Italian and Finnish older men found that those who maintained or increased their physical activity over a period of 10 years had less mental decline.

### Get a good night's rest

Sleep is one of life's necessities, right along with air, food and drink. A good night's sleep leaves you feeling refreshed, alert and ready to tackle the day ahead of you.

Sleep deprivation can lead to forgetfulness and problems with concentration. You may feel less alert and less vigorous, and more confused, irritable and fatigued.

A good night's sleep sounds great, you may say, but as you get older, sleep just doesn't seem to come as easily as it once did. Sleep tends to decrease and become less restful as you age. For more information on changes in sleep that occur with age and what you can do about them, see Chapter 4.

# Opening new doors

If Jim has plans of slowing down, you wouldn't know it. A long and successful career at IBM as a marketing executive turned out to be a beginning — not an end.

Faced with the decision of whether to keep on working every day for full pay or retire early with half pay and the income from his pension, Jim opted for the latter, but with a twist of his own. Together, he and a partner formed a computer consulting company that employed a dozen programmers who had faced the same retirement decision. In short order, the business became a success and was bought out by another consulting firm.

After working briefly for the new owners, followed by a short stint with a manufacturer of data storage devices, Jim decided to shift gears completely — to pursue other interests and challenge himself in new ways.

At age 58, he entered, as he calls it, "the second part of my life." Having always been part of the Roman Catholic Church but lacking the time to become more involved, Jim enrolled in a three-year program with the church's Institute of Lay Ministry — a program designed to prepare laypeople to help fulfill the mission of the church.

Around the same time, he became involved in a local Boys & Girls Club that was undergoing growth pains. Recognizing Jim's talents for leadership, club officials quickly drafted him to bring the organization up to speed. A year of fundraising, locating new facilities and developing the group's efforts followed.

This brings us to the present. Asked what he's currently up to — and with no doubt that his response won't be short — Jim launches into a description of two new business startups: a retail venture selling monogrammed luggage labels and another venture working on a hand-held computer about the size of a business envelope that features a fully functional operating system, a cellular phone and GPS capabilities.

It's not that everything has come easily for Jim. His first marriage ended in the midst of his IBM career, leaving him a single parent with two adolescent daughters and a young son. But armed with a creative approach and the help of friends, they made it work. Not one to flout his blessings, Jim says that he and his children have a much closer relationship today than they might have had otherwise. Another blessing is his current wife of 17 years.

More than anything, Jim's secret elixir seems to be his genuine love affair with life and learning. When asked what keeps him going, Jim replies, "I've always enjoyed everything I've done, and it's always been fun." One of the keys to this, he says, was never staying with any one project for too long. Even within IBM, Jim moved around frequently. "You can't say, 'I'm going to go through 30 years of drudgery, so at the end of 30 years of drudgery I can do anything I want.' You're going to kill yourself in the process."

"My philosophy is that it's always more difficult to hit a moving target. Life is too short to do something you don't like." He sums up his advice in bullet points: "Don't get stagnant. Keep on exploring new things. And keep a positive attitude."

### Limit alcohol

Limiting the use of alcoholic beverages is important to the health of your brain. Excessive alcohol consumption can have immediate effects on your mental state, causing impaired concentration, memory and judgment, and motor skills. But heavy drinking can also have long-term consequences. People who drink to excess for years can experience permanent brain damage due to poor nutrition. They're also at higher risk of developing memory problems and dementia.

While it's true that moderate alcohol consumption can provide some health benefits, such as reducing your risk of heart disease, drinking too much can negate any of these benefits. For more information on the benefits and risks of alcohol use, see Chapter 5.

### Manage stress

Several studies show that chronic stress — the feeling of being constantly overwhelmed by one or more of life's challenges — can result in shrinkage (atrophy) of the hippocampus, an area of the brain important to the creation and storage of memories. This can affect your ability to remember.

Research also suggests that it's how you respond to stress that influences its impact on you. Stress itself isn't necessarily good or bad; the positive or negative effects of stress depend on the amount of stress you're able to tolerate.

A tolerable amount of stress can make a task challenging and exciting. Short-lived stress that has an end in sight (acute stress) can be mentally stimulating. Lack of stress, on the other hand, can be boring.

Chronic stress — stress with no end in sight — is the stuff that can be harmful. Not only does it impair mental processes, it can dampen your immune system and lead to fatigue, depression, anxiety, anger and irritability.

One way to prevent chronic stress is to choose positive and meaningful activities over those that saddle you with an unnecessary emotional load. Another way to cope with stress is to exercise regularly. Exercise helps boost feel-good endorphins, releases tension in your muscles and improves your sleep. For more on stress, see Chapter 5.

## Putting it all together

You're not expected to incorporate these seven strategies into your routine overnight. You might find that some

## Doing nothing can be deadly

An inactive lifestyle is a prominent risk factor for cardiovascular disease. One study found inactivity to be a more important gauge of death than any other cardiovascular disease risk factor. The least fit men and women in the study were nearly twice as likely to die of cardiovascular disease as were their fit counterparts. Poor physical fitness was a greater cardiovascular risk factor than was high blood pressure, high cholesterol, obesity and family history.

Increased physical fitness was also shown to counter the negative effects of other risk factors. Moderately fit smokers with high cholesterol, for instance, lived longer than did healthy but inactive nonsmokers.

In addition, the benefit of the exercise lasted longer.

### Improves mood and self-esteem

When you start an exercise program, you're being proactive — you're taking control of your life and health. You'll improve your strength, endurance and appearance. You may even lose weight. As a result, you'll feel better about yourself. This new confidence will carry over into your everyday life — improving your outlook.

### Enhances sleep

A good night's sleep helps maintain both your physical and mental health. Exercise can help you get much-needed rest. Studies show that moderate exercise, when done at least three hours before bedtime, can help you relax and sleep better at night.

### Prevents disease

One of the greatest myths about health is that illness is an inevitable part of aging. This isn't true. Although illness and disease do occur more often as people get older, this is as much a result of inactivity and other lifestyle factors as it is age. Regular exercise helps you reduce, prevent or slow many diseases and disorders.

# The right exercises to meet your goals

**Goal: Stay healthy and increase longevity.** If your goal is to ward off disease, improve your heart health, maintain a healthy weight, have increased energy and live longer, aim for at least 150 minutes of moderate aerobic activity — or 75 minutes of vigorous aerobic activity — spread out over the course of a week, along with strength training exercises at least twice a week. The more active you are, the more you'll benefit.

**Goal: Lose weight.** To lose weight, it's important to exercise five to six times a week. Aerobic exercise is key because it burns calories. To burn fat calories, choose an activity that's of low to moderate intensity, such as brisk walking, swimming or square-dancing. Exercise duration, and not necessarily intensity, is important to weight loss. Aim for at least 150 minutes of moderately intense activity a week — keep in mind that you may need to do more than this to keep burning calories. Strength training also can aid in losing fat by building muscle and is beneficial for overall health, but strength training alone is not the best form of exercise for weight loss.

**Goal: Reduce blood pressure.** Regular aerobic exercise can reduce blood pressure by an average of 10 millimeters of mercury (mm Hg), which in turn can reduce your risk of cardiovascular disease and stroke. Your goal should be to get at least 30 minutes of moderately intense aerobic activity most, if not all, days of the week.

**Goal: Avoid or manage diabetes.** Try to exercise at least 30 minutes a day most days of the week. Low to moderately intense aerobic activity, such as walking, bicycling or swimming, is best. Strength training can aid in losing fat and building muscle tissue, which can have a positive effect on blood sugar levels and insulin sensitivity.

**Goal: Build strength.** Strength training exercises, such as lifting free weights, using weight training machines or resistance bands, or doing exercises using your own body weight for resistance, are the key to building strength. Do these two to three times a week, and try to do 12 to 15 repetitions of each exercise, if possible.

**Goal: Prevent or minimize osteoporosis.** To achieve this goal, it's best to combine strength training, weight-bearing and flexibility exercises. Do strength training exercises up to three times a week, and weight-bearing and flexibility exercises most days of the week. If you have osteoporosis, talk with your doctor before beginning an exercise program.

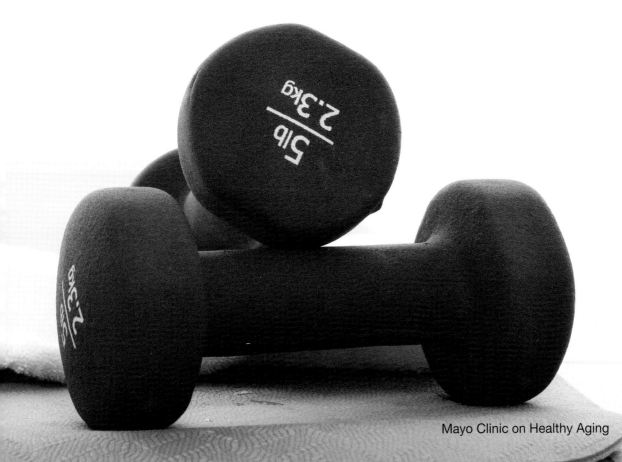

## Cardiovascular disease

Cardiovascular disease refers to many types of heart and blood vessel diseases. Hardening of the arteries, heart attack, stroke, heart failure and coronary artery disease all fall under this umbrella. Cardiovascular disease develops when the arteries that supply the heart with blood slowly become clogged from a buildup of cells, fat and cholesterol. When blood flow gets blocked, a heart attack or stroke can occur.

Regular exercise reduces the amount of low-density lipoprotein (LDL, or "bad") cholesterol in your blood, and it increases the concentration of high-density lipoprotein (HDL, or "good") cholesterol that helps prevent clogging of blood vessels. Exercise also strengthens your heart muscle so that it can pump more efficiently.

## High blood pressure

Regular exercise reduces the risk of developing high blood pressure. Most studies have found that exercise has a relatively early effect on blood pressure. Noticeable decreases in blood pressure are often seen within three weeks to three months after the start of a regular exercise program.

If you already have high blood pressure, exercise can help lower your blood pressure and reduce your risk of dying of the disease. If you take medication, daily exercise may decrease the amount of medication you need to take.

## Diabetes

There are two forms of diabetes. Type 1 diabetes results from the body's failure to produce the hormone insulin. Type 2 diabetes occurs when the body doesn't use insulin properly, allowing a high concentration of blood sugar (glucose) in blood. A significant relationship exists among type 2 diabetes, obesity and the lack of physical activity.

Regular physical activity and a healthy diet reduce your risk of developing type 2 diabetes, and they help control diabetes in individuals who already have the disease.

Mild to moderate exercise helps insulin work better, lowering blood sugar levels, and it helps muscles convert glucose into energy. In addition, exercise helps achieve and maintain a healthy weight, an important factor in the risk and management of type 2 diabetes.

## Obesity

Obesity has become an epidemic in the United States and carries with it serious health risks. People who are obese have an increased risk of premature death, type 2 diabetes, cardiovascular disease, stroke, high blood pressure, gallbladder disease, a deterioration of the cartilage and bone in joints (osteoarthritis), sleep apnea, asthma, certain cancers, high cholesterol, menstrual irregularities and stress incontinence.

Coupled with a healthy diet, exercise can help individuals who are obese lose weight and achieve a healthy weight. People who are overweight can even reap some of the benefits of exercise without losing weight. In one study, overweight women who increased their daily physical activity improved their health by lowering their blood pressure — without weight loss.

### Osteoporosis

Physical activity is likely the single most important influence on maintaining bone density and makeup. It plays several roles in preventing and treating osteoporosis.

Exercise strengthens your bones. Bones, like muscles, grow stronger when they're physically stressed through exercise. Weight-bearing exercises, such as walking and jogging, and strength training exercises, such as lifting weights or working with resistance bands, increase bone density and protect against the decline of bone mass.

## Before you begin

You can exercise at any age — even if you've never exercised before. However, before you jump into an exercise program, it may be wise to pay a visit to your doctor. He or she may perform a physical exam and can recommend certain exercises that would be best for you. This is also a good time to ask whether any medications you're taking may affect your exercise plan. Seeing your doctor is especially important if:

- You've been inactive for some time
- You have a family history of heart disease
- You have heart disease or lung disease
- You have high blood pressure, diabetes, arthritis or asthma
- You smoke
- You're unsure about your health status

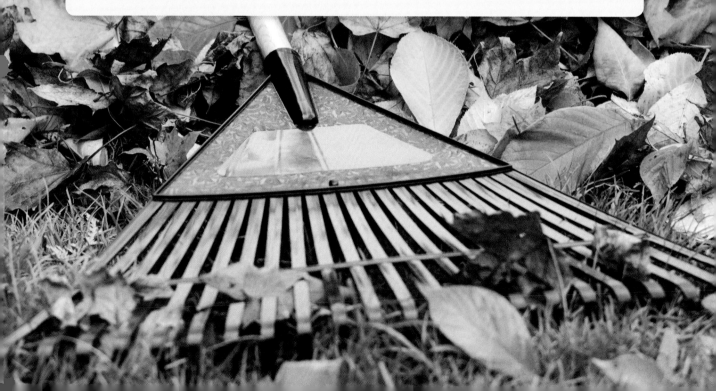

## 10 ways to add more activity to your day

In addition to a regular exercise program, you can also make small lifestyle changes that add more physical activity to your daily routine. Consider these activities as other ways to give your day an activity boost:

1. Walk or bike to do short errands instead of driving your car.
2. Do some gardening. Planting seeds, pulling weeds and tending the soil work your joints, muscles and heart.
3. Do your own yardwork. Mow your lawn, rake your leaves and shovel your walk, but remember to protect your back during shoveling.
4. Put aside kitchen appliances or power tools whenever you can. Instead of using an electric mixer, mix ingredients by hand. Instead of a power saw, use a handsaw.
5. Wash your car in the driveway instead of taking it to the carwash.
6. Avoid restaurant drive-thus. Park the car and walk inside.
7. Park at a distance from your destination and walk the rest of the way.
8. Use the stairs instead of taking the elevator. If you work or live on a high floor, take the elevator only partway up.
9. While golfing, walk instead of riding in a cart.
10. Take your dog for a walk.

### Arthritis

With appropriate, regular physical activity, people with osteoarthritis and rheumatoid arthritis — the two most common forms — generally experience significant reduction in joint swelling and pain. Regular physical activity has also been found to raise the pain threshold and improve the energy level of people with osteoarthritis.

Contrary to what some people believe, moderate physical activity isn't associated with joint damage or the development of osteoarthritis. On the contrary, a lack of physical activity can aggravate osteoarthritis. This is because weak muscles around joints can lead to further joint distress.

### Cancer

Regular exercise may help lower the incidence of some cancers, in particular, cancers of the colon, prostate, uterine lining (endometrium) and breast.

Exercise has been shown to strengthen your immune system, improve circulation and speed digestion — all of which play a role in cancer prevention.

Exercise combats colon cancer by helping digested food move through the colon more quickly. When food remains in the colon for an extended period of time, it can cause irritations that can lead to cancer.

Exercise also lowers the risks of cancer by reducing body fat. Body fat produces the female hormone estrogen. Estrogen, in turn, has been shown to support the growth of some female cancers, including breast and endometrial cancers.

## Increases life expectancy

In an extensive 20-year study of the lifestyles and exercise habits of 17,000 male Harvard University alumni, researchers established the importance of regular exercise to increased longevity. The study showed that regular, moderately intense exercise — equivalent to jogging about 3 miles a day — not only promoted good health but added years to the lives of the participants. Here are some of the results:

- Men who exercised at the equivalent of a light sport activity had a higher life expectancy than did sedentary men.
- Regular exercise countered the life-shortening effects of cigarette smoking and excess body weight.
- Men with high blood pressure who exercised regularly had half the death rate of sedentary men.

- Men who walked 9 or more miles over the course of each week showed more than a 20 percent lower mortality rate than did men who walked 3 miles or less each week.

- Regular exercise countered genetic tendencies toward early death. People with one or both parents who died before age 65 reduced their death risk by 25 percent with a lifestyle of regular exercise.

## What's moderately intense?

Perceived exertion refers to the total amount of effort, physical stress and fatigue that you experience during a physical activity. It's how hard you feel you're working. A rating of 6 on the Borg ratings of perceived exertion scale is the equivalent of sitting in your chair, reading a book. A rating of 20 may be compared to jogging up a very steep hill. Ratings of 11 to 14 constitute a moderately intense activity.

**Borg ratings of perceived exertion scale**

- 6 No exertion at all
- 7 Extremely light
- 8
- 9 Very light
- 10
- 11 Light
- 12
- 13 Somewhat hard

- 14
- 15 Hard (heavy)
- 16
- 17 Very hard
- 18
- 19 Extremely hard
- 20 Maximal exertion

Borg G. Borg's Perceived Exertion and Pain Scales. Champaign, Ill.: Human Kinetics; 1998.

Another way to determine if you're exercising at the appropriate level is if you're able to talk while exercising. If you're working your body but can still carry on a conversation with an exercise partner, you're likely exercising at a moderately intense level. This is commonly referred to as the "talk test."

- Men with the most active lifestyles — those who completed vigorous regular exercise — had the greatest life expectancies. This was due largely to fewer deaths from cardiovascular disease.

# Getting started

It's good to adopt an active lifestyle, but it's also important to develop a regular physical activity routine. Combine the two, and you can't go wrong. Use information in the rest of this chapter to help you determine what kinds of activities are best for you and to learn about some important considerations that will help shape how you exercise.

Hundreds of activities are available to help you become more physically fit. Some are exercises designed to strengthen your heart, some to strengthen the biceps in your arms, some to build your endurance, and some to enhance your flexibility. Other exercises can help you stay balanced, and still others help build bone mass. Each may have a place in your activity routine depending on your goals.

If your goal is simply to get more active, you might start out concentrat-

ing on just one form of exercise, such as walking. If your goal is to reach optimal fitness, you'll want to include these five types of exercise in your program:

- Aerobic
- Strength (resistance)
- Core stability
- Flexibility
- Balance

## How much exercise is enough?

A friend says her doctor told her 30 minutes of exercise three days a week is effective. A magazine you picked up last week claims you need to be physically active at least five days a week. And a story on the news last night said everyone should get 90 minutes of physical activity every day.

The answer to the question, "How much is enough?" will change over the course of your lifetime. The amount of exercise you need is based on some widely accepted guidelines and your specific goals.

The Department of Health and Human Services released today's most comprehensive recommendations in its 2008 Physical Activity Guidelines for

Americans. This report points out that most health benefits occur with at least 150 minutes a week of moderate-intensity physical activity (such as brisk walking) or 75 minutes a week of vigorous-intensity activity (such as running). Ideally, this activity should be spread throughout the week and can be broken down into intervals as small as 10 minutes.

The guidelines also recommend that adults do strength training activities at least twice a week.

The 2008 Guidelines acknowledge that additional benefits occur with more physical activity beyond 150 minutes a week — this is especially true for adults trying to lose weight or getting control of certain chronic health conditions, such as diabetes or high blood pressure.

# Aerobic exercise

Aerobic exercise includes activities during which oxygen plays an important role in the release of energy in your muscles. Aerobic exercise involves some of the most popular and fun exercises you'll do. Examples include walking, dancing, biking and swimming at a low to moderately intense pace.

No matter what your age, aerobic exercise will help you in your daily activities. It will help your heart, blood vessels, lungs and muscles complete routine tasks and rise to unexpected challenges. It will improve your stamina and endurance so that you can do the things you want to, whether it's training for a marathon or playing hide-and-seek with your grandchildren.

Most any activity you do — whether it's taking a walk, doing the dishes or mowing the lawn — requires oxygen. When your aerobic capacity is high, your heart, lungs and blood vessels efficiently transport and deliver large amounts of oxygen throughout your body. As a result, you don't fatigue as quickly. If you don't get enough aerobic exercise, your aerobic capacity is reduced and you fatigue easily.

Aerobic exercise also burns calories to help you lose weight or maintain a healthy weight, and it can increase your life span and improve the overall function of your body.

## Examples of aerobic activities

The key to enjoying and maintaining aerobic activities is to select activities that you enjoy and can do regularly. You don't need to limit yourself to a single activity. Go ahead and take part in a variety of activities.

The idea is to start slowly with exercises that you enjoy, then work up to a more intense pace as you feel ready.

## Walking

A brisk walk lasting 30 to 60 minutes most days of the week can provide many of the benefits of aerobic exercise. Even walking at a slow pace can lower your risk of heart disease, although faster, farther and more frequent walking offers even greater health benefits. Plus, walking is easy to do.

## Jogging

Like walking, jogging also is an excellent form of aerobic exercise. And like walking, jogging doesn't have to be strenuous to have a positive effect. Even when done at low intensity, jogging is a good way to increase cardiovascular fitness.

Jogging for 30 minutes three times a week can help achieve cardiovascular fitness, but it won't prepare you to complete a marathon. If your goal is to run a marathon, a more vigorous, structured training program is necessary.

## Hiking

Hiking can be as intense a workout as you want it to be. A beginner can stick to short, level trails, and an advanced hiker can attempt a trek through miles of hilly terrain. Hiking helps to increase your endurance and muscle strength. Depending on your route, it works different muscles than does walking.

## Bicycling

Bicycling revs up your cardiovascular fitness while strengthening your leg muscles. Biking offers a great deal of freedom, it offers a welcome change of scenery from one session to the next, and it's a good low-impact activity.

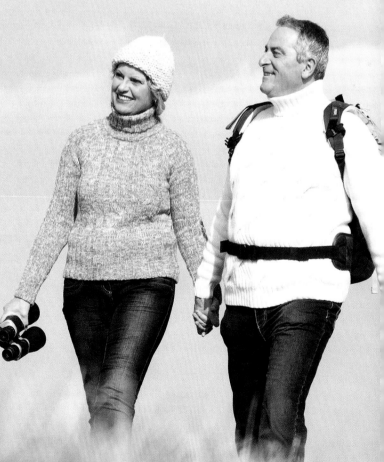

# Getting started on a walking program

Walking is an excellent relatively low-impact exercise. It's simple, inexpensive, versatile and requires no equipment other than a good pair of shoes.

If you're a seasoned walker, keep doing what you're doing. If you've been inactive and tire easily, it's best to start slow and easy. At first, walk only as far or as fast as you find comfortable. For example, you might try short daily sessions of 10 minutes and slowly build up to 15 minutes twice a week. Then gradually increase the pace of your workout over a period of four to six weeks.

For the first few weeks, walk on paths over flat, level ground. As you progress, try adding routes that include hills to increase the intensity of your workout.

Use the chart below as a guide to increasing the intensity of your walking program.

| | Distance | Time |
|---|---|---|
| Week 1 | 1-2 miles | 15-30 min./mile |
| Week 2 | 1-2 miles | 15-30 min./mile |
| Week 3 | 2-2½ miles | 13-25 min./mile |
| Week 4 | 2-2½ miles | 13-25 min./mile |
| Week 5 | 2½-3 miles | 13-20 min./mile |
| Week 6 | 2½-3 miles | 13-20 min./mile |
| Week 7 | 3-4 miles | 13-20 min./mile |
| Week 8 | 3-4 miles | 13-20 min./mile |
| Week 9 | 4-5 miles | 13-20 min./mile |
| Week 10 | 4-5 miles | 13-20 min./mile |
| Week 11 | 5-6 miles | 13-20 min./mile |
| Week 12 | 5-6 miles | 13-20 min./mile |

# Getting started on a jogging program

Many people enjoy the challenge of training for local fun runs and road races, while others enjoy the benefits of jogging in weight management.

The key is to start slowly. Advance one step in this starter program every two to seven days, as you feel able. If you're in step 1, jog for one minute, then walk for one minute. Repeat this until you've jogged and walked for a total of 24 minutes (12 repetitions). When you're comfortable with this portion of the program, move up to step 2. Continue moving up in steps as you're able. By step 10, you'll be able to jog through an entire workout.

The whole program looks like this:

|  | Time | | Repetitions | | Total time |
|---|---|---|---|---|---|
|  | Jog | Walk | Jog | Walk |  |
| Step 1 | 1 min. | 1 min. | 12 | 12 | 24 min. |
| Step 2 | 2 min. | 1 min. | 8 | 8 | 24 min. |
| Step 3 | 3 min. | 1 min. | 6 | 6 | 24 min. |
| Step 4 | 4 min. | 1 min. | 5 | 5 | 25 min. |
| Step 5 | 5 min. | 1 min. | 4 | 4 | 24 min. |
| Step 6 | 7 min. | 1 min. | 3 | 2 | 23 min. |
| Step 7 | 10 min. | 1 min. | 2 | 2 | 22 min. |
| Step 8 | 12 min. | 1 min. | 2 | 1 | 25 min. |
| Step 9 | 15 min. | 1 min. | 2 | 1 | 31 min. |
| Step 10 | 20 min. | — | 1 | — | 20 min. |
| Step 11 | 25 min. | — | 1 | — | 25 min. |
| Step 12 | 30 min. | — | 1 | — | 30 min. |

## Warming up and cooling down

Whatever your activity, make sure to warm up before exercise and cool down afterward. Warming up and cooling down help reduce the risk of injuries and muscle damage.

A warm-up prepares the body for exercise. It gradually revs up your cardiovascular system, increases blood flow to your muscles and raises your body temperature. Start your workout with a few minutes of low-intensity, whole-body exercise, such as walking or pedaling on a stationary bike.

Immediately after your workout, take time to cool down. This gradually brings down the temperature of your muscle tissue and may help reduce muscle injury, stiffness and soreness. Mild activity after exercise also prevents blood from pooling in your legs. Cooling down is similar to warming up. After your workout, walk or continue your activity at a low intensity for five to 10 minutes.

Like traditional bikes, a stationary bike also provides aerobic exercise. Stationary bikes can be upright or reclining (recumbent). One type of stationary bike isn't inherently better than another, although recumbent bikes may be more comfortable for people with back or neck pain.

### Water exercise

If you want a low-impact activity that exercises your entire body, swimming may be right for you. Swimming is often recommended for people with muscle and joint problems. If lap swimming isn't your style, consider water aerobics or just walking in the pool.

Water exercise is great for working all of your muscles, and it's easy on your joints. The water's buoyancy reduces pressure on your joints. Water exercises, however, aren't the best method for weight loss. If weight loss is one of your goals, consider supplementing your water workout with other forms of exercise, such as walking.

### Aerobic dance

Low-impact aerobic dance exercises the whole body while you move to music. Classes are usually offered for a variety of levels, although at any time you can alter your movements to whatever intensity you choose. Of course, the intensity will determine the benefits you derive.

### Aerobic stepping

Like aerobic dancing, stepping is a popular exercise for people of all abilities. Using a short, stable platform-type bench, exercisers step up and down to music during each session. Low-impact stepping can be a fun, motivating way to exercise — increasing your endurance and lower body muscle strength.

## Aerobic and anaerobic

Aerobic means "with oxygen." Anaerobic means "without oxygen." In reference to physical activity, the terms relate to which of the body's energy systems is the primary supplier of fuel during a given activity.

For most activities, your body blends the use of more than one energy system, depending on the intensity and duration of whatever you're doing. For example, a soccer player may be relying primarily on his or her aerobic energy system while jogging, but the dependence shifts to anaerobic energy for quick bursts or relatively intense runs of a minute or so.

For some activities, though, one system predominates. Distance running is primarily aerobic, while golf (with use of a cart) draws primarily on the anaerobic immediate energy system to power the swing.

Aerobic activities tend to be "steady state" or "pay as you go," meaning that you're able to breathe in enough oxygen to keep up with the rate that oxygen is being used. If your intensity level rises to the point where your breathing can no longer keep up, energy production shifts to anaerobic, and fatigue sets in more quickly. People who have developed strong and efficient cardiovascular and respiratory systems, such as distance runners or cross-country skiers, are able to maintain a fairly intense level of activity for a long duration because of their ability to take in and use oxygen. They have a high aerobic capacity.

# How many calories does it burn?

Burning about 1,000 calories a week with exercise significantly improves your overall health. This chart shows the estimated calories used while performing various activities for one hour. The figures represent a moderately intense level of exercise. The more you weigh, the more calories you use. Note that these figures are estimates — actual calories used vary from person to person.

| Activity (1-hour duration) | Calories used | |
|---|---|---|
| | 140- to 150-lb. person | 170- to 180-lb. person |
| Aerobic dancing | 416-442 | 501-533 |
| Backpacking | 448-476 | 539-574 |
| Badminton | 288-306 | 347-369 |
| Bicycling (outdoor) | 512-544 | 616-656 |
| Bicycling (stationary) | 448-476 | 539-574 |
| Bowling | 192-204 | 231-246 |
| Canoeing | 224-238 | 270-287 |
| Dancing | 288-306 | 347-369 |
| Gardening | 256-272 | 308-328 |
| Golfing (carrying bag) | 288-306 | 347-369 |
| Hiking | 384-408 | 462-492 |
| Jogging, 5 mph | 512-544 | 616-656 |
| Racquetball | 448-476 | 539-574 |
| Rope jumping | 640-680 | 770-820 |
| Running, 8 mph | 864-918 | 1,040-1,107 |
| Skating (ice or roller) | 448-476 | 539-574 |
| Skiing (cross-country) | 512-544 | 616-656 |
| Skiing (downhill) | 384-408 | 462-492 |
| Stair climbing | 576-612 | 693-738 |
| Swimming | 384-408 | 462-492 |
| Tennis | 448-476 | 539-574 |
| Volleyball | 192-204 | 231-246 |
| Walking, 2 mph | 160-170 | 193-205 |
| Walking, 3.5 mph | 243-258 | 293-312 |

## Strength training don'ts

Don't exercise the same muscles two days in a row. Plan to rest at least one full day between exercising each muscle group. Consider developing a plan for working specific muscle groups on given days. For example, on Mondays and Thursdays you work your chest, shoulders, quadriceps and triceps — muscles that push. On Tuesdays and Fridays you can work your back, hamstrings and biceps — muscles that pull.

Don't start with a weight that's too heavy. Initially, select a weight that you can lift comfortably 15 to 20 times. A weight that fatigues your muscles after 12 repetitions is an ideal stimulus for muscle strength and tone. Repetitions refer to the number of times you lift the weight or, if you're using a weight machine, push against the resistance. If you're a beginner, you may discover that you're able to lift only 1 or 2 pounds or less. That's OK. Once your muscles, tendons and ligaments grow accustomed to strength exercises, you'll be surprised at how you progress.

Don't rush your movements. Follow proper technique and lift or push the weight as you count slowly to three. Hold the position for one second, then lower the weight as you slowly count to three. Your movements should be unhurried and controlled.

# Strength training

When it comes to overall fitness, investing in a set of weights or other strength training equipment may pay dividends just as great as those gained with a pair of walking shoes. The more fit your muscles are, the easier your daily tasks become, whether they include lifting a load of wet laundry or shoveling snow.

Strength training involves the use of free weights, your own body weight, resistance bands or a weight (resistance) machine to increase muscle strength and endurance. Adults of all ages can benefit from regular strength training.

## You can be strong at any age

It wasn't that long ago scientists believed that a substantial loss of strength was an inevitable part of aging. After all, some decrease in muscle mass is a normal part of getting older. But it's now clear that if you're dedicated to maintaining your strength, you can make great strides in doing so as you age.

Studies have shown that strength can be maintained and perhaps increased at any age — even in your 80s and beyond. The key is to dedicate yourself to a regular and progressive program of strength exercises.

In one study, people in their late 80s and early 90s performed regular strength training exercises over a 12-week period. The results showed an increase in the strength of the participants' upper thigh muscles (quadriceps) by an average of 175 percent. They also improved their balance and found climbing stairs to be easier.

If you're inactive, you can lose up to 10 percent of your lean muscle mass each decade after age 30. With strength training, you can preserve and enhance your muscle mass.

Strength training can help you:

- Increase the strength of your muscles, help protect your joints and decrease your risk of injury.
- Increase the density of your bones, reducing the risk of osteoporosis. If you already have osteoporosis, strength training can lessen the condition's impact.
- Achieve better balance, coordination and agility.
- Strengthen muscles in your abdomen and lumbar region, reducing chronic low back pain.

## Examples of strength training exercises

You don't need to spend 90 minutes a day lifting weights to benefit from strength training. In fact, it's better that you not lift weights every day. Strength training sessions lasting 20 to 30 minutes and done just two to three times a week are sufficient for most people and can result in significant, noticeable improvements.

Strength training can be done in different ways — with free weights, body weight, machines, and resistance bands or tubing. You can choose one method or combine them for greater variety.

### Free weights

The term *free weights* refers to items such as barbells and dumbbells. These are the basic tools of strength training. Plastic soft drink bottles filled with water or sand also may work for you.

When using weights, your movements should be slow and deliberate. If you experience pain in any of your joints when using weights, reduce the amount of weight or switch to a different exercise.

Just one set of 12 repetitions twice a week produces 85 percent of the total benefit gained from use of free weights.

### Resistance machines and home gyms

These machines typically work different parts of your body with controlled weights and resistance. Some have stacked weights, others have bendable plastic pieces, and still others have hydraulic components. Each of these devices works by providing resistance to motion in one fashion or another. Proper instruction is essential for safe use. Ask a professional how to use the equipment to make sure you're getting the maximum benefit. Resistance machines often must be adjusted to your height and arm and leg lengths in order to ensure proper form during exercises.

### Resistance bands or tubing

These are elastic-like cords, tubing or flat bands that offer progressively increasing resistance when you pull on them. They come in different tensions to fit a range of abilities and are usually color-coded by the manufacturer. Resistance bands are very portable and an inexpensive alternative to a home gym.

# Core stability training

Core stability training is a type of strength training. It works the muscles in the midsection of your body. Additional benefits of core stability training include increased flexibility and balance.

The core of your body — the area around your trunk — is where your center of gravity is located. Your core is your body's foundation, linking together your upper body and lower body. When you have good core stability, the 29 muscles in your abdomen, pelvis, lower back and hips work to-gether, stabilizing the rest of your body and providing support to your spine.

Developing a strong, solid core gives you increased balance. A strong core can also help prevent poor posture and low back pain. For many people, the prevention of low back pain is a compelling argument for exercising core muscles.

Regular aerobic and strength training exercises often don't build core strength because most of them focus on arm and leg strength.

## Examples of core stability exercises

Essentially any exercise that uses the trunk of your body without support is

## Danger signs

If you develop any of the following warning signs, stop whatever physical activity you're doing.

If any of these signs or symptoms persist or become worse, seek medical attention immediately. Even if they go away, tell your doctor before resuming any physical activity.

Danger signs include:

- Severe shortness of breath, that is, you can't talk or carry on a conversation
- Pain, pressure or aching in the chest, arms, jaw, neck, shoulders or back
- Extreme fatigue more than an hour after exercising
- Lightheadedness or dizziness
- Very rapid or very slow heart rate
- Distinct joint or muscle pain
- Visual changes, such as blurred vision

a core exercise. For example, a push-up stresses your core more than does a bench press, during which the bench is supporting your trunk. As a result, nearly any exercise can be modified to increase your core activity.

It's a good idea to get some personal instruction as you begin a core training program because pinpointing your core muscles takes some practice. Taking a class with a certified fitness instructor can help you make sure you're using the correct muscles. Whichever core exercises you choose, aim to do them three times a week or every other day.

Core stability exercises include floor exercises, workouts using a fitness ball, and Pilates.

### Floor exercises

Perhaps the two most important deep core muscles are your transversus abdominis (located deep in a hoop-like ring around your abdomen) and your multifidus (found in your back). You can find and strengthen these key muscles specific exercises that require nothing but your body and the floor.

### Fitness ball workouts

Fitness balls, which look like large, sturdy beach balls, can be used to work the deep core muscles of your abdomen and back. If you're stocking a home gym, fitness balls are versatile investments. They're also called stability balls, physioballs or Swiss balls — because they were first used in Switzerland many years ago to help rehabilitate people with stroke-related disabilities.

These balls not only work the trunk in almost every exercise they're designed for, but also help with balance and flexibility exercises. When strengthening your core with a fitness ball, you want to create a balance between your abdominal muscles and your back muscles by doing exercises that work each equally. This is because if there's imbalance in your abdomen or your back muscles, pain and poor posture can result.

### Pilates

Due to a recent surge in popularity, you might think that Pilates is a hot new exercise fad. In fact, Pilates is a low-impact fitness technique developed back in the 1920s by Joseph Pilates. Designed specifically to strengthen the body's core muscles by developing pelvic stability and abdominal control, Pilates exercises also help improve flexibility, joint mobility and strength. They can help you develop long, strong muscles, maintain a strong back and improve your posture.

# The right way to stretch

Before stretching, take a few minutes to warm your muscles. Stretching muscles when they're cold increases your risk of injury, including pulled muscles. Warm up by walking while gently swinging your arms, or do a low-intensity exercise, such as walking, for at least five minutes.

With the busy schedules and hectic demands of today, if you have time to stretch only once, do it after you exercise. This is when blood flow to your muscles is increased and the tissues are more flexible.

Stretching techniques are fairly simple and easy to learn. Here are some guidelines to consider:

- Hold your stretches for at least 30 seconds and up to a minute for a really tight muscle or problem area. That can seem like a long time, so use a watch or count out loud to make sure you're holding your stretches long enough.
- When you begin a stretch, spend the first 15 seconds in an easy stretch. Stretch just until you feel a mild tension, then relax as you hold the stretch. The tension should be comfortable, not painful.
- Once you've completed the easy stretch, stretch just a fraction of an inch farther until you again feel mild tension. Hold it for 15 seconds. Again, you should feel tension, but not pain.
- Relax and breathe freely while you're stretching. Try not to hold your breath. If you're bending forward to do a stretch, exhale as you bend forward and then breathe slowly as you hold the stretch.
- Avoid bouncing. This can cause small tears in muscle, which leave scar tissue as the muscle heals. The scar tightens the muscle further, making you even less flexible, and more prone to pain.
- Avoid locking your joints. Bend your joints slightly while stretching.

## Yoga variations

Yoga can be as vigorous or as gentle as you choose. Different styles appeal to different people, depending on their goals and ability levels.

- **Hatha yoga**. It is a gentle form of yoga, combining deep breathing with slow stretches and movement through a series of poses.
- **Ashtanga yoga.** Also called power yoga, this fast-paced, aerobic form of yoga is designed to build flexibility, strength and stamina.
- **Bikram yoga.** Also known as hot yoga, this form is practiced in rooms that can be heated to more than 100 F. It's best for people who are already fit and looking for a new challenge.
- **Kundalini yoga.** This type combines poses and breathing techniques with chanting and meditation.
- **Iyengar yoga.** It emphasizes mental clarity and precision in doing yoga postures. It uses benches, ropes, mats, blocks and chairs.
- **Svaroopa yoga.** From a Sanskrit word that means "bliss," this type uses postures that focus on the spine and hips.

Many Pilates exercises are done with special machines. The earliest Pilates machine, known as the Reformer, was a wooden device outfitted with cables, pulleys, springs and sliding boards. Using their own body weight as resistance, exercisers used the Reformer to perform a series of range-of-motion exercises that worked the abdominals, back, upper legs and buttocks.

Although machines are still used, many Pilates programs offer floor-work classes as well, designed to stabilize and strengthen the core back and abdominal muscles. Instead of emphasizing quantity, Pilates focuses on quality, meaning that exercisers do very few, but extremely precise, repetitions. Exercises can be adapted according to a person's own flexibility and strength abilities.

It may be a good idea to review the Pilates approach before committing to a class. You can do this by viewing a Pilates videotape or DVD.

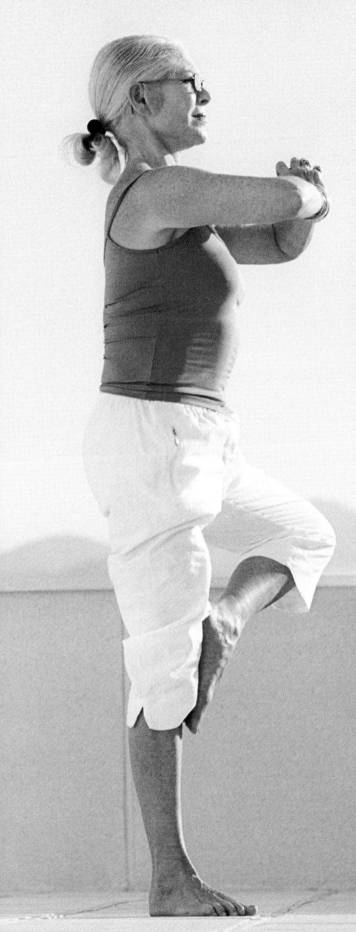

# Flexibility exercises

When you hear the terms *flexible* and *agile*, you may think of Olympic gymnasts or world-class ballerinas. But the truth is that everyone is flexible to some degree, and almost anyone can acquire greater flexibility. Flexibility is the ability to move your joints through their full range of motion.

Like many other indicators of fitness, your flexibility may diminish as you age. But like other effects of aging and inactivity, flexibility can be regained and maintained.

Increased flexibility, which is achieved by regularly stretching muscles, will help improve your daily performance. Routine tasks are easier and less tiring when your muscles and joints have good flexibility. Flexibility exercises also help improve posture and coordination.

## Examples of flexibility exercises

A regular stretching program is the most common way to increase your flexibility, but other activities such as swimming, yoga and tai chi also are effective for improving flexibility.

## Stretching

Stretching is a common way to gain range of motion about a joint, and nearly anyone can do it. Stretching is truly one of the easiest exercises to work into your routine.

A good rule of thumb is to spend five to 10 minutes stretching before your workouts (after a short five-minute warm-up) and another five to 10 minutes afterward. In addition to stretching before and after aerobic and strength training, you may want to adopt a stretching program. If you can, try to stretch three days a week. And each day focus on different muscle groups. One day you might focus on your neck and shoulders, another day on your hips and lower back, and another day on your calves and thighs.

Also stretch any muscles and joints that you routinely use. If you frequently play tennis or golf, working in extra shoulder stretches loosens the muscles around your shoulder joint, making it feel less tight and more ready for action.

## Yoga

Yoga, which combines deep breathing, movement and postures, can reduce anxiety, strengthen muscles, lower blood pressure and help your heart work more efficiently.

Yoga's techniques for stretching and strengthening the body can be practiced by people of all ages. However, adults with osteoporosis, older adults or those with stiff joints may have to eliminate and adapt some of the traditional poses. If you've had joint replacement surgery, especially hip replacement, some yoga positions may put you at risk of injury and joint dislocation. If you've had such surgery, be sure to talk with your doctor before starting yoga.

## Tai chi

This ancient form of martial arts involves gentle, circular movements combined with deep breathing. Tai chi helps strengthen muscles, improve balance and flexibility, and reduce stress. Health clubs and community centers frequently offer classes with experienced instructors.

## Feldenkrais Method

The Feldenkrais Method uses gentle movements to develop increased flexibility and coordination. Though similar to yoga, the Feldenkrais Method doesn't strive for correct positions, but instead aims for more dexterous, painless and efficient body movements.

The goal is to create an awareness and quality of movement through your body feedback rather than through pre-defined postures. These techniques often are used in physical and occupational therapies.

# Balance exercises

Balance is your ability to control your center of gravity over your base of support. It's related to your strength, inner ear balance center (vestibular system), vision and sensory input from your feet, as well as your muscles and tendons. The balance required to complete daily tasks is often taken for granted in adulthood, but the truth is that if you don't use your balancing skills, you may lose them.

Balance exercises — activities you do to hone your balance and coordination skills — are beneficial for all people, but especially so for older adults. Balance exercises can help prevent falls, improve your coordination, give you more confidence in your stability and boost your feelings of security. When combined with strength training, balance exercises can help you build muscles around your joints, making them more stable and your balance more

sure. People who do balance exercises have greater mobility as they age.

## Examples of balance exercises

Almost any activity that keeps you on your feet and moving is helpful in maintaining good balance. Basic exercises that get your legs and arms moving at the same time can help you maintain your balance in addition to stimulating muscle and nerve communication that increases your coordination.

### Walking
Walking can help your balance as well as your cardiovascular health. So while you're out getting your aerobic exercise with a brisk walk, you're also improving your balance. Walking keeps your leg muscles strong and reinforces your basic balance. The more you walk, the better your balance will be and the more practice you'll get at catching yourself when tripping or changing directions quickly.

### Tai chi
Tai chi, mentioned earlier as a way to increase flexibility, is also a popular method of improving balance. Tai chi may also help you build stamina and experience greater relaxation.

# Exercise guide

Your health care team can help identify the best set of exercises for you, based on your health status and fitness goals. You may benefit from some of the exercises illustrated on the following pages.

## Exercises for strength and balance

The following strength training exercises are commonly recommended. Some of these exercises also promote balance.

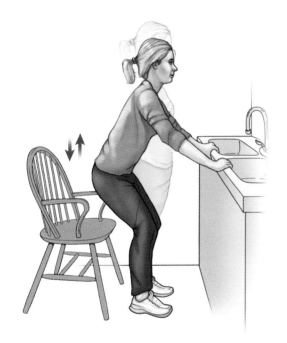 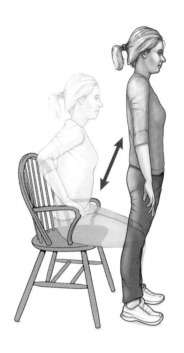

### Squats

Stand with a sturdy chair behind you. Hold on to a counter for support. Breathe out as you squat down as far as you can comfortably go, keeping knees in line with your toes. Hold the position for five seconds. Inhale as you return to standing. Relax and repeat. As you build strength, hold the squat for longer or squat down farther.

### Sit-to-stand

Sit in a sturdy chair with arms. Keeping your spine straight, raise yourself up off the chair without using your arms or hands to assist you. Keep your knees over your toes during the motion. Relax and repeat. If your legs are weak, you may need to push your body up using your arms or hands to assist you. Skip this exercise if it causes pain to your hands, wrists and elbows.

## Biceps strengthening

Sit in a sturdy chair with a length of resistance tubing (left-hand illustration). Grasp one end of the tubing in each hand and place your hands on your knees, with palms up and arms straight. Pull upward with one arm, as shown. Slowly return to the starting position and repeat with the other arm.

## Triceps strengthening

Grasp one end of the resistance tubing in each hand and hold both hands at shoulder height, with thumbs up and elbows bent (right-hand illustration). Straighten one arm toward your knee, keeping your elbow at your side. Slowly return to starting position and repeat with the other arm.

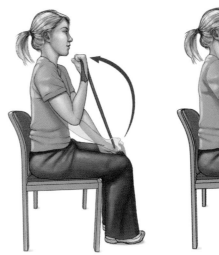
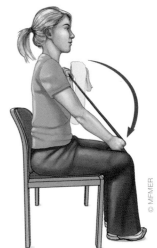

## Toe lift

Stand with your feet as wide as your hips (left-hand illustration). Hold on to a counter for support. Keeping your heels firmly planted, lift your toes as high as you can. Lower your toes and repeat.

## Heel lift

Stand with your feet as wide as your hips (right-hand illustration). Hold on to a counter for support. Keeping your toes firmly planted, lift your heels as high as you can. Lower your heels and repeat.

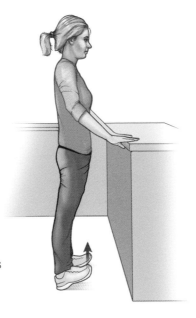
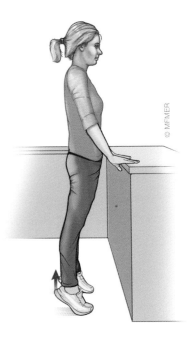

# Exercises for flexibility

The exercises illustrated on the following pages are a sample of the many different stretches you can do to improve flexibility and range of motion in your joints. You may want to get advice from your doctor or physical or occupational therapist to include stretches in your regular exercise routine that address your specific needs.

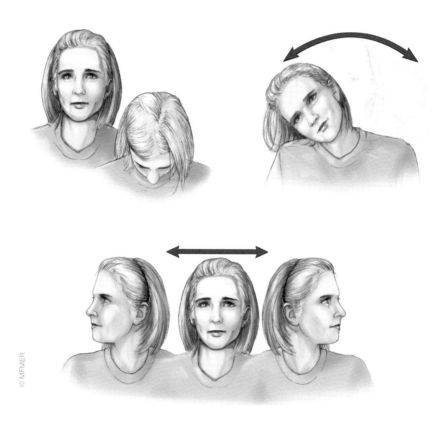

## Neck stretch

Tilt your chin forward and down to your chest (upper left). Next, tilt your ear toward one shoulder and then the other, without raising your shoulders (upper right). Finally, turn your face to the left, keeping your neck, shoulders and spine straight, and then turn your face to the right (lower illustration).

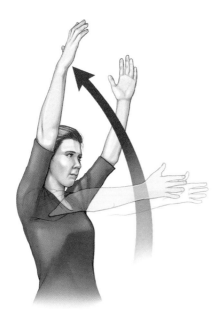

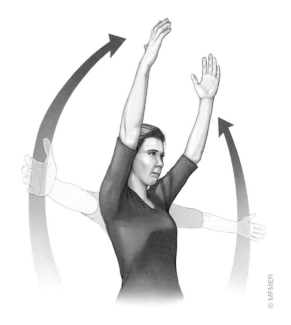

## Overhead arm raise

Stand with your arms straight out at chest height. Gently raise your arms over your head. Lower them back to the starting position. Relax and repeat.

## Overhead side raise

Stand with your arms out to the side at chest height, palms facing forward. Gently raise your arms over your head. Lower them back to the starting position. Relax and repeat.

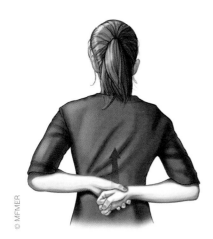

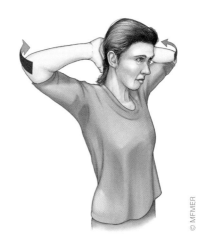

## Behind-the-back stretch

Grasp one wrist behind your back. Gently pull your arm up until you feel a stretch in your shoulders. Relax and repeat. Switch arms.

## Shoulder-blade squeeze

Raise your hands behind your head with your arms out to the side. Pinch your shoulder blades together by moving your elbows back. Hold briefly. Relax and repeat.

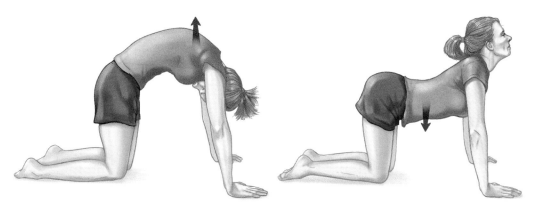

## Cat stretch

Get on your hands and knees. Arch your back away from the floor and then let it sag toward the floor. Focus on your mid- to lower back where the motion should be taking place. Don't arch your head backward too far. Relax and repeat. If you have hand or wrist arthritis, you may not be able to tolerate this position.

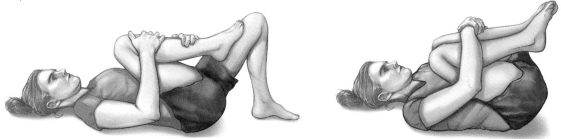

## Lower back stretches

Lie on your back, with your knees bent and feet on the floor. Keeping your lower back on the floor, lift your right knee and hug it toward your chest, using your hands (left). Hold this position for a few deep breaths. Repeat with the left knee. Then hug both knees (right). If knee pain is aggravated by this exercise, place your hands behind the knee joints when pulling your knees toward your chest.

## Lumbar rotation

Lie on your back, with knees bent and feet on the floor. Place your hands behind your head with your elbows out. Gently roll your knees to the left, all the way to the floor if you can. Hold this position for a few deep breaths. Return to the starting position. Then roll to the right. Repeat.

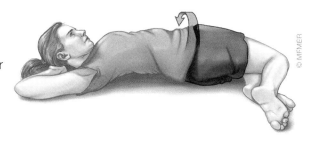

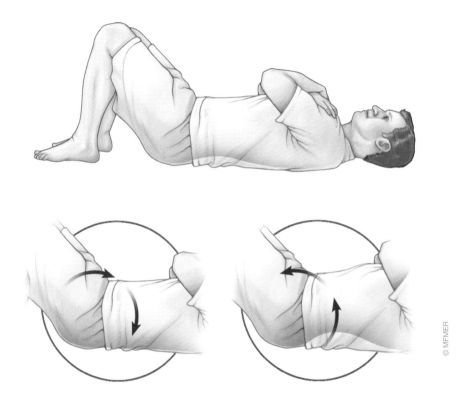

## Pelvic tilt

Lie on a firm, flat surface with your knees bent. Place your hands across your chest. The natural curves of the spine in your neck and lower back may not be touching the underlying surface. Tighten your abdominal muscles to flatten the small of your back against the surface (lower left). Release tension in your abdominal muscles to arch the small of your back (lower right). Slowly return to the starting position.

## Knee bend

Stand with your feet as wide as your hips. You may hold on to a counter for support. Slowly bend one knee, bringing your heel up toward your buttocks, and hold for a few seconds. Return to the starting position and repeat with the other knee. To help improve balance, stand in place for progressively longer periods of time with your knee bent.

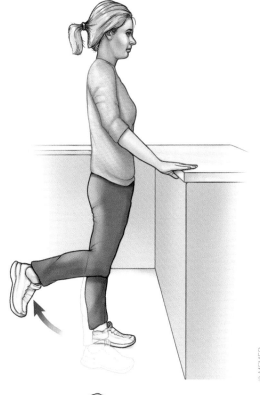

## Hip swing

Stand with your feet shoulder-width apart. You may hold on to a counter for support. Slowly swing one foot off the floor to the side, as far as you can, and hold. Keep your spine neutral and do not allow it to bend, twist or rotate during the hip-swing motion. Return to starting position and repeat with the other foot. To work on balance, remove one hand from the counter.

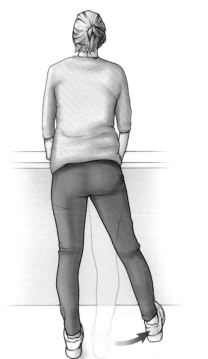

## Calf stretch

Stand with your hands pressing against a wall.
Bring one leg back, keeping the knee straight
and your foot flat on the floor. Lean on your front,
slightly bent leg until you feel a stretch in the calf
of your back leg and hold for a few seconds.
Return to the starting position and repeat with
your other leg.

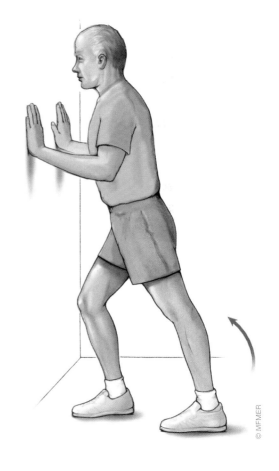

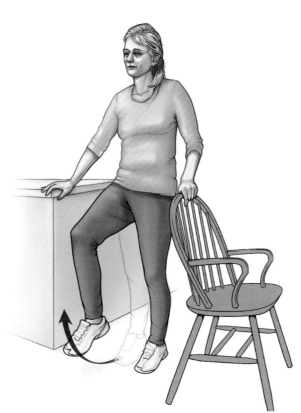

## Standing march

Stand between a counter and a sturdy chair.
Hold on to the counter and chair for support, if needed. Keep your spine straight
and slowly march in place, lifting your feet as
high as you can.

Tai chi consists of a series of graceful movements that help improve your stance and coordination. You learn how to turn your body more slowly and gain more confidence in your movements. Each of these benefits can result in better balance.

Finding an experienced instructor is your best bet for reaping all the benefits of tai chi. If you can't find a class, consider renting or purchasing tai chi videotapes or DVDs. A number of books are available as well, although it may be more difficult to learn the movements that way.

Whether you take a class, rent a video or refer to a book, look for instruction that's geared to your age group or activity level.

### Individual exercises

You can also incorporate balance exercises into your strength training routine. Just add variations to strength exercises, such as standing on one leg, using a weight in only one hand, or standing on a pillow or foam pad while performing an exercise. For each of these variations, if you're worried about losing your balance, make sure someone is nearby to help you should you do so, or put yourself in position to hold on to a rail or stable surface if needed.

# Staying motivated

Starting a fitness program takes initiative, and sticking with it takes commitment. It may help to think of physical fitness as a journey, not a destination. Fitness is not a goal you simply achieve one day and then are done with. It's something you strive for, for the rest of your life.

As with any journey, you may encounter some roadblocks and setbacks. For some people, getting started is the hardest step. Others begin with tremendous enthusiasm and go at it so vigorously that they get hurt and stop.

To have the best chance of success — a lifelong commitment to physical activity — you need to get and stay motivated. Exercise has to be as natural and ingrained a habit as is brushing your teeth or taking a shower. As explained earlier in this chapter, it's worth it.

With the right frame of mind, anyone can get and stay motivated to exercise. If you don't feel motivated right now, it's not because you don't have what it takes or are destined to fail. You just haven't identified and activated your own motivational process.

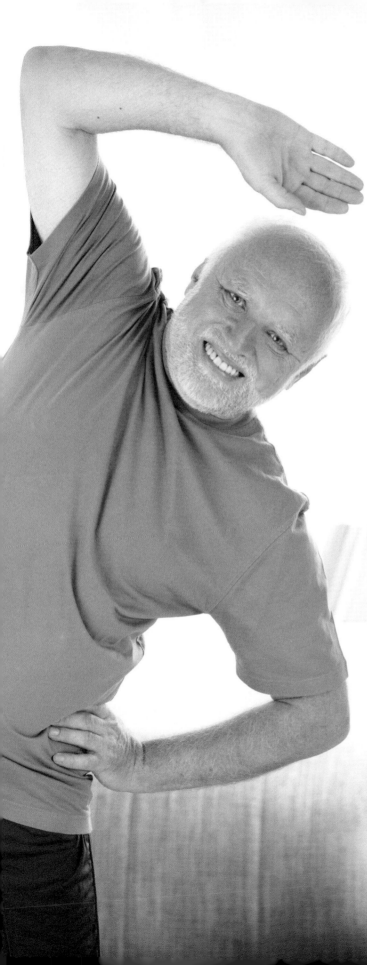

## Understanding what motivates you

People who are self-motivated are more likely to stick with an exercise program than are those who rely solely on external forms of motivation. If your motivation is internally based, you're doing the activity for yourself — because you enjoy it, because you want to look or feel better, or because you want to become healthier.

External motivation, in contrast, comes from outside — you're exercising to please someone else or to reach a particular goal, such as a 10-pound weight loss, or reward, such as new clothes. You're more focused on the outcome than the process.

That's not to say that external motivators have no place. An occasional tangible reward, such as a new pair of shoes, may be just the boost you need to keep going. But if you're constantly focusing on such rewards, you may lose some of your intrinsic motivation, exercising less for the enjoyment and more for the rewards.

The bottom line is that you'll be more motivated if you can embrace the activity as something you want to do for yourself over the long term.

# Creating an action plan

For a majority of people, getting started on a fitness program is the hardest step. If you've been dragging your feet about getting more active, you're not alone.

You may have a million excuses for not exercising. You just don't like to exercise, or you find it boring. You're already too busy and don't have time for a new activity. Your family and friends want more of your free time. Exercise equipment and health club memberships cost too much.

As soon as you start thinking about exercising, a host of negative thoughts may pop up: "I know I'll never be able to keep this up." "I don't have time for this." "I'll hurt my knees."

Lots of people have started from this same place, with the same excuses and have come not only to tolerate physical activity but to enjoy it. It's possible to change the beliefs that are keeping you stuck and to mobilize your motivation.

So how do you change your thinking and behaviors? Follow these 10 steps.

1. **Take some time to recognize what does or doesn't motivate you.** Think about your previous experiences with changes you've tried to make. What worked and what didn't? What can you learn from your past experiences? What might help you this time around?

2. **Ask for support.** Your odds of success are greater if you have the support of those around you. Work on developing friendships with physically active people.

3. **Start slowly.** The most common mistake that people make is starting a fitness program at too high an intensity and progressing too quickly. If your body isn't accustomed to vigorous exercise, your joints, ligaments and muscles are more vulnerable to injury. The resulting pain and stiffness can be very discouraging. It's better to "start low and progress slow" than to push too hard.

4. **Choose activities you enjoy.** Boredom is a major reason people stop exercising. If you have to drag yourself to aerobics class or you find walking on a treadmill mind-numbingly dull, then you're going to seize on any possible excuse to avoid these activities. Find activities you like doing.

5. **Focus on the process and take small steps.** Set realistic, attainable goals and continue to evaluate them. It's easy to get frustrated and give up on goals that are too ambitious.

For example, if you're currently inactive, a goal of running a marathon in three months isn't realistic. Your goals should also be specific and measurable. Rather than saying something general like, "I will be more active this month," you might set a specific goal of taking the stairs instead of the elevators three times this week.

Some of your goals should be short term, some intermediate and some long term. For example, a short-term goal might be to walk five minutes once or twice a day just to establish a comfortable tolerance level. An intermediate goal might be to work up to 20 to 30 minutes most days of the week.

A long-term goal might be to complete a 10-kilometer (10K) race after you complete 12 weeks of training. Other long-term goals may include things like feeling healthier, looking better, improving your fitness level, losing weight, or toning or strengthening your muscles. Over time your long-term goals may shift.

Write down your goals and place them where you can see them, such as on the refrigerator. Seeing your goals can help keep you motivated.

6. **Monitor your progress.** Keep track as you go along. Monitoring progress is a great way to reinforce your new habit, feel good about what you've accomplished and help set your goals for the future.

7. **Accept some ambivalence.** Everyone who embarks on a major lifestyle change feels ambivalent about it sometimes. Even regular, committed exercisers occasionally have days when they'd rather stay in bed than get up and work out. However, ambivalent thoughts don't have to be more than a passing detour.

8. **Plan for exercise.** Reserve a time slot each day for physical activity, and protect that time. If you wait to find the time, you probably won't do it. Schedule an exercise appointment on your calendar just as you would a haircut appointment or an important meeting.

9. **Reward yourself.** Work on developing an internal reward system that comes from feelings of accomplishment, self-esteem and control of your behavior. After each exercise session, take a few minutes to sit down and relax. Savor the good feelings that exercise gives you, and reflect on what you've just accomplished. This type of internal reward can help you make a long-term commitment to regular exercise.

**10. Remember how good it feels.**
When you find yourself dragging your feet, call to mind the thought of how great you feel after an exercise session. Use images of successful experiences that remind you of how good physical activity makes you feel.

# Avoiding aches and pains

Forget the old saying, "No pain, no gain." Exercising shouldn't be painful. Still, everyone who's physically active is bound to feel some soreness, stiffness, or occasional minor aches and pains.

Muscle soreness that follows a day or two after exercise is normal, especially if you've been inactive or you're starting a new workout routine or trying a new activity. This type of soreness, called delayed-onset muscle soreness, is also common after a bout of heavy exercise, even if you've been regularly active. The soreness means that your muscles are growing stronger.

On the other hand, pain during exercise can be a warning sign of impending injury. Excessive exercise can cause muscle injury. Injured muscle fibers will need time and occasionally medical treatment to rebuild and recover. Pay attention to what your body is telling you. If you're feeling pain, you're overdoing it.

Another common cause of aches and pains is doing the same activities over and over without variation. Regular exercisers tend to focus on one or two activities. This can lead to overuse injuries, caused by repeated stress on a particular area of the body. Cross-training, which is performing a variety of exercise, can help prevent overuse or stress injuries.

## Heading off muscle soreness

The following steps can help prevent or reduce muscle soreness that can accompany physical activity.

- **Warm up.** Before an activity, warm up your muscles by walking or doing your activity at a slow and gentle pace. Once your muscles are limbered up, gently stretch the muscles if you feel the need to do so. Gentle activity enhances blood flow within the muscle, reducing the risk of injury. See page 172 for more on warming up.

# Running for the fun of it

If you think your physical fitness peaked at the age of 22 and is never to return, you might want to think again. Dick began training for his first marathon at the age of 56. After retiring from a career as a senior engineer in 1993 and accepting an academic position at a local university, Dick's friends convinced him that now was the perfect time to enter a marathon.

"I had always thought that it was just too much effort. So I always used the excuse while I was working that I was just too busy, that I couldn't find the time to train for it. But as good friends are, when I retired, they said, 'OK, Dick, you no longer have that excuse. You're going to run with us.'"

The marathon was just over 26 miles long, and after completing it Dick vowed to never do it again. "When I crossed the finish line, I was just completely exhausted and sore. I could hardly lift my legs."

He held to his word for about a year. But with time, the memories of that first experience receded, and soon enough, he was back on the pavement. And this time, he has no plans to stop. Since 1993, Dick has run a total of 30 marathons in his home state of Minnesota and around the country.

Dick began running in his mid-30s, after a three-on-three basketball game left him feeling so out of shape that he considered it a wake-up call.

At first, he thought running would be too boring, but a six-week stay in Manhattan for a seminar, where he started running in Central Park during his spare time, gave him his start. Since then he has kept up his routine at home, following a path that takes him past a lake and extends just short of 4 miles.

He runs this route most days of the week and tries to include a longer run on the weekends.

Dick attributes running to helping him keep his blood pressure down and his weight at a healthy level. He says it also provides him a way to relax.

"For me, running not only is a good source of fitness, but mentally it's a great re-laxer. It gives me time to think about problems at work and also just enjoy the out-doors. I still have a tendency to gain weight, but over the last couple of years I've lost 30 pounds, so I'm actually running faster."

Running is also a source of camaraderie and friendship. Once a week, he runs with his "runner" friends. "I've met the nicest people. Over the years, we've developed a small group that has decided to run together on weekends at least 10 miles. That's important to me, too, because it keeps me in a minimum condition. Then when it comes time to run a marathon, I don't have to train quite as hard. And this group of friends has pretty much stuck together over the years. We've kept very close."

At 68, Dick is dismissive of the notion that age might hold him back. "So far my age has not significantly slowed me down at all," he says. "I'm feeling better and better."

- **Exercise smart.** When exercising, use proper form and technique, wear proper shoes and protective equipment, and take appropriate precautions for the weather conditions. Also make sure to drink plenty of water to keep your body well hydrated.
- **Stretch afterward.** After an activity is when your muscles are the most limber. This is the best time to stretch your muscles. Stretching helps to reduce muscle soreness (see page 180).
- **Pay attention to warning signs.** Sometimes, your body may be telling you to take a break from exercise. If you have a flare-up of a bone or joint condition, rest until it subsides. If your pain is beyond normal achiness, it persists for longer than two weeks or you have swelling, back off from your fitness activities and consider seeing a doctor.

# The payoff

Longevity is affected by some things that you simply can't control, such as your genes. But of those factors that you can control, being physically active is one of the most important steps that you can take to both extend and improve the quality of your life.

Consider this: Nearly 1 million people in the United States die of cardiovascular diseases each year. More than one-third of adult Americans are obese. Worldwide, more than 200 million people have the bone-thinning disease osteoporosis. And that's just the beginning of a very long list.

Regardless of your age, the time you invest now in becoming more physically active and staying fit will pay off in the years to come.

Before you know it, you'll have a well-developed, personalized plan that makes exercise a regular part of your life. Remember, fitness is for everybody.

# Chapter 9

# Eat as if your life depended on it

The decisions you make each day as you select and prepare food for your meals go beyond just satisfying your appetite. They affect how well you'll live now and in the years ahead. That's because you really are what you eat!

The evidence is overwhelmingly clear that good food is crucial to good health. Your health is greatly influenced by the interaction of nutrients and genes — a continual interplay in which certain foods enhance the action of protective (or harmful) genes, while other foods try to suppress them. People who regularly enjoy meals made with a variety of healthy ingredients generally are at less risk of developing many diseases, including heart disease, diabetes, many kinds of cancer, osteoporosis, digestive disorders and more.

Variety is key. Because your body is a complex machine, it needs a variety of foods in order to operate at its best. A diet that emphasizes a smorgasbord of vegetables, fruits and whole grains results in a rich supply of nutrients, fiber and other healthy substances.

The bottom line: If you want to live well, you have to eat well.

## How to eat well

Eating well means enjoying great taste as well as great nutrition. The pages that follow contain the latest information about how the food you eat can help keep you healthy. By learning more about how your body uses the different nutrients found in food, you'll

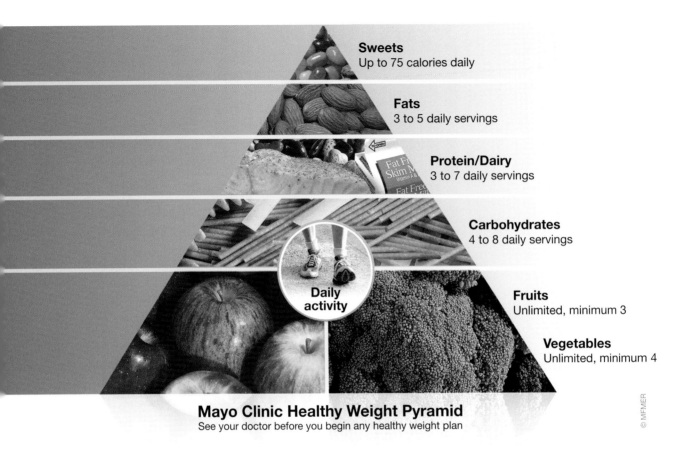

**Sweets**
Up to 75 calories daily

**Fats**
3 to 5 daily servings

**Protein/Dairy**
3 to 7 daily servings

**Carbohydrates**
4 to 8 daily servings

**Daily activity**

**Fruits**
Unlimited, minimum 3

**Vegetables**
Unlimited, minimum 4

**Mayo Clinic Healthy Weight Pyramid**
See your doctor before you begin any healthy weight plan

© MFMER

better understand how what you eat everyday affects how you function today and in the years to come.

The eating approach that we recommend for better health and great nutrition is the Mayo Clinic Healthy Weight Pyramid. This pyramid is a guide to healthy eating that focuses on vegetables, fruits and whole grains as the basis of good health. That's because vegetables, fruits and whole grains are endowed with many nutrients and health-enhancing compounds called phytochemicals, which experts believe work together to fight disease.

# The Mayo Clinic Healthy Weight Pyramid

The Mayo Clinic Healthy Weight Pyramid includes six sections, representing six food groups. Foods are

## The reasoning behind the name

The Mayo Clinic Healthy Weight Pyramid was developed not only to help people eat more nutritiously but also to help individuals who are overweight achieve a weight that's more healthy.

If you're already at a healthy weight, the pyramid can help you maintain that weight and ensure you're getting the nutrients your body needs. If you're overweight, the pyramid can help you lose weight. Weight loss based on the principles of the Mayo Clinic Healthy Weight Pyramid is discussed later in this chapter.

grouped according to common health benefits that they share and their levels of energy density. All foods contain a certain number of calories (energy) within a given amount (volume). Some foods contain many calories in just a small portion, such as fats. They're described as high in energy density. Foods with fewer calories in a larger volume, such as vegetables and fruits, are low in energy density.

Foods high in energy density are at the top of the pyramid — you want to eat less of these. Those low in energy density are at the bottom of the pyramid — you want to eat more of these. Foods low in energy density are generally healthier, and you get a lot more food for the calories.

## Vegetables

It's hardly news that vegetables and fruits are good for you. The real news is why. More and more is being learned about how fresh produce can supply us with substances that ward off many illnesses and diseases.

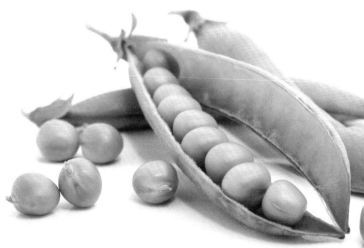

# 10 ways to eat more vegetables and fruits

1. Add a banana, strawberries or another favorite fruit to your cereal or yogurt at breakfast.

2. Include a small salad with one or more of your meals.

3. When eating a full meal, eat your vegetable portions right away, rather than reserving them for the end after you've finished other items.

4. Stir-fry vegetables with a small portion of poultry, seafood or meat.

5. Use fresh fruit or fruit sauces as toppings on desserts and pancakes.

6. Have ready-to-eat frozen vegetables handy as a quick addition to a meal.

7. Liven up your sandwiches with lettuce and tomato, onion, pepper, and cucumber slices.

8. When you have a craving for chips, have a small handful with lots of salsa.

9. For dessert, have baked apples or grilled pineapple.

10. Experiment. Try vegetables and fruits that you're unfamiliar with — perhaps mango, papaya, tomatillo and jicama.

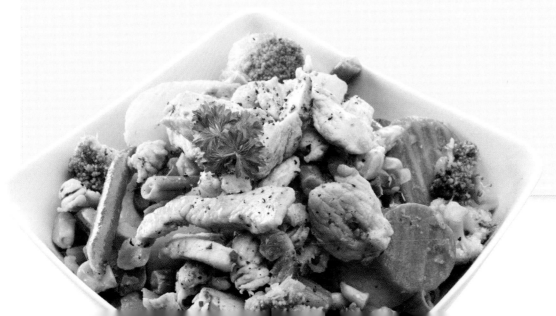

Strong evidence is stacking up that people who eat generous helpings of vegetables — a variety of vegetables — run a lower risk of developing heart disease, a leading killer of American adults. In addition, researchers have identified substances in vegetables — called phytochemicals — that appear to offer some protection against cancer.

Most vegetables are loaded with the antioxidants beta carotene and vitamin C. Antioxidants can be important because these substances play a role in inhibiting molecules called oxygen free radicals, which can damage healthy cells in the body. Vegetables are also key sources of essential vitamins and minerals, including folate, potassium, magnesium and selenium. Many are rich in health-enhancing fiber, and some even have calcium. Vegetables also contain no cholesterol, and they're naturally low in fat and calories.

## Fruits

Fruits, like many vegetables, have an abundance of vitamins, minerals and fiber, not to mention a long list of healthy antioxidants, including vitamin C. Some fruits, as well as vegetables, contain the antioxidants lutein and zeaxanthin, which may guard against certain conditions related to aging, such as macular degeneration, a disease that affects vision.

Researchers have also discovered that many fruits contain generous amounts of flavonoids, substances that apparently work together to lower the risk of cancer and heart disease. Oranges and avocados, for instance, are rich in a flavonoid compound called beta-sitosterol, which is believed to help lower blood cholesterol.

As with vegetables, because different fruits provide different nutrients, variety is vital.

## Carbohydrates

Envision every kind of food containing carbohydrates laid out in a line. At one end are whole wheat, oats and brown rice. In the middle sit white bread, white rice, potatoes and pasta. And at the far end are cookies, candies and soft drinks. The foods in this spectrum incorporate all three kinds of carbohydrates: fiber, starch and sugar.

It's not hard to determine the healthy and unhealthy ends — unrefined whole grains on one end and refined sugar on the other. The foods in the middle —

## Carbs: Setting the record straight

Carbohydrates don't make you fat — excess calories do. Many diets have promoted low-carbohydrate foods for weight loss. These diets claim that carbohydrates stimulate insulin secretion, which promotes body fat. So, the logic goes, reducing carbohydrates will reduce body fat. As a matter of fact, carbohydrates do stimulate insulin secretion immediately after they're consumed, but this is a normal process that allows carbohydrates to be absorbed into cells and used as energy. People who gain weight on high-carbohydrate diets do so because they're eating excess calories. Excess calories from any source, whether it contains a lot of carbohydrates or only a few, will cause weight gain.

Furthermore, some low-carbohydrate diets restrict grains, fruits and vegetables and emphasize the consumption of protein and dairy products, which can be high in calories and loaded with saturated fat and cholesterol. Plant-based foods not only are low in saturated fat and cholesterol-free but also are loaded with vitamins, minerals and other nutrients. These nutrients play a protective role in fighting serious diseases such as cancer, osteoporosis, high blood pressure and heart disease.

Be skeptical of the low-carbohydrate claims. Many carbohydrate-containing foods are healthy and are an important part of a weight-control plan.

rice, pasta, bread and potatoes — are all nutritious, but can lose some of their health benefits depending on how they're processed and prepared.

Whole grains are the types of carbohydrates that you should eat the most of. Some are rich in vitamin E, an antioxidant with many health benefits. Others contain lignans — estrogen-like substances that may help protect against some forms of cancer. All contain fiber that's good for digestive health. That's why it's important to purchase products made from whole grains rather than foods made from refined carbohydrates.

## Protein and dairy

Protein is essential to human life. But despite what you may have heard, it's not necessary or even desirable to eat meat every day. Although rich in protein, many cuts of beef, pork, lamb, chicken and turkey are too high in saturated fat and cholesterol.

There are other ways to get protein than eating meat. Foods that also provide protein include low-fat dairy products, seafood and many plant foods. Legumes — namely beans, lentils and peas — are excellent sources of protein. That's because they have no cholesterol and very little fat. In addition, the fiber in beans actually helps lower the "bad" form of blood cholesterol, and the minerals they contain help control blood pressure.

It's also important that you include fish and shellfish in your diet. Not only do they provide protein, but some supply omega-3 fatty acids. Omega-3 fats help lower triglycerides, fat particles in the blood that appear to raise heart disease risk. Omega-3s may also improve immune function and help regulate blood pressure. Research suggests that most people would benefit from eating at least two servings of fish a week.

## Lovable legumes

The term *legume* refers to a large family of plants, including beans, lentils and peas, whose seeds develop inside pods and are usually dried for ease of storage.

Legumes are low in fat and high in fiber, protein, folate, potassium, iron, magnesium and phytochemicals. The fiber in legumes is mostly soluble, which studies show may help lower cholesterol and help regulate blood sugar levels. In addition, legumes — which include soybeans, peanuts, lima beans, chickpeas, black-eyed peas, split peas and lentils — are versatile and inexpensive. They're a healthy substitute for meat, which has more fat and cholesterol. If you use canned legumes, rinse them well to eliminate salt that may have been added during processing.

## Getting your omega-3s

Omega-3 fatty acids are most abundant in fatty, cold-water fish, but some freshwater fish also are good sources. Examples of fish high in beneficial omega-3s include anchovies, bass, herring, salmon, sardines, trout (rainbow and lake) and tuna (especially white, albacore and bluefin).

Omega-3s are also present in some plants. Good plant sources include canola oil, flaxseed (ground and oil), soybeans (whole and oil), tofu and walnuts (whole and oil).

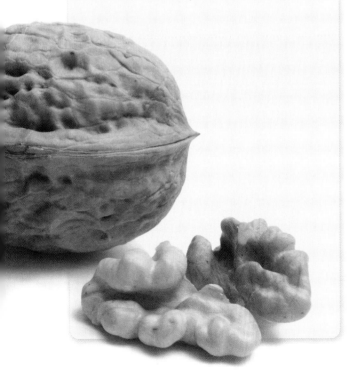

## Fats

Not all fat is bad for you. Some kinds are actually beneficial. Therefore, it's important that you include some fat in your diet. The keys are not to eat too much and to eat the right kinds.

High-fat plant foods, such as avocados, olives, seeds and nuts, and some cooking oils, such as canola and olive oils, are good for you. Nuts, for instance, contain monounsaturated fat, which helps keep harmful deposits from accumulating in blood vessels and lowers the risk of a heart attack. They also deliver many other key nutrients.

But even though nuts and vegetable oils may be beneficial, you want to use them in moderation. A tablespoon of peanut butter weighs in at nearly 100 calories; a tablespoon of olive oil, 140. In other words, the goal is to eat enough of these foods to gain their health benefits but not too much that you consume too many calories. Most nutrition experts recommend no more than three to five servings daily.

## Sweets

Foods in the sweets group include candies, cookies and other desserts.

# Fats: The good and the bad

Not all fats are created equal. There are different kinds of fat in the food you eat, and some are better for you than are others.

- **Monounsaturated fat.** This type of fat is found in olive, canola and nut oils, as well as in nuts and avocados. Monounsaturated fat is considered a "good" fat. It helps lower blood cholesterol, and it's more resistant to oxidation. Oxidation is a process that promotes the buildup of fat and cholesterol deposits in the arteries. However, because all fat — even monounsaturated fat — is high in calories, you want to limit how much you eat.
- **Polyunsaturated fat.** Polyunsaturated fat is found in plant oils such as safflower, corn, sunflower, soy and cottonseed. It helps lower "bad" blood cholesterol, but it also lowers "good" blood cholesterol, and it seems susceptible to oxidation.
- **Saturated fat.** Saturated fat is an unhealthy fat that can raise your blood cholesterol and increase your risk of cardiovascular disease. It's found in meats and dairy products (including butter), as well as coconut, palm and other tropical oils.
- **Trans fat.** This type of fat is found in stick margarine, shortening and the processed products made from them, such as pastry and other baked goods, crackers, candy, and other snack foods. Trans fat — short for trans-fatty acids — raises blood cholesterol, and it may lower "good" cholesterol, increasing your risk of cardiovascular disease. If you use margarine, look for products labeled as trans fat-free or that are made from canola oil. Stick margarines are generally higher in trans fat than are tub varieties.

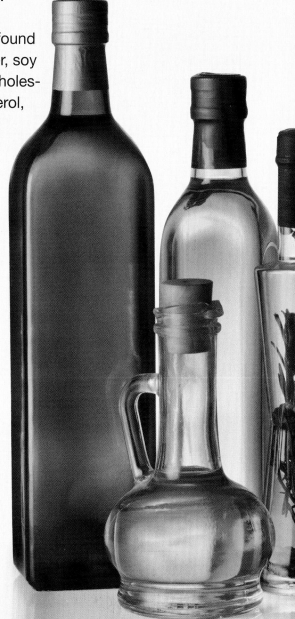

And don't forget the sugar you may add to your cereal or beverages. Sweets are high in energy density and calories, and they offer little to nothing in terms of nutrition.

# Do you need to lose weight?

Whether you would benefit from losing weight shouldn't be determined by your desire to fit into a certain clothing size. Rather, it should be based on what's healthiest. A question often asked is,

"How do I know if I'm at a healthy weight — one that's good for me?"

Perhaps the best way to assess your weight is to compare it with standards established by doctors, dietitians and other health professionals who help individuals determine whether their weight is putting their health at risk.

## What's a healthy weight?

Simply put, a healthy weight means you have the right amount of body fat in relation to your overall body mass. A healthy weight is one that reduces

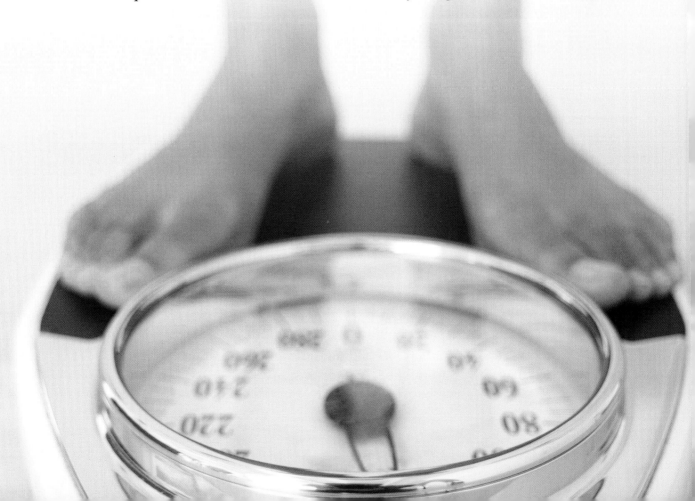

health risks, helps prevent premature aging, maintains energy levels and improves your quality of life. Stepping on the scale only tells you your total weight — including bone, muscle and fluid — not how much of your weight is fat. The scale also doesn't tell you where you're carrying fat. In determining health risks, both of these factors are more important than weight alone.

The most accurate way to determine how much fat you're carrying is to have a body fat analysis. This requires a professional using a reliable method of estimation, such as weighing a person underwater, using a procedure called dual energy X-ray absorptiometry or using bioelectric impedance analysis. These methods can be expensive and fairly complicated.

The most common method to determine if you're at a healthy weight is to consider three key components:

- Your body mass index
- Your waist measurement
- Your medical history

## Body mass index

Body mass index (BMI) is a tool for indicating your weight status. The calculation involved takes into account both your weight and height and relates them to health (see page 216).

Although a BMI number tends to correlate well with an approximate measure of body fat, it's not always a good match. Some people may have a high BMI but relatively little body fat. Many athletes have BMIs that would seem to classify them as overweight, but they're not overweight because athletic training has turned most of their weight into lean muscle mass. By the same token, there may be people with a BMI in the "healthy" range but who carry a high percentage of body fat.

For most people, though, the BMI provides a fairly accurate approximation of body fat as it relates to their total weight.

## Waist measurement

Many conditions associated with excess weight, such as high blood pressure, abnormal levels of blood fats, coronary artery disease, stroke, diabetes and certain types of cancer, are influenced by the location of fat on your body. If you carry most of your weight around your waist, most of your fat is located in and around your abdominal organs. This increases your risk of disease.

## Limit dried fruit and fruit juice

One of the basic premises of the Mayo Clinic Healthy Weight Pyramid is unlimited servings of fresh vegetables and fruits. You can basically eat as much as you want. This, however, doesn't apply to dried fruit, such as raisins and dates, or to fruit juice, such as orange or apple juice. That's because these items are less filling and higher in energy density. Unlimited servings could cause a significant increase in daily calories.

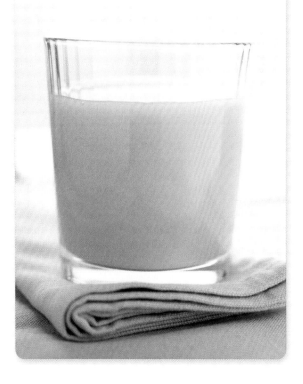

To determine whether you're carrying too much weight around your middle, you'll need to measure your waist.

There are differences of opinion among health organizations as to what's an unhealthy waist size. Some organizations suggest men with a waist measurement greater than 35 inches (89 centimeters) are at increased risk of weight-related diseases — others say a measurement greater than 40 inches (102 centimeters). Among women, a waist measurement greater than 32 inches (81 centimeters) may pose an increased risk of disease, according to some groups — a measurement greater than 34 inches (86 centimeters), according to others.

## Medical history

A complete evaluation of your medical history also is important to get a complete picture of your weight status.

- Do you have a health condition, such as high blood pressure or diabetes, that would improve if you lost weight?
- Do you have a family history of obesity, cardiovascular disease, diabetes, high blood pressure or sleep apnea? This may mean increased risk for you.

- Have you gained considerable weight since high school? Even people with normal BMIs may be at increased risk of weight-related conditions if they've gained more than 10 pounds since young adulthood.
- Do you smoke cigarettes or engage in little physical activity? These risk factors can compound the risks of excess weight.

## Adding it up

If your BMI indicates that you're not overweight (BMI under 25), if you're not carrying too much weight around your abdomen, and if you answered no to all of the medical history questions, there's probably little health advantage to changing your weight. The weight you're at now appears to be healthy.

If your BMI is between 25 and 29 or your waist circumference exceeds healthy guidelines and you answered yes to one or more of the medical history questions, you may benefit from losing a few pounds. Discuss your weight with your doctor at your next checkup.

If your BMI is 30 or more, you weigh too much. Losing weight will improve your health and reduce your risk of weight-related illnesses.

# The right way to lose weight

An effective diet — that is, one that works — is a diet in which you consume fewer calories each day than you burn up in physical activity. However, cutting calories shouldn't come at the cost of good health, taste and practicality.

A diet that's also enjoyable and satisfying is vital to the long-term success of any weight-loss program. In addition, shopping, cooking and eating practices should be simple and inexpensive. Otherwise, you won't stay with the plan.

The Mayo Clinic Healthy Weight Pyramid can help you lose weight safely, and keep it off. The pyramid is based on a plant-based diet (as represented by the vegetable and fruit groups at the base of the pyramid) and on the concept of energy density (eating foods with fewer calories per volume).

The pyramid also addresses the importance of regular physical activity as a key component to your weight. It's easier to lose weight and to keep it off when you're physically active.

The Mayo Clinic Healthy Weight Pyramid can help you improve your health

## Where calories come from

Carbohydrates, fats and proteins all contain calories and are the main energy sources for your body. The amount of energy each of these nutrients provides varies.

During digestion, carbohydrates are broken down into sugar (glucose) and absorbed into your bloodstream. When there's an energy demand, the glucose is absorbed immediately into your body's cells to provide energy. If there's no immediate demand, the glucose is stored in your liver and muscles. When these storage sites become full, excess glucose is converted into fatty acids and stored in fat tissue for later use. Carbohydrates contain 4 calories a gram.

Fats are an extremely concentrated form of energy and pack the most calories. When digested, they're broken down into fatty acids, which can be used immediately for energy or for other body processes. If there's an excess of fatty acids, a small quantity can be stored in your muscles, but most of them are stored in fat tissue. Fat has 9 calories a gram.

Proteins have many responsibilities in your body, including supplying energy for physical activity if your body runs out of carbohydrate power. This can happen if you consume too few calories or if you're involved in prolonged physical activity. Any excess calories from protein also are stored in fat tissue. Protein has 4 calories a gram.

Empty calories is a term applied to sugar and alcohol. They contribute calories, but no other essential nutrients. Sugar, a carbohydrate, has 4 calories a gram, whereas alcohol has almost twice as many — 7 calories a gram.

and achieve your weight goal. It's a common-sense approach to better health that encourages healthy behaviors. By following the guidelines recommended, you'll lose weight slowly and safely — about 1 to 2 pounds a week — and keep it off.

To get started, you need to follow four simple steps.

## 1. Establish your weight-loss goal

How much weight would you like to lose? Perhaps you'd like to lose 10 to 20 pounds. Or maybe your goal is more ambitious.

Now ask yourself if your goal is realistic. If you think your goal may be unrealistic, decide on a number that you feel confident you can achieve. For many people, a reasonable goal is to lose about 10 percent of their body weight over several weeks to months. That amount is generally achievable. And many people experience noticeable improvements in their health when they lose just 10 percent of their body weight.

Remember that weight control is an ongoing process. Once you reach your goal, you can set another, until you achieve the weight you want to be at. What you don't want are expectations that are too high and that set you up for disappointment.

## 2. Determine your calorie goal

To meet your weight-loss goal, how many calories should you eat each day? If you eat 500 calories fewer than the number of calories you burn, you should lose about 1 pound a week. Five hundred fewer calories each day for seven days is 3,500 fewer total calories, which equals 1 pound of body fat. But if you don't know how many calories you consume each day, this may be difficult to determine.

Here's a simpler approach. If you weigh 250 pounds or less and you want to lose weight, a daily calorie goal of 1,200 calories generally works best for women, and 1,400 calories works best for men. If you feel exceptionally hungry at this calorie level, or you lose weight too quickly, you may consider jumping to the next higher calorie level.

Getting less than 1,200 daily calories for women and 1,400 daily calories for men generally isn't recommended for

# What's your BMI?

You can determine your body mass index (BMI) by finding your height and weight on this chart. A BMI of 18.5 to 24.9 is considered the healthiest. People with a BMI under 18.5 are considered underweight. People with a BMI between 25 and 29.9 are considered overweight. People with a BMI of 30 or greater are considered obese.

| | Normal | | Overweight | | | | | Obese | | | | |
|---|---|---|---|---|---|---|---|---|---|---|---|---|
| **BMI** | **19** | **24** | **25** | **26** | **27** | **28** | **29** | **30** | **35** | **40** | **45** | **50** |
| Height | | | | | | | | Weight in pounds | | | | |
| 4'10" | 91 | 115 | 119 | 124 | 129 | 134 | 138 | 143 | 167 | 191 | 215 | 239 |
| 4'11" | 94 | 119 | 124 | 128 | 133 | 138 | 143 | 148 | 173 | 198 | 222 | 247 |
| 5'0" | 97 | 123 | 128 | 133 | 138 | 143 | 148 | 153 | 179 | 204 | 230 | 255 |
| 5'1" | 100 | 127 | 132 | 137 | 143 | 148 | 153 | 158 | 185 | 211 | 238 | 264 |
| 5'2" | 104 | 131 | 136 | 142 | 147 | 153 | 158 | 164 | 191 | 218 | 246 | 273 |
| 5'3" | 107 | 135 | 141 | 146 | 152 | 158 | 163 | 169 | 197 | 225 | 254 | 282 |
| 5'4" | 110 | 140 | 145 | 151 | 157 | 163 | 169 | 174 | 204 | 232 | 262 | 291 |
| 5'5" | 114 | 144 | 150 | 156 | 162 | 168 | 174 | 180 | 210 | 240 | 270 | 300 |
| 5'6" | 118 | 148 | 155 | 161 | 167 | 173 | 179 | 186 | 216 | 247 | 278 | 309 |
| 5'7" | 121 | 153 | 159 | 166 | 172 | 178 | 185 | 191 | 223 | 255 | 287 | 319 |
| 5'8" | 125 | 158 | 164 | 171 | 177 | 184 | 190 | 197 | 230 | 262 | 295 | 328 |
| 5'9" | 128 | 162 | 169 | 176 | 182 | 189 | 196 | 203 | 236 | 270 | 304 | 338 |
| 5'10" | 132 | 167 | 174 | 181 | 188 | 195 | 202 | 209 | 243 | 278 | 313 | 348 |
| 5'11" | 136 | 172 | 179 | 186 | 193 | 200 | 208 | 215 | 250 | 286 | 322 | 358 |
| 6'0" | 140 | 177 | 184 | 191 | 199 | 206 | 213 | 221 | 258 | 294 | 331 | 368 |
| 6'1" | 144 | 182 | 189 | 197 | 204 | 212 | 219 | 227 | 265 | 302 | 340 | 378 |
| 6'2" | 148 | 186 | 194 | 202 | 210 | 218 | 225 | 233 | 272 | 311 | 350 | 389 |
| 6'3" | 152 | 192 | 200 | 208 | 216 | 224 | 232 | 240 | 279 | 319 | 359 | 399 |
| 6'4" | 156 | 197 | 205 | 213 | 221 | 230 | 238 | 246 | 287 | 328 | 369 | 410 |

Source: National Institutes of Health, 1998

Asians with a BMI of 23 or higher may have an increased risk of health problems.

## Your daily calorie goal

| | Weight in pounds | Starting calorie level | | | |
|---|---|---|---|---|---|
| | | 1,200 | 1,400 | 1,600 | 1,800 |
| **Women** | 250 or less | X | | | |
| | 251 to 300 | | X | | |
| | 301 or more | | | X | |
| **Men** | 250 or less | | X | | |
| | 251 to 300 | | | X | |
| | 301 or more | | | | X |

weight loss. This is because you may not get enough of the nutrients you need daily. If you weigh more than 250 pounds, you'll need higher calorie goals (see the chart above.

## 3. Determine your daily servings

Once you've established a calorie goal, you can control your daily calories by consuming the number of servings recommended for that calorie level (see the chart on pages 218-219).

Spread these servings out over a day's worth of meals and snacks. If you eat the recommended number of servings daily, you should be getting about

the right number of calories to meet your weight goal. You don't have to count calories, except for when you eat sweets.

The serving recommendations for the carbohydrates, protein and dairy, and fats groups are limits — you shouldn't exceed them. Servings for the vegetables and fruits groups, on the other hand, are minimums. Eat at least the recommended number of fresh vegetables and fruits listed for your calorie level.

## 4. Get started

You now have the basic information that you need to get started. The next step is just to do it. Before you begin, however, you may want to plan out your menus for the week and put together a grocery list. Try to keep your menus practical and simple, but at the same time don't exclude good flavor and fun.

Stock up on items that you'll need for your meals and snacks. Having healthy foods in your house is a big step in your commitment to get and stay fit.

# Sizing up servings

Estimating your servings at meals is important to controlling calories. Unfortunately, the eye can be deceiving. Most people habitually, and unintentionally, underestimate the number of servings they eat. This means they

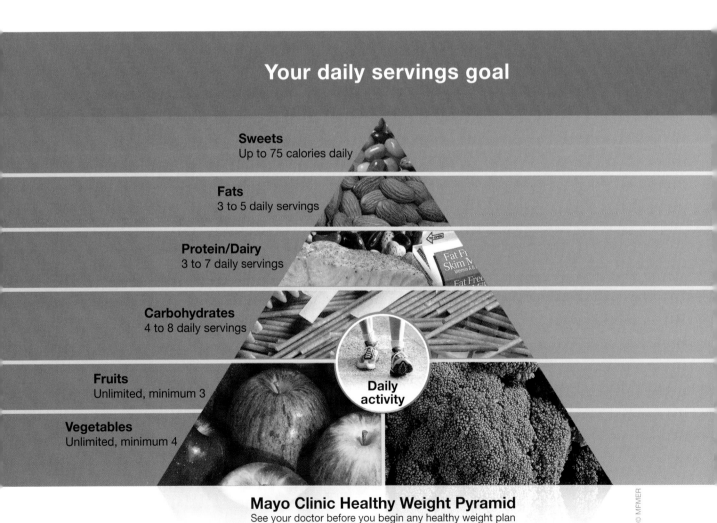

## Your daily servings goal

**Sweets**
Up to 75 calories daily

**Fats**
3 to 5 daily servings

**Protein/Dairy**
3 to 7 daily servings

**Carbohydrates**
4 to 8 daily servings

**Fruits**
Unlimited, minimum 3

**Daily activity**

**Vegetables**
Unlimited, minimum 4

**Mayo Clinic Healthy Weight Pyramid**
See your doctor before you begin any healthy weight plan

© MFMER

consume more calories than they think, and they can't understand why they're gaining weight, or not losing any.

A serving isn't the amount of food you choose to eat or that's put on your plate. The Mayo Clinic Healthy Weight Pyramid defines how big a serving is by common measurements such as cups, ounces, tablespoons or pieces — for example, a medium apple or a large egg.

Serving sizes in the Mayo Clinic Healthy Weight Pyramid are based on calories. All foods within each group are relatively equal in calories a serving. The total number of servings you eat each day from each food group will determine the total calories you consume.

## Daily serving recommendations for various calorie levels

| 1,200 | 1,400 | 1,600 | 1,800 | 2,000 |
|-------|-------|-------|-------|-------|
| 3 | 3 | 3 | 4 | 5 |
| 3 | 4 | 5 | 6 | 7 |
| 4 | 5 | 6 | 7 | 8 |
| 3 or more | 4 or more | 5 or more | 5 or more | 5 or more |
| 4 or more | 4 or more | 5 or more | 5 or more | 5 or more |

# Quick guide to serving sizes

An important part of eating healthy is understanding how much of a particular food makes up a serving. Many people envision servings to be larger than they are, and they eat more than they should.

| Vegetables | Calories | Visual cue |
|---|---|---|
| 1 cup broccoli | 25 | 1 baseball |
| 2 cups raw, leafy greens | 25 | 2 baseballs |

| Fruits | Calories | Visual cue |
|---|---|---|
| ½ cup sliced fruit | 60 | Tennis ball |
| 1 small apple or medium orange | 60 | Tennis ball |

| Carbohydrates | Calories | Visual cue |
|---|---|---|
| ½ cup pasta or dried cereal | 70 | Hockey puck |
| ½ bagel | 70 | Hockey puck |
| 1 slice whole-grain bread | 70 | Hockey puck |
| ½ medium baked potato | 70 | Hockey puck |

| Protein/Dairy | Calories | Visual cue |
|---|---|---|
| 3 ounces of fish | 110 | Deck of cards |
| 2–2½ ounces of meat | 110 | ⅔ deck of cards |
| 1½–2 ounces of hard cheese | 110 | ⅓ deck of cards |

| Fats | Calories | Visual cue |
|---|---|---|
| 1½ teaspoons peanut butter | 45 | 2 dice |
| 1 teaspoon butter or margarine | 45 | 1 die |

**These visual cues can help you use the food lists on pages 221 to 225.**

# Vegetables (25 calories in a serving)

| Best foods | Amount in 1 serving | Other foods | Amount in 1 serving |
|---|---|---|---|
| Artichoke | 1/2 bud | Canned vegetables | 1/2 cup |
| Asparagus | 1/2 cup or 6 spears | Marinara sauce | 1/4 cup |
| Bamboo shoots | 1/2 cup | Pickle, sour | 1 large |
| Bean sprouts | 1 cup | Pizza sauce | 1/4 cup |
| Beets | 1/2 cup sliced | Salsa | 1/4 cup |
| Bell pepper | 1 medium | Sauerkraut | 2/3 cup |
| Broccoflower | 1 cup | Tomato sauce | 2 tablespoons |
| Broccoli | 1 cup florets or spears | Vegetable juice | 1/3 cup |
| Brussels sprouts | 4 sprouts | | |
| Cabbage, cooked | 1/2 cup | | |
| Cabbage, raw | 1 cup | | |
| Carrots | 1 medium or 1/2 cup baby | | |
| Cauliflower | 1 cup florets | | |
| Celery | 4 medium stalks | | |
| Cherry tomatoes | 8 or about 1 cup | | |
| Cucumber | 1 or 1 cup sliced | | |
| Eggplant, cooked | 1 cup pieces | | |
| Green beans | 2/3 cup | | |
| Green onions | 3/4 cup | | |
| Kale, cooked | 2/3 cup | | |
| Lettuce | 2 cups shredded | | |
| Mushrooms | 1 cup whole | | |
| Okra | 1/2 cup | | |
| Onions | 1/2 cup sliced | | |
| Radishes | 12 medium | | |
| Scallions | 3 large | | |
| Spinach, cooked | 1/2 cup | | |
| Spinach, raw | 2 cups | | |
| Squash, summer | 3/4 cup sliced | | |
| Tomatillo | 1/2 cup diced | | |
| Tomato | 1 medium | | |
| Water chestnuts | 3/4 cup | | |
| Zucchini | 3/4 cup | | |

# Fruits (60 calories in a serving)

| Best foods | Amount in 1 serving | Other foods | Amount in 1 serving |
|---|---|---|---|
| Apple | 1 small | Apple juice | ½ cup |
| Apricots | 4 whole | Applesauce, unsweetened | ⅓ cup |
| Banana | 1 small or ½ large | Cranberry juice | ½ cup |
| Berries, mixed | ¾ cup | Dates | 3 |
| Blackberries | 1 cup | Figs, dried | 2 small |
| Blueberries | ½ cup | Grapefruit juice | ½ cup |
| Cantaloupe | 1 cup cubed | Juice bar, frozen | 3-ounce bar |
| Cantaloupe wedge | ⅓ small melon | Orange juice | ½ cup |
| Cherries | 1 cup or about 15 | Pineapple juice | ½ cup |
| Figs, fresh | 2 small | Prunes | 3 |
| Grapefruit | ½ cup or ½ large | Raisins | 2 tablespoons |
| Grapes | 1 cup | | |
| Honeydew melon | 1 cup cubed | | |
| Kiwi | 1 large | | |
| Mandarin oranges | ½ cup sections | | |
| Mango | ½ cup diced | | |
| Melon balls | 1 cup or 8 | | |
| Mixed fruit | ½ cup | | |
| Nectarine | 1 | | |
| Orange | 1 medium | | |
| Papaya | ½ medium | | |
| Peach | 1 large | | |
| Pear | 1 small | | |
| Pineapple | ½ cup cubed or 2 rings | | |
| Plums | 2 | | |
| Raspberries | 1 cup | | |
| Strawberries | 1½ cups whole | | |
| Tangerine | 1 large or ¾ cup | | |
| Watermelon | 1¼ cups cubed or small wedge | | |

# Carbohydrates (70 calories in a serving)

| Best foods | Amount in 1 serving | Other foods | Amount in 1 serving |
|---|---|---|---|
| Bagel, whole-grain | 1/2 | Animal crackers | 6 |
| Barley, cooked | 1/3 cup | Baked chips, low-fat | 10 chips (about 1 ounce) |
| Bread, sourdough | 1 slice | Breadsticks, crispy | 2, 6- to 8-inch |
| Bread, whole-grain | 1 slice | Corn | 1/2 cup |
| Bulgur, cooked | 1/2 cup | Corn on the cob | 1/2 large ear |
| Cereal, whole-grain | 3/4 cup | Corn tortillas | 1 |
| English muffin, whole-grain | 1/2 | **Crackers** | |
| Grits, cooked | 1/2 cup | • Cheese | 14 small |
| Kasha (buckwheat groats), cooked | 1/2 cup | • Snack | 15 bite-sized, 5 round |
| Oatmeal, cooked | 1/2 cup | • Rye (crispy) | 1 (triple cracker) |
| Pasta, whole-grain, cooked | 1/3 cup | • Wheat | 8 |
| Pita bread, whole-grain | 1/2 circle, 6-inch diameter | Melba rounds | 6 |
| Pumpkin, cooked | 1 1/2 cups | Muffin, any flavor | 1 small |
| Rice, brown, cooked | 1/3 cup | Orzo, cooked | 3/4 cup |
| Roll, whole-grain | 1 small | Pancake | 1, 4-inch diameter |
| Rutabaga, cooked | 3/4 cup | Popcorn, microwave, low-fat | 3 cups |
| Shredded wheat | 1 biscuit or 1/2 cup spoon-sized | **Potato** | |
| Squash, winter, cooked | 1 cup | • Baby | 3 |
| Sweet potato, baked | 1/2 large | • Baked | 1/2 medium |
| Turnips, cooked | 1/3 cup | • Mashed | 1/2 cup |
| | | Pretzels, sticks | 30 |
| | | Pretzels, twists | 3 |
| | | Rice, white, cooked | 1/3 cup |
| | | Rice or popcorn cakes | 3 |
| | | Soup, chicken noodle | 1 cup |
| | | Waffle | 1, 4-inch square |

# Protein/Dairy (110 calories in a serving)

| Best foods | Amount in 1 serving | Other foods | Amount in 1 serving |
|---|---|---|---|
| Beans | ½ cup | Beef, lean | 2 ounces |
| Chicken | 2½ ounces | **Cheese** | |
| Clams, canned | 3 ounces or about 10 | • Cheddar, low-fat | 2 ounces |
| Crab | 4 ounces | • Colby, low-fat | 2 ounces |
| Egg whites | 4 | • Cottage, low-fat | ⅔ cup |
| Fish | 3 ounces | • Feta | ¼ cup |
| Garbanzos | ⅓ cup | • Mozzarella, part-skim | ½ cup shredded |
| Lentils | ½ cup | • Parmesan, grated | 4 tablespoons |
| Milk, skim or 1% | 1 cup | • Ricotta, part-skim | ⅓ cup |
| Peas | ¾ cup | • Swiss, low-fat | 2 ounces |
| Pheasant | 3 ounces | Duck, breast | 2½ ounces |
| Shrimp | 4 ounces | Egg | 1 medium |
| Soybeans, green (edamame) | ½ cup | Egg substitute | ½ cup |
| Tofu | ½ cup | Lamb, lean cuts with no fat | 2 ounces |
| Tuna, canned in water | 3 ounces or ½ cup | Milk, 2% | 1 cup |
| Turkey | 3 ounces | Pork, lean cuts with no fat | 3 ounces |
| Vegetarian burger, black bean | 3-ounce pattie | Veal | 3 ounces |
| Venison | 3 ounces | Yogurt, fat-free, reduced-calorie | 1 cup |

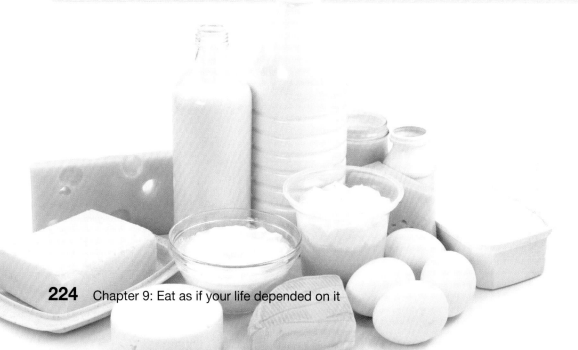

# Fats and Sweets (Fats 45 calories in a serving • Sweets 75 calories in a serving)

| Best fats | Amount in 1 serving | Other fats | Amount in 1 serving |
|---|---|---|---|
| Avocado | 1/6 | Butter, regular | 1 teaspoon |
| **Nuts** | | **Cream** | |
| • Almonds | 7 whole | • Half-and-half | 2 tablespoons |
| • Cashews | 4 whole | • Heavy (whipping) | 1 tablespoon liquid or 4 tablespoons whipped |
| • Peanuts | 8 whole | • Nondairy topping, whipped | 1/4 cup |
| • Pecans | 4 halves | • Sour | 2 tablespoons |
| • Walnuts | 4 halves | • Sour, fat-free | 4 tablespoons |
| **Oil** | | **Cream cheese** | |
| • Canola | 1 teaspoon | • Fat-free | 3 tablespoons |
| • Olive | 1 teaspoon | • Regular | 1 tablespoon |
| Olives | 9 large | Margarine, tub | 2 teaspoons |
| Peanut butter | 1 1/2 teaspoons | **Mayonnaise** | |
| **Seeds** | | • Reduced-calorie | 1 tablespoon |
| • Sesame | 1 tablespoon | • Regular | 2 teaspoons |
| • Sunflower | 1 tablespoon | **Salad dressing** | |
| | | • Low-calorie | 2 tablespoons |
| | | • Regular | 2 teaspoons |

| Sweets | Amount in 1 serving |
|---|---|
| Angel food cake | 1 small slice |
| Frozen yogurt | 1/2 cup |
| Fruit spread | 2 tablespoons |
| Gelatin dessert | 1/2 cup |
| Honey | 1 tablespoon |
| Ice cream, soft serve | 1/2 cup |
| Jam | 1 1/2 tablespoons |
| Maple syrup | 1 1/2 teaspoons |
| Sorbet/sherbet | 1/3 cup |

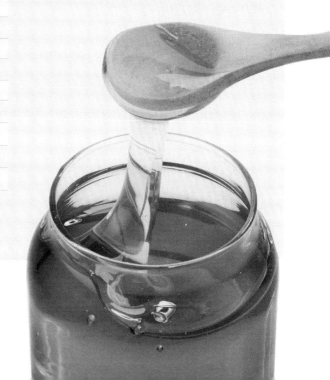

You don't need the mind of a mathematician to estimate serving sizes, and there's no need to carry measuring cups and spoons with you to make sure that your calculations are exact. It's important, though, that you understand the crucial role serving sizes play in successful weight control. To lose weight, you need to make sure that you're eating the right amount.

The chart on page 220 provides some visual clues to help you gauge serving sizes. When trying to determine what constitutes a serving, keep these clues in mind.

To further help you control food portions and calories, pages 221-225 contain listings of serving sizes for a number of common foods. Use these serving lists to help you develop your daily menus.

# Shaking your salt habit

You've been trying to eat less sodium — just a pinch of salt on your baked potato and a dash on your eggs. But a pinch here and a dash there can quickly add up. Consider that just 1 teaspoon of table salt has 2,325 milligrams (mg) of sodium — more than what experts recommend daily. And it's not just table salt you have to worry about.

## Essential in small amounts

Your kidneys naturally balance the amount of sodium stored in your body for optimal health. When your sodium levels are low, your kidneys essentially hold on to the sodium. When sodium levels are high, your kidneys excrete the excess in urine.

But if for some reason your kidneys can't eliminate enough sodium, the sodium starts to accumulate in your blood. Because sodium attracts and holds water, your blood volume increases. Increased blood volume makes your heart work harder to move more blood through your blood vessels, which increases pressure in your arteries. If this becomes chronic, it can lead to heart disease, stroke, kidney disease and congestive heart failure.

## Main dietary sources of sodium

The average American gets about 3,600 mg of sodium a day — much more than recommended. Here are the main sources of sodium in a typical diet:

- **Processed and prepared foods.** This is where the vast majority of sodium in the typical American diet comes from. Processed foods include bread, prepared dinners such as pizza, pasta, meat and egg dishes, cold cuts and bacon, cheese, soups, and fast foods. It's estimated that about 75 percent of your daily sodium intake comes from foods that have salt or sodium-containing compounds added when they're processed.
- **Natural sources.** Some unprocessed foods — including vegetables, milk, eggs, fresh meat and shellfish — naturally contain sodium. While they don't have an abundance of sodium, eating these foods does add to your overall sodium intake.
- **In the kitchen and at the table.** Many recipes call for salt, and many people also salt their food at the table. Condiments also may contain sodium. One tablespoon of soy sauce, for example, has about 900 mg of sodium.

## How much do you need?

The Dietary Guidelines for Americans, 2010, recommends limiting sodium to less than 2,300 mg a day — or 1,500 mg if you're age 51 or older, if you are black, or if you have high blood pressure, diabetes or chronic kidney disease.

Keep in mind that these are upper limits, and less is usually best, especially if you're sensitive to the effects of sodium. If you aren't sure how much sodium your diet should include, talk to your doctor.

## Be a savvy shopper

Taste alone may not tell you which foods are high in sodium. For example, you may not think a bagel tastes salty, but a typical 4-inch oat-bran bagel has about 620 mg of sodium, and even a slice of whole-wheat bread contains 132 mg of sodium.

So how can you tell which foods are high in sodium? Read food labels. The Nutrition Facts label found on most packaged and processed foods lists the amount of sodium in each serving. The ingredient list will also indicate salt or sodium-containing compounds, such as:

- Monosodium glutamate (MSG)
- Baking soda
- Baking powder
- Disodium phosphate
- Sodium alginate
- Sodium nitrate or nitrite

## More tips to cut back

Virtually all Americans can benefit from reducing the sodium in their diet. Here are more ways you can cut back on sodium:

- **Eat more fresh foods.** Most fresh fruits and vegetables are naturally low in sodium. Also, fresh meat is lower in sodium than are luncheon meat, bacon, hot dogs, sausage and ham. Buy fresh and frozen poultry or meat that hasn't been injected with a sodium-containing solution. Look on the label or ask your butcher. Buy plain whole-grain rice and pasta instead of ones that have added seasonings. Make your own soups from scratch.
- **Opt for low-sodium products.** If you do buy processed foods, choose those that are labeled "low sodium" or that contain less than 140 mg of sodium a serving. Don't be misled by labels such as "reduced sodium" or "light in sodium" — these products may still contain a lot of salt. For example, regular canned chicken noodle soup contains about 900 mg of sodium a cup. By law, a "reduced sodium" product has 25 percent less sodium than does the regular variety. So the reduced sodium soup still has a whopping

675 mg of sodium a cup. The same holds true for products labeled "lite" or "light in sodium."

- **Remove salt from recipes whenever possible.** You can leave out the salt in many recipes, including casseroles, stews and other main dishes that you cook. Baked goods are generally an exception since leaving out the salt could affect the leavening quality. Use cookbooks that focus on lowering risks of high blood pressure and heart disease to help guide you to sparing the salt without spoiling taste or quality.
- **Limit use of sodium-laden condiments.** Soy sauce, salad dressings, sauces, dips, ketchup, mustard and relish all contain sodium.
- **Use herbs, spices and other flavorings to enhance foods.** Use fresh or dried herbs, spices, onion or garlic, zest from citrus fruit, and fruit juices to jazz up your meals. And remember that sea salt has about the same amount of sodium as table salt.
- **Use salt substitutes wisely.** Some salt substitutes or light salts contain a mixture of table salt and other compounds. To achieve that familiar salty taste, you may use too much of the substitute — and get too much sodium. Also, many salt substitutes contain potassium

chloride. Although potassium can lessen some of the problems from excess sodium, too much potassium can be harmful if you have kidney problems or if you're taking medications for congestive heart failure or high blood pressure that cause potassium retention.

## Cut back gradually

Your taste for salt is acquired, so you can learn to enjoy less. Decrease your use of salt gradually, and your taste buds will adjust. After a few weeks of cutting back on salt, you probably won't miss it, and some foods may even taste too salty. Start by using no more than ¼ teaspoon of salt daily — at the table and in cooking. Then after a week or two, throw away the saltshaker. As you use less salt, your preference for it diminishes, allowing you to enjoy the taste of the food itself, with heart-healthy benefits.

# Stay off the SoFAS

One of the main focuses of the Dietary Guidelines for Americans, 2010, was

# Winning the war

Roseann wasn't quite ready to tolerate the thought of turning 50 and being overweight. It seemed that every article she read pointed out the dangers of obesity and how it could lead to heart disease, diabetes and even cancer. Instead of ignoring the warnings, she finally decided to do something.

First came a list of reasons why she thought she should lose weight. Then, the question of how she would do it.

After waking up every morning and thinking that today would be the day she'd start on a diet, but with no results, she opted to join Weight Watchers. With no food restrictions, except for the number of points she was allowed each day in terms of calories, Roseann felt it was an easy program to follow. "I didn't tell anyone in the beginning I had joined Weight Watchers because I didn't want people watching everything I ate. Then, if I didn't lose weight, no one would know the difference."

Along the way, though, she gained the support of friends and family. And from the program she learned a lot of tricks for eating better and reducing calories, such as munching on vegetables to fill herself up and using spray butter instead of whole pats.

Roseann also thought of joining a health club, but she quickly reminded herself that a gym just wasn't her style. Instead, she decided to walk during her lunch hour and work breaks. During the cold months, she sticks to walking inside the subways and skyways that connect the various buildings where she works. But as the weather becomes nicer, she takes her walks outdoors. "It's nice. You really start getting to know the people that you see every day." In all, Roseann walks about 40 to 60 minutes on workdays and then throws in some walks on weekends for something different.

"A lot of the changes I've made are simple and easy," she says.

And not only did the changes fit well into her lifestyle, they worked! Over the course of two years, Roseann has lost more than 100 pounds! Previous problems with her knees have improved dramatically, and she no longer requires blood pressure medications. While shopping for clothes, she often has to do a double take at the person she sees in the mirror.

"Am I happier?" She responds, "Much more so. I'm willing to try more things activitywise. It's more fun to do things when you feel good. I'm able to do stairs, walk more, and also I like how I look and what I'm able to wear."

Though the changes she's made have been "simple" lifestyle adjustments, that doesn't mean the process has been easy. Roseann still battles food cravings on a regular basis, and she works to maintain her positive attitude. She admits she enjoys eating just as much as ever and has a sweet tooth to boot.

"I still read articles on obesity and feel I am part of that. By reading articles, I feel it might help in keeping me on track. It's so easy to get off your eating plan and then be back to square one again, which I don't want!"

Roseann knows, though, that if she blows it one day, she can get back on track the next day and start fresh. You can't go on vacation, she says, and not indulge yourself somewhat. "I treat myself and blow it usually. But then, next day it's back to reality." This ability to forgive herself for losing an occasional small battle is what enables Roseann to win the war.

These days, Roseann is working on conquering the 18 flights of steps to her office. She's already up to walking nine flights. She doesn't know if she'll make it the full 18, but she's willing to give it a try.

# 10 easy steps to healthier eating

You don't need to turn your life upside down to eat for better health. A few simple changes can make a big difference in your daily diet.

1. Have at least one serving of fruit at each meal and another as a snack during the day.
2. Switch from a low-fiber breakfast cereal to a higher fiber cereal or other breakfast food.
3. Lighten your milk by moving one step down in fat content — from 2 to 1 percent, for instance, or from 1 percent to fat-free (skim).
4. Whenever you can, cook with olive, canola or another vegetable oil instead of butter or margarine.
5. Choose whole-grain breads instead of white bread and switch from white rice to brown rice.
6. Include at least two servings of vegetables at lunch.
7. Include at least two servings of vegetables at dinner.
8. Have fish as a main course at least twice a week.
9. Serve fresh fruit for dessert in place of foods rich in calories and fat.
10. Instead of high-calorie sweetened beverages, drink water or unsweetened beverages.

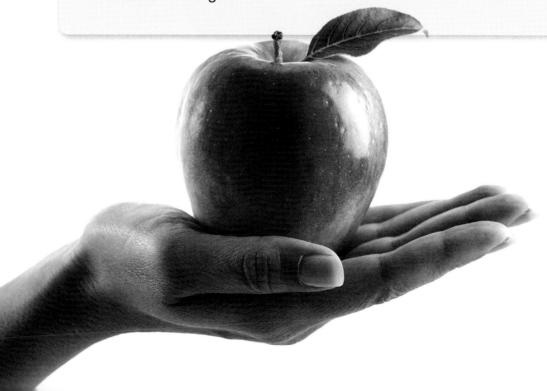

the role of solid fats and added sugars (SoFAS) in the U.S. diet. SoFAS are high in calories and low in nutrients — contributing to unwanted pounds. But the potential health concerns go beyond excess calories. Solid fats include naturally occurring saturated fats and man-made trans fats — both major contributors to heart disease.

For most people, SoFAS make up a whopping 35 percent of their total calories. That's not surprising considering the top food sources of SoFAS:

- Grain-based desserts such as cakes, cookies, doughnuts, pies, crisps, granola bars
- Dairy desserts and cheese
- Candy
- Soda, fruity drinks, energy and sports drinks
- Pizza and fried potatoes
- Sausage, franks, bacon, ribs

Foregoing one or more of the foods high in SoFAS might be a good strategy for cutting fat and sugar calories — many of these are also high in sodium. To get people off the SoFAS, the guidelines recommend that Americans:

Cut back on calories from solid fats and added sugars. Health experts recommend that SoFAS account for no more than five to 15 percent of your daily calories.

Choose foods that don't have sugar added. Drink fewer calorie-containing beverages and more water.

Use oils — such as olive oil, canola oil or nut oils — to replace solid fats whenever possible.

# Small changes add up

We tend to be comfortable with our behaviors and habits, even if they're not always beneficial — they're familiar. They give order and stability to our lives. That means most of us are reluctant to change the way we're used to doing things. It may feel overwhelming.

Although change can be difficult, it's not impossible. Most people underestimate their ability to change. And changing behaviors in small ways can add up to a big difference in your health.

Here's a common dietary example: Many people have switched from drinking whole milk to skim milk. Maybe they tapered off gradually, or maybe

## The Mayo Clinic Diet

The Mayo Clinic Diet is a lifelong approach to help you improve your health and maintain a healthy weight. This weight-loss and lifestyle program, designed by Mayo Clinic health experts, uses the Mayo Clinic Healthy Weight Pyramid as a guide to making smart-eating choices and encouraging daily activity. The healthy changes it promotes in diet and exercise can reduce your risk of weight-related health problems, such as diabetes, heart disease, high blood pressure and sleep apnea.

The Mayo Clinic Diet has two main parts:

**Lose It!** is a two-week phase that allows you to jump-start your weight loss, losing as much as 6 to 10 pounds in a healthy way. In this phase, you focus on lifestyle habits. You learn how to add five healthy habits, break five unhealthy habits and adopt another five bonus healthy habits. This phase also includes getting at least 30 minutes of physical activity or exercise every day.

**Live It!** is a lifelong approach to diet and health. In this phase, you learn more about food choices, portion sizes, menu planning and sticking to healthy habits. You continue steady weight loss of 1 to 2 pounds a week until you reach your goal weight. By continuing the healthy lifestyle habits you adopted, you can maintain your goal weight permanently. In this phase, you also learn how to set a goal weight and how to develop long-term healthy-eating patterns. Regular physical activity remains a central part of this phase.

To learn more about the Mayo Clinic Diet, visit *store.mayoclinic.com* or call Customer Service at 800-291-1128.

they switched from one to the other in one bold leap. Either way, they made what they thought was an impossible change. Skim milk probably seemed watered down at first, but once used to skim, whole milk tasted too thick and rich. It's a small change, but if you drink 2 cups of milk a day, over the course of a year the simple step of switching from whole to skim can result in a loss of about 13 pounds!

As you take steps to eat healthier and control your weight, here are some strategies to consider:

## Have a plan

Try to plan what you're going to eat for the day at least one day in advance. Base your decisions on your daily calorie goal. Planning ahead means you'll have the ingredients on hand at mealtimes and can start preparing food without delays. This helps keep you from making something unhealthy because you don't have nutritious food in the house.

Of course, the best plans can go astray. A good rule of preparedness is always to have something ready that's healthy to munch on, such as low-calorie popcorn, cut-up vegetables or fruit.

## Shop from a list

The practice of making a shopping list goes along with planning meals ahead of time. Following a list will help keep you from impulse buying. Along the same lines, don't shop when you're hungry — you'll be tempted to grab anything that looks vaguely appetizing. While you're at it, read the labels on food packages. Don't assume something's healthy just because it appears to be. Compare similar products and choose the one that's lowest in calories or fat and highest in vitamins and other nutrients.

## Don't tempt yourself

You might trick yourself into believing that bag of chocolate-covered peanuts you tossed into your shopping cart is for a special occasion, but once it's in the house, can you resist sampling them? Do yourself a favor. Don't buy high-calorie foods that tempt you. That doesn't mean you have to give up sweets and junk food entirely. Just purchase them in small amounts or consider not having them in your home.

If you have time, look for recipes in cookbooks that are healthy and lower in calories. Cookbooks can stimulate creative ideas for meals and keep you dedicated to your plan.

Keep in mind that as you acquire new eating habits, your tastes will change. Foods that once seemed dreamy eventually may taste too sweet or too fatty. You can "unacquire" a taste.

## Stick to a schedule

Having a meal schedule can give you a better sense of control. This doesn't necessarily mean the traditional three meals of breakfast, lunch and dinner. Just don't go for longer periods without eating. Build a schedule with fairly flexible time frames for eating rather than sticking to exact times.

You may find that eating three meals and two snacks works best for you. Or perhaps six minimeals suit your schedule better. The important thing is to stick with a routine. But don't go more than four or five hours without eating because you could become extremely hungry, tempting you to overeat.

## Enjoy your food

When you eat, keep your mind focused on the pleasure of what you're doing.

Be aware of every bite. Don't read or watch television during a meal or snack, just savor your food. Remember, eating should give you pleasure, not just fuel your body.

Eating with awareness may take practice, but it's worth the effort. You'll enjoy food more and be satisfied with eating less.

## Eat from hunger

Many people reach for food as a form of comfort — not because they're hungry. Don't try to console yourself with food. If you're tired, then rest or meditate. If you're thirsty, drink a glass of water. If you're anxious, take a walk. Here's a clue: If you can't decide what you want to eat, chances are you're not very hungry.

## Stop when you're full

No matter what you heard from your parents as a child, you don't have to finish all the food on your plate. Eat slowly, savor every bite and stop when you're full. It takes time for your stomach and the processes of digestion to signal your brain that you're full. Meals should take 20 to 30 minutes.

If you belong to the clean-plate club, try to change this behavior by leaving a dab of food on your plate at every meal — just to signal your brain that doing so is OK. As you become more adept at identifying when you're hungry and when you're satisfied, it will become easier not to overeat.

## Keep a food diary

It helps to understand what causes a behavior before you try to change it. One of the best ways to do that is to keep a diary that records what you eat and what triggers your eating.

Keeping a diary takes some effort, but it's often one of the success tools used by people who reach and maintain their weight goals. Several studies suggest that keeping a food diary causes people to reduce their food intake, likely by increasing their awareness of what and how much they eat — and why.

In addition to recording the types of food and amounts of food you eat, your diary may include:

- Feelings (bored, anxious, stressed)
- Social interaction (with friends, alone)

- Environment (potluck at work, passed by a bakery)
- Level of hunger (from extremely hungry to not hungry at all)
- Rate of eating (fast, slow, moderate)

After several days, you may be able to discern behaviors that affect your weight. Whatever the patterns, you can work on changing them.

# You can do it

Perhaps you've heard or read the statistic about the likelihood of keeping weight off permanently — 95 percent of individuals who lose weight regain it within five years. This doesn't mean you're doomed to failure.

Here are some more figures to ponder. The National Weight Control Registry conducted a study involving 629 women and 155 men who had been overweight for years. The participants changed their eating and exercise habits, and they lost an average of 66 pounds each.

What were the long-term results? Some individuals eventually did gain some of the weight back, but they kept a minimum of 30 pounds off for at least five years. Most of them did it through a combination of exercise and restricting fat and calories — in other words, by changing their lifestyle.

A big surprise of the study was that 42 percent claimed that maintaining a healthy weight was easier than their initial weight loss. The participants also stated their weight loss improved their quality of life, including their mood, health and self-confidence.

This group is living testimony that when you lose weight the right way — by making lifelong changes in your eating and exercise habits — you can be successful.

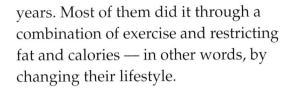

# Chapter 10

# Use supplements wisely

You can't help but notice them — the endless bottles of supplements that line the shelves of grocery and discount stores and drugstores, all promising to improve your health in various ways. The question is, do they actually work? Some may. Some don't. And for most, we simply don't know.

Vitamin, mineral and herbal supplements are all considered dietary supplements by the Food and Drug Administration. Unlike prescription and over-the-counter medications, which are tested rigorously to prove their benefits and identify their risks, most dietary supplements aren't. And the fact is, you're far more likely to improve your diet and protect your health with good lifestyle habits than from dietary supplements — pills, capsules and other forms.

It may seem easier to take a few pills than to prepare a balanced meal. The trouble is, if you depend on supplements for nutrition, you miss out on the potential benefits of antioxidants, phytochemicals, fiber and other nutrients that only foods can provide. For example, you can get vitamin C from a pill or from an orange. Sure, the pill is easy. But the orange is a better choice because it also supplies carotene, calcium, fiber, flavonoids and simple sugars for energy — all important components of a healthy diet.

That said, this doesn't mean vitamins, minerals and other supplements don't play a role in good health. In some cases they're highly recommended. Just remember that their purpose is to "supplement" a healthy lifestyle, not be a substitute for one.

# Vitamin and mineral supplements

Having the right balance of vitamins and minerals in your body is essential. Deficiencies in certain vitamins or minerals can lead to specific diseases or conditions, such as pernicious anemia (vitamin B-12 deficiency) or anemia (iron deficiency).

However, too much of some vitamins and minerals isn't good either.

## Vitamins

You need vitamins for normal body functions, mental alertness and resistance to infection. They enable your body to process proteins, carbohydrates and fats. Certain vitamins also help you produce blood cells, hormones, genetic material and chemicals found in your nervous system.

There are 14 vitamins, which fall into two categories:

- **Fat soluble.** These include vitamins A, D, E and K. They're stored in your body's fat. Some excess fat-soluble vitamins, such as vitamins A and D, can accumulate in your body, cause problems and reach toxic levels.
- **Water soluble.** These include vitamin C, choline, biotin and the seven B vitamins: thiamin (B-1), riboflavin (B-2), niacin (B-3), pantothenic acid (B-5), pyridoxine (B-6), folic acid (folate, also known as B-9) and cobalamin (B-12). They're stored to a lesser extent than are fat-soluble vitamins.

## Minerals

Your body also needs minerals. Major minerals — those needed in larger amounts - - include calcium, phosphorus, magnesium, sodium, potassium and chloride. Calcium, phosphorus and magnesium are important in the development and health of bones and teeth. Sodium, potassium and chloride, known as electrolytes, are important in regulating the water and chemical balance in your body.

In addition, your body needs smaller amounts of the minerals chromium, copper, fluoride, iodine, iron, manganese, molybdenum, selenium and zinc. These are all necessary for normal growth and good health.

# Should you take supplements?

The best way to get the vitamins and minerals you need is through a nutritionally balanced diet. However, even if you don't have a vitamin or mineral deficiency, a vitamin or mineral supplement may be appropriate if:

- **You're older than age 50.** As you get older, especially if you've reached age 65, your body may not be able to absorb calcium and vitamins B-12 and D like it used to, making supplementation necessary. Health problems also can contribute to a poor diet, making it difficult to get the vitamins and minerals you need. In addition, there's evidence that a multivitamin may improve your immune function and decrease your risk of some infections.

- **You're a postmenopausal woman.** For some women, it can be difficult to obtain the recommended daily amounts of calcium and vitamin D without supplementation. With age, bone loss accelerates, calcium requirements increase, and your body's ability to absorb calcium and metabolize vitamin D decrease. Both calcium and vitamin D supplements have been shown to help protect against osteoporosis.

- **You don't eat well.** If you don't eat the recommended daily servings of fruits, vegetables and other healthy foods, taking a multivitamin-mineral supplement may be reasonable. But your best course of action is to adopt better eating habits.

- **You smoke.** Smoking may be associated with a poor diet — a diet lacking in essential nutrients. In addition, smoking increases your requirement for the antioxidant vitamin C. However, because some high-dose antioxidant supplements have been associated with increased risk of lung cancer, it's important to talk with your doctor before taking such a supplement if you smoke.

- **You drink alcohol excessively.** Long-term excessive alcohol consumption can impair digestion and absorption of thiamin, folic acid and some vitamins, as well as increase the loss of minerals such as zinc and magnesium. If you drink excessively and substitute alcohol for food, your diet will lack most nutrients. However, supplements aren't a substitute for food, and in some cases they can be dangerous. Alcoholics with liver disease may actually be harmed by taking certain supplements.

- **You eat a special diet.** If your diet has limited variety because of food allergies or intolerance to certain

# Daily Values for vitamins and minerals

If you decide to take a supplement, choose one that doesn't exceed 100 percent of the Daily Value for each vitamin and mineral, unless your doctor advises otherwise. Daily Values are listed on supplement labels. They're based on a daily intake of 2,000 calories and meet or exceed recommended vitamin and mineral needs for most people.

| Vitamin | 100% Daily Value |
| --- | --- |
| Vitamin A* | 5,000 international units (IU) |
| Vitamin C | 60 milligrams (mg) |
| Vitamin D | 400 IU |
| Vitamin E | 30 IU |
| Vitamin K | 80 micrograms (mcg) |
| Thiamin (vitamin B-1) | 1.5 mg |
| Riboflavin (vitamin B-2) | 1.7 mg |
| Niacin (vitamin B-3) | 20 mg |
| Pantothenic acid (vitamin B-5) | 10 mg |
| Pyridoxine (vitamin B-6) | 2 mg |
| Folic acid/folate (vitamin B-9) | 0.4 mg (400 mcg) |
| Cobalamin (vitamin B-12) | 6 mcg |
| Biotin | 0.3 mg (300 mcg) |

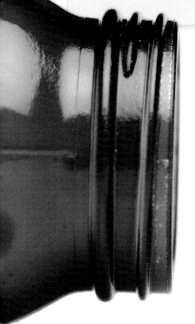

| Mineral | 100% Daily Value |
| --- | --- |
| Calcium | 1,000 mg, or 1 gram (g) |
| Chloride | 3,400 mg |
| Chromium | 120 mcg |
| Copper | 2 mg |
| Iodine | 150 mcg |
| Iron** | 18 mg |
| Magnesium | 400 mg |
| Manganese | 2 mg |
| Molybdenum | 75 mcg |
| Phosphorus | 1,000 mg |
| Potassium | 3,500 mg |
| Selenium | 70 mcg |
| Zinc | 15 mg |

*For vitamin A, the Food and Nutrition Board of the Institute of Medicine recommends a lower amount: 3,000 IU a day for men and 2,330 IU a day for most women.

**For iron, it's probably wise for men and postmenopausal women who take a multivitamin to use a pill with little (8 mg a day or less) or no iron. Too much iron can be toxic.

foods, you may benefit from a vitamin-mineral supplement. If you're a vegetarian who eliminates all animal products from your diet, you may need vitamin B-12. In addition, if you don't eat dairy products and don't get 15 minutes of sun on your skin two to three times a week, you may need to supplement your diet with calcium and vitamin D.

- **Your body can't use nutrients properly.** If you have a disease of your liver, gallbladder, intestine, pancreas or kidney or if you've had surgery on your digestive tract, you may not be able to digest or absorb nutrients properly. In such cases, your doctor may recommend that you take a vitamin or mineral supplement. A supplement may also be prescribed if you take antacids, antibiotics, laxatives, diuretics or other medications that interfere with how your body uses nutrients.

## Choosing and using supplements

If you wish to take a vitamin or mineral supplement, here are some recommendations to keep in mind:

- **Avoid supplements that provide megadoses.** Most cases of nutrient toxicity stem from high-dose supplements. In general, choose a multivitamin-mineral supplement that provides about 100 percent Daily Value (DV) of all the vitamins and minerals. Taking significantly more than the recommended amount of some vitamins and minerals (megadoses) can be dangerous. The exception to the 100 percent DV recommendation is calcium. You may notice that calcium-containing supplements don't provide 100 percent DV. If they did, the tablets would be too large to swallow.
- **Beware of gimmicks.** Don't give in to the temptation of added herbs, enzymes, amino acids or unusual "special" ingredients — they add nothing but cost.

- **Look for expiration dates.** Supplements can lose potency over time, especially in hot and humid climates. If a supplement doesn't have an expiration date, don't buy it.
- **Store supplements in a dry, cool place.** Avoid hot, humid storage locations, such as the bathroom or above your stove.
- **Play it safe.** Before taking anything other than a standard multivitamin-mineral supplement of 100 percent DV or less, check with your doctor, pharmacist or a registered dietitian. This is especially important if you have a health problem or are taking one or more medications. High doses of niacin, for example, can result in liver problems. In addition, supplements may interfere with certain medications.

## An overview of 15 vitamins and minerals

Here's what you need to know about 15 popular vitamins and minerals — how much you need, good food sources, what they do for your body, and cautions and side effects.

### Vitamin A
**Recommended Dietary Allowance (RDA) for Adults**

*Men*

Age 19 or older: 3,000 international
units (IU), or 900 micrograms
(mcg) a day

*Women*

Age 19 or older: 2,330 IU (700 mcg)
a day

**Maximum daily intake.** Maximum
intake from both food and supplements
that's unlikely to pose a risk of side
effects for adults: 10,000 IU or 3,000
mcg a day.

**Food sources.** Animal sources include
whole milk, fat-free milk fortified with
vitamin A, whole eggs, liver, beef and
poultry. Plant sources of beta carotene,
which converts into vitamin A, include
dark green leafy vegetables and orange
and yellow fruits and vegetables, such
as carrots, sweet potatoes, spinach,
broccoli, cantaloupe, mangos and
apricots. Vegetable soup and tomato
juice also contain good amounts of
beta carotene.

**What it does.** Vitamin A is a fat-soluble
vitamin that plays a role in healthy
vision, bone and tissue growth, and reproduction. It's needed for the maintenance of your vital organs. It also helps
to regulate your immune system, which
prevents and fights infections.

**What the research says.** Two national
surveys in the 1990s indicated that some
Americans don't eat enough foods rich
in vitamin A. However, vitamin A deficiency is rare in the United States — it's
more often associated with malnutrition in developing countries. But people
with certain diseases who have trouble
absorbing vitamin A may take supplements recommended by their doctors.
Surveys suggest a link between diets
rich in vitamin A and beta carotene from
food — not supplements — and a lower
risk of some types of cancer.

**Cautions.** Too much vitamin A stored
in the body may increase the risk of
liver abnormalities as well as reduce
bone mineral density, leading to osteoporosis. Long-term high vitamin
A intake from supplements and fortified foods may increase the risk of
hip fractures.

**Side effects.** Signs and symptoms of
vitamin A toxicity may include nausea
and vomiting, headache, dizziness,
blurred vision, and problems with
muscular coordination. Vitamin A
toxicity usually results from excess use
of supplements.

## Vitamin B-6 (Pyridoxine)
**Recommended Dietary Allowance
(RDA) for Adults**

*Men*
Ages 19 to 50: 1.3 milligrams (mg) a day
Age 51 or older: 1.7 mg a day

*Women*
Ages 19 to 50: 1.3 mg a day
Age 51 or older: 1.5 mg a day

**Maximum daily intake.** Maximum intake from all sources that's unlikely to pose a risk of side effects for adults: 100 mg a day.

**Food sources.** Poultry, fish, pork, potatoes, soybeans, oats, whole-grain products, fortified cereals, nuts, seeds and bananas.

**What it does.** Vitamin B-6 is a water-soluble vitamin that's essential for protein metabolism, energy production and brain function. It's also involved in immune function

**What the research says.** Vitamin B-6 works with vitamin B-12 and folic acid (folate) to reduce blood levels of homocysteine, an amino acid that builds and maintains tissues. Elevated homocysteine may increase your risk of heart attack or stroke or cause loss of circulation in your hands and feet. Studies evaluating vitamin B-6 as a remedy for premenstrual syndrome (PMS) show conflicting results.

**Cautions.** See your doctor before taking vitamin B-6 if you have intestinal problems, liver disease, an overactive thyroid, sickle cell disease, or if you've been under severe stress as a result of illness, burns, an accident or recent surgery.

**Side effects.** High daily doses of vitamin B-6, especially more than 250 mg a day, may cause nerve damage.

## Vitamin B-12 (Cobalamin)
**Recommended Dietary Allowance (RDA) for Adults**

*Men and women*
Age 19 or older: 2.4 mcg a day

**Maximum daily intake.** Maximum intake from all sources that's unlikely to pose a risk of side effects in adults: There's no known toxicity in humans from vitamin B-12.

**Food sources.** Meat, fish, shellfish, poultry, eggs, dairy products and some fortified breakfast cereals.

**What it does.** This is a water-soluble vitamin that plays essential roles in red blood cell formation, cell metabolism and nerve function.

**What the research says.** Vitamin B-12 supplements containing 100 percent of the Daily Value (6 mcg a day) help prevent deficiency in vegetarians who eliminate all animal foods from their diets — plant foods don't contain vitamin B-12. Injections of vitamin B-12 are used to prevent and treat deficiency in people whose digestive tracts can't absorb this vitamin, because of surgery, bowel disease or a hereditary problem. In addition, with age, it can become harder to absorb vitamin B-12 from animal foods. If you're older than age 50, you may need to get vitamin B-12 through supplements or fortified foods.

**Cautions.** Talk to your doctor before taking vitamin B-12 supplements if you have anemia with no known cause.

**Side effects.** Studies don't indicate adverse health effects in healthy people from excess intake of supplements or food containing vitamin B-12.

## Vitamin C (Ascorbic acid)
**Recommended Dietary Allowance (RDA) for Adults**

*Men*
Age 19 or older: 90 mg a day
Adult smokers: 125 mg a day

*Women*
Age 19 or older: 75 mg a day
Adult smokers: 110 mg a day

**Maximum daily intake.** Maximum intake from all sources that's unlikely to pose a risk of side effects for adults: 2,000 mg a day.

**Food sources.** Citrus juices and fruits, berries, tomatoes, potatoes, green and red peppers, broccoli, and spinach.

**What it does.** Vitamin C maintains skin integrity, heals wounds and is important in immune functions. It also has antioxidant properties, helping to prevent cell damage by neutralizing free radicals — molecules associated with aging and certain diseases.

**What the research says.** Studies indicate that people who eat foods high in

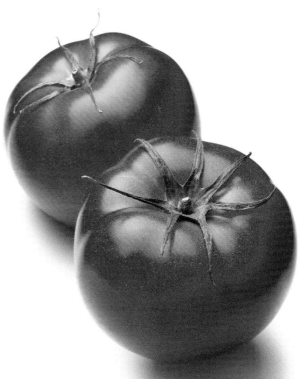

vitamin C have lower rates of cancer and heart disease, though it's unclear whether taking vitamin C supplements produces similar benefits. A 2001 study indicates that supplementation with vitamin C, other specific antioxidants and zinc may slow the progression of age-related macular degeneration. A doctor's supervision is important to determine proper doses. The Institute of Medicine states there aren't any established benefits for consuming more than the recommended amount of vitamin C. Other research has suggested that 200 mg/day may be the optimal daily dose.

**Cautions.** See your doctor before taking vitamin C if you have gout, kidney stones, sickle cell anemia or iron storage disease.

**Side effects.** Taking excessive amounts of vitamin C (more than 2,000 mg/day) may cause mild diarrhea and may interfere with blood sugar (glucose) testing, stool tests for blood and other laboratory tests.

## Vitamin D (calciferol)
### Recommended Dietary Allowance (RDA) for Adults

*Men and women*
Age 19 or older: 600 IU (15 mcg) a day

**Maximum daily intake.** Maximum intake from all sources that's unlikely to pose a risk of side effects for adults: 4,000 IU (100 mcg) a day.

**Food sources.** Vitamin D-fortified milk, vitamin D-fortified cereal, cod-liver oil, and fatty varieties of fish such as salmon, mackerel and sardines.

**What it does.** Vitamin D is necessary for effective absorption of dietary calcium and helps deposit calcium in your bones and teeth. It's also important for muscle and nerve function and for the immune system to work effectively.

**What the research says.** Your body gets vitamin D from dietary sources, but it can also generate its own when sunlight converts a chemical in your skin into a usable form of the vitamin. Some people don't get enough vitamin D naturally, due to lack of exposure to sunlight, less efficient conversion of the vitamin in their skin, or reduced liver or kidney function. If you don't drink milk, have dark skin, are at risk of osteoporosis, live in a cloudy environment or rarely go outside, consider taking a vitamin D supplement. Studies show that people who supplement their diets with a combination of vitamin D and calcium slow bone loss and reduce the incidence of fractures.

**Cautions.** See your doctor before taking vitamin D if you have heart or blood vessel disease, disease of the kidney, liver or pancreas, intestinal problems, or the immune system disorder sarcoidosis.

**Side effects.** Prolonged intake of vitamin D above 4,000 IU/day poses the risk of toxic effects. Side effects can include nausea, headache, excessive urination, high blood pressure, deposits of calcium in soft tissues, kidney damage and other problems.

## Vitamin E (Tocopherol)
### Recommended Dietary Allowance (RDA) for Adults

*Men and women*
Age 19 or older: 15 mg (22.5 IU) a day

**Maximum daily intake.** Maximum intake from supplements and fortified foods that's unlikely to pose a risk of side effects for adults: 1,500 IU or 1,000 mg a day. Important note: A recent review of multiple studies questions the safety of these upper limits. The analysis concludes that high daily intake — 400 IU or more — of vitamin E may pose health risks and should be avoided. It also found that harmful effects might occur at more than 150 IU daily for some people.

**Food sources.** Vegetable oils, wheat germ, whole-grain products, avocados and nuts, especially almonds.

**What it does.** Vitamin E is a fat-soluble vitamin that protects red blood cells and plays an important role in reproduction. It also has antioxidant properties, helping to prevent cell damage by neutralizing free radicals — molecules believed to be associated with aging and certain diseases.

**What the research says.** A 2001 study indicates that supplementation with vitamin E and certain other antioxidants may slow the progression of age-related macular degeneration, but a doctor's supervision is important to determine proper doses. Although research results conflict, recent studies show no benefit for individuals with high-risk heart disease who took vitamin E supplements. Recent studies also found vitamin E supplements had no impact on preventing progression from mild to

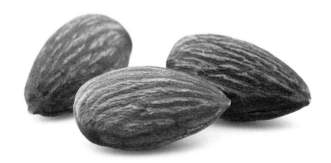

moderate memory impairment among people with Alzheimer's disease.

Most important, a high daily intake of vitamin E supplements may harm your health. Researchers analyzed 19 studies that involved almost 136,000 people (most with chronic diseases) who took vitamin E alone or in a multivitamin. People who took about 400 IU a day or more of vitamin E for at least one year died at a higher rate than did those who didn't take the supplements, but the reason why isn't clear. Some studies involved individuals who were taking a number of other supplements in addition to vitamin E. This further complicates interpretation of the data.

**Cautions.** Check with your doctor first before taking vitamin E if you're taking blood-thinning (anticoagulant) medications. Vitamin E can hinder the control of blood thinning. Also see your doctor before taking vitamin E if you have iron deficiency anemia, bleeding or clotting problems, cystic fibrosis, intestinal problems, or liver disease.

**Side effects.** In rare cases, people who take vitamin E may develop dizziness, fatigue, headache, weakness, abdominal pain, diarrhea, flu-like symptoms, nausea or blurred vision. In addition to the risks previously noted, high doses

of vitamin E can cause side effects that can include bleeding — especially for people on blood-thinning medications — and gastrointestinal complaints.

## Folic acid (folate, or vitamin B-9)
### Recommended Dietary Allowance (RDA) for Adults

*Men and women*
Age 19 or older: 400 mcg a day

**Maximum daily intake.** Maximum intake from supplements and fortified foods that's unlikely to pose a risk of side effects for adults: 1,000 mcg a day.

**Food sources.** Citrus juices and fruits, beans, nuts, seeds, liver, dark green leafy vegetables, and some fortified grain products.

**What it does.** Folate, also called vitamin B-9, occurs naturally in certain foods. Folic acid is the synthetic form of folate. Folic acid is found in supplements and in fortified breads and cereals. This water-soluble vitamin is important in red blood cell formation, protein metabolism, growth and cell division.

**What the research says.** Folic acid has been shown to work together with vitamin B-6 and vitamin B-12 to reduce blood levels of homocysteine, an amino acid that builds and maintains tissues. Elevated homocysteine levels may increase your risk of heart attack, stroke, or loss of circulation in your hands and feet. If you don't get adequate folate in your diet, talk with your doctor about taking a folic acid supplement.

**Cautions.** See your doctor before taking folic acid if you have anemia. Intake of folic acid from supplements and fortified foods shouldn't exceed 1,000 mcg a day, to prevent folic acid from covering up the symptoms of a vitamin B-12 deficiency. Follow your doctor's recommendation if you're taking folic acid for any medical reasons.

**Side effects.** People who take folic acid may develop bright yellow urine, fever, shortness of breath, a skin rash or, very rarely, diarrhea. Doses higher than 1,500 mcg a day can cause nausea, appetite loss, flatulence and abdominal distention.

## Niacin (Vitamin B-3)
**Recommended Dietary Allowance (RDA) for Adults**

*Men*
Age 19 or older: 16 mg a day

*Women*
Age 19 or older: 14 mg a day

**Maximum daily intake.** Maximum intake from supplements and fortified foods that's unlikely to pose a risk of side effects for adults: 35 mg/day.

**Food sources.** Lean meats, poultry, fish, organ meats, brewer's yeast, peanuts and peanut butter.

**What it does.** Niacin is a water-soluble B vitamin that is important in converting food to energy.

**Cautions.** Don't take niacin if you have impaired liver function or an active peptic ulcer. See your doctor before taking niacin if you have diabetes, gout, gallbladder or liver disease, or glaucoma.

**Side effects.** At doses higher than 2,000 mg a day, niacin has potentially serious side effects that can include liver damage, high blood sugar and irregular heartbeats. As little as 50 mg a a day can cause flushing, itching, headaches, cramps and nausea.

## Beta carotene
**Recommended Dietary Allowance (RDA) for Adults:** None established at this time.

The Food and Nutrition Board of the Institute of Medicine states that beta carotene supplements are not advisable for the general population.

**Maximum daily intake.** Maximum intake from all sources that's unlikely to pose a risk of side effects for adults: None established.

**Food sources.** Carrots, cantaloupe, pumpkin, winter squash, sweet potatoes and dark leafy vegetables, such as spinach, kale, turnip greens and collards.

**What it does.** Beta carotene is one of more than 600 carotenoid compounds found in animals, plants and microorganisms. Your body converts beta carotene into vitamin A.

**What the research says.** Some studies indicate that diets high in beta carotene and other carotenoids obtained from food are associated with a lower risk of chronic diseases such as heart disease and some cancers. However, this beneficial effect may be due to other substances found in carotenoid-rich foods, not only beta carotene.

Several well-designed studies have shown that beta carotene supplements offer no protection against heart disease. Three large clinical trials found the supplements didn't protect against cancer. Two studies found an increased risk of lung cancer among smokers who took beta carotene supplements, and one found an increased risk of prostate cancer among men who took the supplements and also drank alcohol. A large Finnish study of male smokers found that daily beta carotene supplements had no effect on the incidence of cataract surgery.

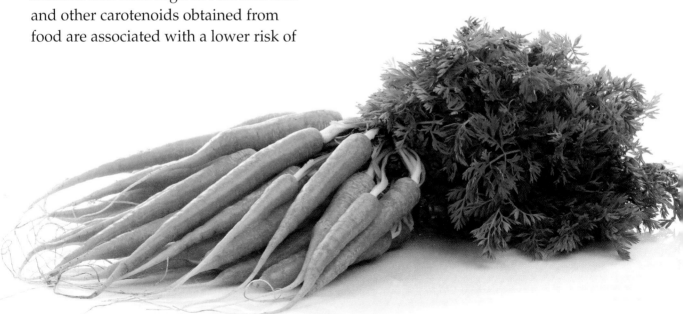

## Understanding antioxidants

Antioxidants are vitamins, minerals and enzymes that protect the body by neutralizing "free radicals." Free radicals are byproducts of normal cell activity. The damage done to cells by free radicals is thought to contribute to aging and to disorders such as coronary artery disease and cancer.

Vitamins C and E are antioxidants. Some people take large amounts of these vitamins in the hope of slowing the aging process. Other antioxidants include beta carotene (a form of vitamin A), the mineral selenium and coenzyme Q10, an antioxidant produced by the body, which is also found in meat and seafood.

While the use of antioxidants to prevent aging makes sense, no studies have proved that they actually do. In addition, taking large doses of some antioxidants, such as vitamin E, may be harmful.

Another study indicates that a small amount of beta carotene taken with certain other antioxidants and zinc may slow the progression of age-related macular degeneration. However, a doctor's supervision is important to determine proper doses, to lower the risk of side effects.

**Cautions.** Avoid taking beta carotene supplements because of the potential risks, unless your doctor advises otherwise. If you're seeking the potential benefits of beta carotene, eat more red, yellow and dark green leafy vegetables.

**Side effects.** People who take beta carotene may develop an orange color to their skin, which is reversible.

Calcium
**Recommended Dietary Allowance (RDA) for Adults**

*Men*
Ages 19 to 70: 1,000 mg a day
Age 71 or older: 1,200 mg a day

*Women*
Ages 19 to 50: 1,000 mg a day
Age 51 or older: 1,200 mg a day

**Maximum daily intake.** Maximum intake from all sources that's unlikely to pose a risk of side effects for adults: 2,500 mg a day for adults ages 19 to 50; 2,000 mg a day for adults 51 or older.

**Food sources.** Milk and milk products, fish with bones that are eaten, calcium-fortified tofu, calcium-fortified orange juice, calcium-fortified cereals, greens (collards, spinach, turnips, kale), green soybeans (edamame), and broccoli.

**What it does.** Calcium is a mineral important for strong teeth and bones and for muscle and nerve function.

**What the research says.** Studies suggest that calcium supplements, if taken regularly, help prevent osteoporosis by reducing bone loss. The question is how much calcium you need to achieve this. Although the suggested intake for calcium is 1,200 mg a day for women age 51 or older and men age 71 or older, some people may need more, such as those with osteoporosis or osteopenia or postmenopausal women not taking estrogen. If you don't get enough calcium in your diet, consider a supplement. In addition, a 14-year study of 86,000 women found that those who had a relatively high intake of calcium, whether through diet or use of supplements, had a reduced risk of stroke.

**Cautions.** Don't take calcium if you have sarcoidosis or a high blood-calcium level. See your doctor before taking calcium if you have kidney disease, chronic constipation, colitis, diarrhea, stomach or intestinal bleeding, irregular heartbeat, or heart problems. Although studies conflict, the American Cancer Society (ACS) notes that a high calcium intake, primarily through supplements, may increase the risk of aggressive prostate cancer in some men. The ACS advises men at risk to get calcium through low-fat and fat-free food sources. Follow your doctor's advice about using supplements, especially if you have osteoporosis or you don't get enough calcium in your diet.

Avoid calcium supplements made from bone meal, dolomite or oyster shell, often advertised as "natural." These may contain toxic substances, such as lead, mercury and arsenic. If you take an iron supplement, don't take it at the same time as your calcium supplement. Calcium can interfere with the absorption of iron.

**Side effects.** People who take calcium supplements may experience constipation and headache. Potential serious side effects include confusion, muscle or bone pain, nausea, vomiting, and slow or irregular heartbeat.

## Iron

### Recommended Dietary Allowance (RDA) for Adults

*Men*\*
Age 19 or older: 8 mg a day

*Women*
Ages 19 to 50: 18 mg a day\*\*
Age 51 or older: 8 mg a day\*

\*For men and postmenopausal women who take a multivitamin, it's probably wise to take a pill with little or no iron — 8 mg a day or less.

\*\*Women who are menstruating.

**Maximum daily intake.** Maximum intake from all sources that's unlikely to pose a risk of side effects for adults: 45 mg a day.

**Food sources.** There are two types of dietary iron:

- Heme iron, which the body usually absorbs well, is found in meat, seafood and poultry. A portion (3 ounces) of beef, pork, lamb or veal contains 2 to 3 mg of iron.
- Nonheme iron, which isn't absorbed as well as heme iron, is found in iron-fortified cereals, whole grains, beans, peas and dark green leafy vegetables. Because absorption of nonheme iron is lower, vegetarians who don't consume animal products may require higher amounts of dietary iron. The body better absorbs nonheme iron from plant foods when they're consumed along with a source of vitamin C, such as citrus fruits or tomato products.

**What it does.** Iron is a mineral that is an essential constituent of blood and muscle and important for the transport of oxygen.

**What the research says.** When there isn't enough iron in your diet, too few red blood cells are made to adequately carry oxygen. This condition is called iron deficiency anemia. It can affect women of childbearing age and people with conditions that cause internal bleeding, such as ulcers or intestinal diseases. For men who are healthy and postmenopausal women, iron deficiency is rare. If you want to make sure you're getting enough iron, your best bet is to eat a balanced diet containing iron-rich foods.

**Cautions.** Don't take iron if you have acute hepatitis, hemosiderosis or hemochromatosis (conditions involving excess iron in the body), hemolytic anemia or if you've had repeated blood transfusions. See your doctor before taking iron if you've had peptic ulcer disease, enteritis, colitis, pancreatitis or hepatitis. Also see your doctor if you have kidney disease, intestinal disease or you consume excessive alcohol. And if you're older than age 55 and have a family history of heart disease, consult your doctor before taking iron.

**Side effects.** In some people, iron supplements can cause side effects such as nausea, vomiting, constipation, diarrhea, dark-colored stools or abdominal pain. Taking the supplement in divided doses and with food may help avoid or limit these signs and symptoms. Liquid iron can stain your teeth.

## Magnesium
### Recommended Dietary Allowance (RDA) for Adults

*Men*
Ages 19 to 30: 400 mg a day
Age 31 or older: 420 mg a day

*Women*
Ages 19 to 30: 310 mg a day
Age 31 or older: 320 mg a day

**Maximum daily intake.** Maximum intake from supplements only that's unlikely to a pose risk of side effects for adults: 350 mg a day.

**Food sources.** Nuts, legumes, whole grains and dark green vegetables.

**What it does.** Magnesium is a mineral necessary in many enzyme processes. It helps your nerves and muscles function.

**What the research says.** Low magnesium levels are linked with a variety of diseases, including high blood pressure, heart disease, osteoporosis and poorly controlled diabetes, as well as alcohol abuse. Using certain diuretics and other medications can increase the loss of magnesium through urination and requires monitoring of magnesium levels by a doctor. Your doctor will likely recommend eating more foods that contain magnesium if your levels are mildly depleted. Supplements may be recommended when normal levels can't be achieved through dietary changes.

**Cautions.** Don't take magnesium supplements if you have kidney failure or heart block (unless you have a pacemaker) or have had an ileostomy. See your doctor before taking magnesium if you have stomach or intestinal bleeding, symptoms of appendicitis, or chronic constipation, colitis or diarrhea. Laxatives and antacids often contain magnesium, so check the label. Because older adults usually have decreased kidney function, those who routinely take large amounts of magnesium-containing laxatives may increase their risk of toxicity.

**Side effects.** People who take magnesium supplements may experience abdominal cramps, appetite loss, diarrhea, irregular heartbeat, mood changes, fatigue, nausea, vomiting or pain when urinating. When taken with food, magnesium supplements are less likely to cause diarrhea, nausea and abdominal cramps.

## Potassium
### Adequate Intake (AI) for Adults*

*Men and women*
Age 19 or older: 4,700 mg (4.7 grams) a day

*AI levels are used because the Recommended Dietary Allowance (RDA) has not been established.

**Maximum daily intake.** Maximum intake from all sources that's unlikely to pose a risk of side effects for adults: None established.

**Food sources.** Citrus fruits (such as oranges), apples, bananas, apricots, cantaloupe, potatoes (especially with skin), tomatoes, spinach, Brussels sprouts, mushrooms, beans, peas and almonds.

**What it does.** Potassium is one of the minerals responsible for maintaining the electrical stability of the cells of your heart and nervous system. It's also called an electrolyte. Potassium is important for cell and muscle growth and for maintaining normal fluid balance in the body.

**What the research says.** Most people in the U.S. get only about half the recommended amount of potassium daily. It's important to eat adequate fruits and vegetables, which are naturally good sources of potassium. If you don't get enough potassium because of a medical condition or certain medications, your doctor may recommend a potassium supplement. For example, chronic diarrhea may cause potassium deficiency. Some studies indicate that low potassium may contribute to high

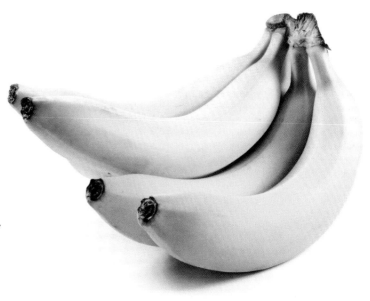

blood pressure and that increasing potassium intake through diet may help prevent or help treat high blood pressure. Some studies indicate that increased potassium intake is linked with a lower risk of stroke, but more research is needed.

**Cautions.** Don't take potassium supplements unless your doctor specifically recommends them. Too much or too little potassium can lead to serious health effects. Your blood levels will likely be monitored if you're taking potassium or a medication that affects blood potassium. Some high blood pressure medications (diuretics) increase urination, which could lead to potassium deficiency. However, potassium-sparing diuretics cause the kidneys to retain potassium. Follow your doctor's recommendations. Too much potassium may be a concern.

**Side effects.** Side effects can include nausea, vomiting, upset stomach, diarrhea and gas. Confusion and an irregular heartbeat are less common.

## Selenium
### Recommended Dietary Allowance (RDA) for Adults

*Men and women*
Age 19 or older: 55 mcg a day

**Maximum daily intake.** Maximum intake from all sources that's unlikely to pose a risk of side effects for adults: 400 mcg a day.

**Food sources.** Milk, poultry, fish, seafood, organ meats, Brazil nuts and whole-grain products.

**What it does.** Selenium is a mineral that has antioxidant properties, helping to prevent cell damage by neutralizing free radicals — molecules believed to be associated with aging and certain diseases. Selenium also helps regulate thyroid function.

**What the research says.** Some studies suggest that selenium may help prevent cancer and, possibly, heart disease. One small study found that those taking 200 mcg of selenium a day had lower rates of prostate and colon cancers than did those taking an inactive pill (placebo). Another small study confirmed the prostate cancer finding. In 2001, a large study was launched to determine if selenium and vitamin E can help protect against prostate cancer. However, results released in 2011 showed no benefit in using this combination of supplements or in taking selenium alone. Participants in this study continue to be followed to see if results change over time.

**Cautions.** See your doctor before taking selenium in high doses.

**Side effects.** Excessive amounts of selenium may cause hair and nail loss, gastrointestinal disturbance, skin rash, fatigue, tooth decay, and nervous system abnormalities.

## Zinc

**Recommended Dietary Allowance (RDA) for Adults**

*Men*
Age 19 or older: 11 mg a day

*Women*
Age 19 or older: 8 mg a day

**Maximum daily intake.** Maximum intake from all sources that's unlikely to pose a risk of side effects for adults: 40 mg a day.

**Food sources.** Meat, fish, poultry, liver, milk, oysters, crab, lobster, beans, nuts, wheat germ, whole-grain products and fortified cereals.

**What it does.** Zinc is a mineral involved in wound healing, immune function, sense of taste and smell, growth, and sexual maturation. Zinc is also contained in enzymes that regulate metabolism.

**What the research says.** Studies have conflicted on the use of zinc to ease cold symptoms. Most-recent data suggest that zinc (as lozenges or syrup) is beneficial in reducing the duration and severity of the common cold in healthy people when taken within 24 hours of the onset of symptoms. However, because different dosages and preparations were used for different lengths of time, it's not clear what the effective dose and treatment schedule would be.

In addition, a 2001 study indicates that supplementation with zinc and certain antioxidants may slow the progression of age-related macular degeneration, but a small percentage of participants had side effects. A doctor's supervision is important.

**Cautions.** Don't take zinc if you have stomach or duodenal ulcers. It's better not to exceed the RDA, although vegetarians may need more because of lower absorption of zinc from plant sources. If you take zinc lozenges for a cold, stop taking them once your cold is gone. Be aware that lozenges may cause nausea or a bad taste in the mouth. See your doctor before taking zinc in higher doses or if you're taking a calcium supplement or tetracycline drugs. Zinc may interfere with absorption of these medicines.

## Other hormone supplements

Hormones are chemicals made by your body to regulate the activities of vital organs. Because hormone levels decline with age, some scientists speculate that hormones play a role in the aging process. According to proponents of hormone products, you can set back your body's clock by restoring your hormone levels to those of your youth. Studies generally don't support such thinking. Hormone supplements include:

- **Testosterone.** Declining levels of this male sex hormone have been linked with common complaints of aging, such as decreased energy and sex drive.

  Anti-aging enthusiasts say increasing your testosterone level — often beyond the normal range of testosterone in your body — will improve your energy, well-being, complexion and sex drive. You can find a number of products that claim to be "testosterone boosters" on the Internet. Most claims regarding testosterone remain unproved, and so-called testosterone boosters are just a ploy.

  In high doses, testosterone can result in prostate problems, elevated cholesterol and fertility problems.

**Side effects.** Long-term, high doses of zinc (50 to 100 mg/day) can lower high-density lipoprotein (HDL, or "good") cholesterol, suppress immune system function and interfere with the absorption of copper, which may result in microcytic anemia. Other side effects may include diarrhea, heartburn, nausea, vomiting and abdominal pain.

# An overview of other popular supplements

In addition to vitamins and minerals, many people look to other supplements to improve their health. Research on

- **Melatonin.** This hormone, produced in the brain, helps regulate sleep and may help with jet lag. But claims that melatonin, also a type of antioxidant, can slow or reverse aging, fight cancer, and enhance sexuality are far from proved. Supplements sold in stores typically contain many times the melatonin produced by your body. If taken improperly, melatonin can actually disrupt your sleep cycle.
- **Human growth hormone (HGH).** This hormone, responsible for growth spurts in children, tapers off after adolescence. It's available by prescription to treat adults with true growth hormone deficiency. Proponents say HGH injections burn fat, build muscle and renew energy.

A few small studies suggest some benefit from HGH. However, most doctors say it's too early to draw solid conclusions from them. Strength training with weights or other equipment is a cheaper and more effective way to boost muscle mass and strength. Possible side effects of growth hormone include fluid retention, joint pain and high blood pressure.

Some websites claim to sell a pill form of growth hormone that produces similar results as the injected form. The pills are sometimes called human growth hormone releasers. They're completely ineffective.

herbal and other dietary supplements is ongoing. The best approach here is a cautious one. Use such supplements with care — if you use them at all. Do your homework and don't be afraid to ask questions.

Following are some of the more popular products. Some additional supplements are discussed in Part 4 of this book.

### DHEA

Dehydroepiandrosterone (DHEA) is a steroid hormone produced by the adrenal glands that's converted into sex hormones, such as estrogen and testosterone.

# Anti-aging therapies: Beware of the hype

Ponce de León never did find the fountain of youth. But the lure of an ultimate elixir of life continues to beckon. These days, however, people are more likely to search on the shelves of a drugstore for a magic potion than in the swamps of Florida. Who wouldn't want to look and feel years younger simply by taking a pill?

Anti-aging products range from dietary supplements to wrinkle creams. Can they really slow down or even stop the aging process? When evaluating claims made about such remedies, some old advice is good advice — if it sounds too good to be true, it probably is.

Aging is an intricate, complex process that involves many areas of your body. It's unlikely that a product, pill or potion could cure all of the changes age brings. One technique that does seem to increase life span — in lab animals, anyway — is to radically cut daily calories, by nearly half. But how many people want to go through life in a constant state of hunger? The strategies that do help are the sensible ones outlined in this book.

Despite tempting claims, there's no product out there that's scientifically proved to prevent or reverse aging. Even worse, many have potentially dangerous side effects. The safety of anti-aging supplements also isn't guaranteed. As you take steps to stay active and vibrant in your later years, stick with good health practices proved by time — not quick fixes with a lot of glitz but no real results.

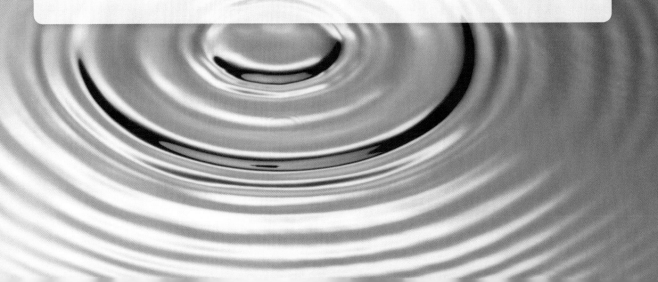

**Other names.** Prasterone

**Popular uses.** DHEA is taken to improve memory, mood, energy and a sense of well-being. Many athletes claim DHEA supplements build muscle, and there are also claims that DHEA may reverse the effects of aging, stimulate the immune system, treat depression, lupus and a variety of other conditions, and improve functioning in people with Parkinson's disease or Alzheimer's disease.

**What the research says.** A two-year Mayo Clinic study published in 2006 found that DHEA has no effect on anti-aging indicators such as endurance, muscle mass, fat mass and insulin sensitivity and no effect on quality of life. DHEA may be useful for treating depression and lupus, but strictly under the guidance of a specialist.

**Cautions.** When DHEA is used for a long time or in large amounts, it may stimulate the growth of some prostate, breast, ovarian and other hormone-sensitive cancers. The supplements may also reduce the level of high-density lipoprotein (HDL, or "good") cholesterol in blood in people with diabetes and liver problems. However, none of these potential negative effects has been confirmed.

Generally, individuals with a history of abnormal heart rhythms (arrythmias), blood clots and liver disease should avoid DHEA supplements.

**Side effects.** The most common complaints are fatigue, nasal congestion and headache. The supplements may result in breast enlargement in men and excess hair growth in women. The supplements may also lead to hair loss. Other potential side effects include insomnia, agitation, delusions, nervousness and mania.

## Echinacea

You may know echinacea by its common name, the coneflower. The roots and herbs from three echinacea species are prepared for medicinal use as pills, applications and teas.

**Popular uses.** Echinacea is taken to stimulate the immune system and is typically used for colds and influenza. It's also used to help heal wounds.

**What the research shows.** Despite all of the claims, latest study results suggest echinacea isn't an effective method for cold prevention or treatment. If you have a cold, it won't hurt you to try echinacea for a few days, but there's no guarantee that it will help. Some studies have found that taking echinacea orally in combination with a topical antifungal cream seems to help prevent recurrent vaginal yeast infection.

**Cautions.** It's best to use echinacea for eight weeks or less because some studies have suggested that chronic use actually leads to diminished immune function. You shouldn't take echinacea if you have diabetes, multiple sclerosis, leukemia, HIV or autoimmune diseases, such as rheumatoid arthritis or lupus, because it can stimulate your immune system. Avoid taking echinacea if you're allergic to the daisy family, including ragweed, chamomile and chrysanthemum.

**Side effects.** Side effects can include intestinal upset, diarrhea, skin rash (if used topically) and a suppressed immune system (with habitual use).

## Fish oil

Fish oil contains both docosahexaenoic acid (DHA) and eico-sapentaenoic acid (EPA). Supple-ments vary in the amounts and ratios of DHA and EPA. A common amount of omega-3 fatty acids in fish oil capsules is .18 grams (180 mg) of EPA and .12 grams (120 mg) of DHA.

**Popular uses.** Fish oil supplements are typically taken to protect against heart and blood vessel (cardiovascular) disease. They may also ease symptoms of depression in some people.

**What the research shows.** Fish oil has been shown to reduce triglycerides (a type of blood fat) as well as deaths from heart attack. Omega-3 fatty acids found in fish also have been shown to reduce heart disease and other problems related to blood vessel disease. Some evidence also suggests fish oil may help lower blood pressure slightly, reduce the risk of artery re-blockage following angioplasty, increase exercise capacity in people with clogged arteries, reduce strokes in people with cardiovascular disease and may possibly reduce the risk of irregular heartbeats.

The American Heart Association recommends getting omega-3 fatty acids in your diet, mainly from fish and plant sources. However, some people with high triglycerides or known cardiovascular disease may benefit from taking fish oil supplements to get more omega-3 fatty acids than they can get from diet alone.

**Cautions.** High doses of fish oil may have harmful effects, such as increased risk of bleeding. Don't take more than the recommended amount.

**Side effects.** Fish oil supplements can cause gastrointestinal upset, nausea and vomiting, or bleeding in some people. But for most people they're considered safe.

## Garlic

In addition to the fresh garlic found in grocery stores, garlic is also available as an oil and in the form of a tablet or capsule.

**Other names.** *Allium sativum*

**Popular uses.** Garlic is used to lower blood cholesterol and to reduce blood clot formation in narrowed arteries. It's also used to relieve symptoms of upper respiratory infection because of its antibiotic effect.

**What the research shows.** Several studies suggest garlic may modestly lower cholesterol and reduce blood clot formation. However, long-term effects remain unknown. Some studies suggest consuming garlic as a regular part of your diet may lower the risk of certain cancers, including gastric and colon cancers. However, no clinical trials have examined this. Research also suggests garlic may slow hardening of the arteries (atherosclerosis), a condition that can lead to heart disease, as well as reduce blood pressure.

**Cautions.** You shouldn't use garlic supplements if you're taking anti-clotting medications. This includes taking aspirin regularly. If you take garlic tablets, make sure they contain allicin, the active ingredient in garlic.

**Side effects.** Side effects can include stomach upset, heartburn, intestinal problems, and bad breath or body odor.

## Ginger

The ginger plant has played a significant role in Chinese, Japanese and Indian medicine since the 1500s.

**Other names.** *Zingiber officinale*; Amomum zingiber; African ginger

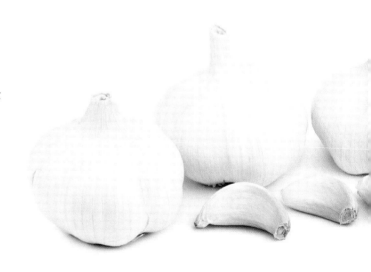

**Popular uses.** Ginger is taken to reduce nausea, motion sickness and seasickness, and may help with nausea from chemotherapy when combined with standard anti-nausea medications. Ginger may also be used to treat pain associated with arthritis. The medicinal part of the plant is the root.

**What the research shows.** There's mixed evidence regarding ginger's effect on nausea associated with motion sickness, seasickness, chemotherapy and anesthesia. Some small studies found it had no effect, while other research found it reduced vomiting, but not nausea. It's unclear whether ginger is effective in treating osteoarthritis, rheumatoid arthritis, or joint or muscle pain — results of a few small studies have been mixed.

**Cautions.** Ginger supplements shouldn't be taken by individuals who are allergic to ginger. Individuals who've had ulcers, inflammatory bowel disease, blocked intestines and gallstones should use caution when taking ginger supplements and should avoid large quantities of fresh-cut ginger. Ginger increases the production of digestive juices and bile.

**Side effects.** There are few side effects when ginger supplements are taken at low doses. The most common side effects include a bad taste in the mouth, heartburn, bloating and gas, especially with the powdered forms. Fresh ginger that's swallowed without enough chewing can cause blockage of the intestines.

### Ginkgo

Ginkgo comes mainly from the fan-shaped leaves of the Ginkgo biloba (maidenhair) tree.

**Other names.** *Ginkgo biloba*

**Popular uses.** Ginkgo is used to treat symptoms connected with decreased blood flow to the brain, particularly in older adults. These include short-term memory loss, dizziness, ringing in the ears, headache, depression and anxiety. Ginkgo is also used to relieve circulation problems in the legs.

**What the research shows.** Numerous studies suggest ginkgo improves circulation to the brain, arms and legs. More studies are needed on the effect of its long-term use. Recent large studies indicate that ginkgo doesn't reduce the risk of Alzheimer's disease or other dementias, nor does it seem to improve memory or brain function. A 2009 study of 3,000 people found no difference in attention, memory or other cognitive functions between those who took ginkgo and those who didn't. This was true for both those who had mild cognitive impairment at the start of the study and for those that didn't.

**Cautions.** You shouldn't take ginkgo if you're taking an anti-clotting medication. Mayo Clinic doctors also recommend that you avoid ginkgo if taking a thiazide diuretic. If used with this drug, ginkgo may raise blood pressure.

**Side effects.** Possible side effects can include muscle spasms, mild digestive problems, allergic skin reactions and bleeding.

## Ginseng

Ginseng is made from the root of the ginseng plant. Look for products that contain ginsenosides, the active chemical found in ginseng. Some so-called ginseng products don't contain ginseng at all.

**Other names.** *Panax ginseng, Panax quinquefolius, Panax japonicus and Panax notoginseng*

**Popular uses.** Ginseng is used to increase energy and sexual stamina, reduce stress and improve mental performance. It may also be used for people with diabetes.

**What the research shows.** It's unclear how much benefit ginseng provides with exercise performance — study results have been mixed. Studies report that gingeng can modestly improve the performance of thinking and learning tasks. It may also improve mood and enhance sleep. Several studies report that ginseng may lower blood sugar levels in people with type 2 diabetes. However, more studies are needed, and ginseng shouldn't be substituted for proven therapies.

**Cautions.** It's best not to take ginseng for more than three months or exceed the recommended maximum dosage. Some studies suggest ginseng may raise estrogen levels in women. Don't take it if you have an estrogen-related disease, such as breast cancer. You also shouldn't take ginseng if you have uncontrolled high blood pressure because ginseng may raise blood pressure.

**Side effects.** With proper use, ginseng typically doesn't cause side effects. If you experience any adverse reactions, see your doctor.

## Glucosamine

Glucosamine is a natural compound found in healthy cartilage. Glucosamine sulfate is the most studied form of glucosamine.

## Herb and drug interactions

Herbal supplements contain ingredients that may not mix safely with prescription or over-the-counter medications. Here are two examples, but many other herbs also can interact with medications.

- **Ginkgo.** If you regularly take aspirin or warfarin (Coumadin), use of ginkgo may cause spontaneous and excessive bleeding.

- **St. John's wort.** This herb can cause serious problems by altering the effects of many prescription medications, including antidepressants, digoxin, warfarin and cyclosporine. St. John's wort is discussed further on page 270.

Herbal supplements can also be dangerous when used with anesthesia and surgery. Some herbs can increase your risk of bleeding or affect your heart rate or blood pressure. Be certain to stop taking an herbal supplement at least two to three weeks before surgery, to clear it from your body. If this isn't possible, let medical professionals know what you're taking.

**Popular uses.** Glucosamine is commonly combined with chondroitin sulfate, another naturally occurring substance that gives cartilage its elasticity. These two substances are typically taken in combination as tablets or capsules to decrease pain and inflammation in arthritic joints — primarily the knee joint. Together, the substances appear to strengthen cartilage and improve lubrication in the knee joint.

**What the research shows.** Results of more than 30 studies have produced enough mixed results that researchers aren't able to conclude that glucosamine and chondroitin improve pain and function in people with osteoarthritis of the knee. Glucosamine, though, has shown benefits for osteoarthritis in other joints. In some instances, it appeared to reduce joint pain and tenderness as effectively as did conventional medications and slow progression of the disease. Whether people taking glucosamine for longer periods have less joint damage compared with those taking a placebo is uncertain and requires further study. Early evidence suggests glucosamine may also be beneficial in the treatment of rheumatoid arthritis; however, more study is needed before a conclusion can be drawn.

**Cautions.** Glucosamine can be made from the shells of shrimp, crab and other shellfish. Therefore, people with shellfish allergies or iodine hypersensitivity should avoid the supplement or be very cautious in its use. There's also some evidence suggesting a possible link between glucosamine and chondroitin products and asthma attacks. Until more reliable data exists, it's suggested individuals with a history of asthma avoid these supplements.

**Side effects.** When taken at recommended doses, the supplement is generally well-tolerated. Possible side effects may include upset stomach, insomnia, headache, skin reactions, sun sensitivity and nail toughening.

## Lycopene

Lycopene is an antioxidant found in colorful fruit, such as the tomato. (Tomatoes are technically fruits, although they're generally used as vegetables.)

Lycopene is what gives tomatoes their red color.

**Popular uses.** Lycopene supplements are taken to reduce the risk of cardiovascular disease, macular degeneration and cancer, especially prostate cancer.

**What the research shows.** A number of studies have suggested a link between high intake of foods containing lycopene and reduced risk of cancer, cardiovascular disease and macular degeneration. However, many of these studies have been based on tomato intake, not on the use of lycopene supplements. In addition, since tomatoes are sources of other nutrients, it's not clear that lycopene itself is beneficial, and not one of the other nutrients or a combination of nutrients. Because there hasn't been a well-designed study involving lycopene supplements, whether they're of any benefit is unclear.

**Cautions.** Lycopene supplements shouldn't be taken by individuals who are allergic to tomatoes. The safety of these supplements has not been thoroughly studied.

**Side effects.** A review of available scientific literature finds no reports of serious side effects from use of lycopene supplements.

## Peppermint

Mint plants such as peppermint have a long history of medicinal use, dating back to ancient Egypt, Greece and Rome.

**Other names.** *Mentha piperita*

**Popular uses.** Peppermint supplements (oils and capsules) are taken to relieve indigestion, abdominal cramps, headache and nasal congestion.

**What the research shows.** Studies on the effects of peppermint oil to relieve indigestion haven't been well designed, and it's unclear if the oil is beneficial for this condition. For the treatment of abdominal pain and bloating associated with irritable bowel syndrome, results have been mixed. These trials have been small and more study is needed. For the treatment of headache and nasal congestion, good-quality studies are lacking.

**Cautions.** People with allergies to peppermint should avoid these products. Peppermint oil should be used cautiously by people with gastroesophageal reflux disease (GERD) or gallbladder disease, including gallstones.

**Side effects.** When used on the skin, peppermint oil has been associated with skin rash and hives and with eye irritation. Peppermint products taken by mouth may cause headache, dizziness, heartburn and anal burning. In animals, very large doses of peppermint oil taken by mouth have resulted in muscle weakness, brain damage and seizure.

## St. John's wort

Extracts of *Hypericum perforatum*, the botanical name of the plant, have been used in folk medicine since Hippocrates' time.

**Other names.** *Hypericum perforatum*

**Popular uses.** It's taken to treat depression, anxiety and sleep disorders.

**What the research shows.** Several studies support the therapeutic benefit of St. John's wort in treating mild to moderate depression. It's been proved as effective as some prescription antidepressants and with fewer side effects. Potential benefits in the treatment of other disorders are less clear. A major concern is that studies show St. John's wort may not mix well with various types of prescription drugs, significantly affecting the concentration of the medication in your blood. Results from studies examining its effectiveness on symptoms of anxiety have been mixed.

**Cautions.** If you think you're experiencing depression, talk with your doctor. Depression is a serious illness, and you shouldn't treat it yourself. And don't mix St. John's wort with other antidepressant medications. A good rule of thumb is not to mix St. John's wort with any medication until you've talked with your doctor first.

**Side effects.** Possible side effects include sun sensitivity, itching, fatigue, headache, weight gain, bloating and constipation.

### Soy

Soybeans are legumes, but their popularity and health effects puts them in a category of their own. The protein in soy is unique and has been the source of numerous studies.

**Other names.** Edamame

**Popular uses.** Soy is taken to reduce cholesterol, reduce menopausal hot flashes, prevent some cancers and for a variety of other reasons.

**What the research shows.** The thinking used to be that adding soy to your diet produced a moderate decrease in cholesterol levels. This view changed after the American Heart Association, following an extensive review of research, concluded that soy-based foods don't significantly lower cholesterol.

Components of soy called isoflavones also appear to inhibit the effects of sex hormones, so they may offer some protection from cancers that feed on these hormones, such as some breast cancers. Consuming 20 to 60 grams of soy protein daily seems to modestly decrease the frequency and severity of hot flashes in some women.

**Cautions.** Soy can act as a food allergen similar to milk, eggs, peanuts, fish and wheat. Use of soy is discouraged in people with hormone-sensitive cancers, such as breast or ovarian cancer because of concerns soy's estrogen-like effects could stimulate cancer growth.

**Side effects.** Limited side effects have been reported. When side effects do occur, they generally include bloating, nausea and constipation. It's not known if soy or soy isoflavones share

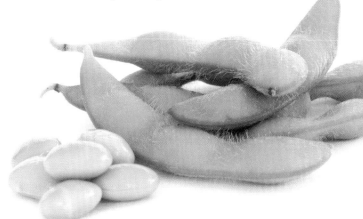

the same side effects as estrogens, such as increased risk of blood clots.

# Be supplement savvy

If you take herbal or other types of supplements — or you're considering doing so — keep these four points in mind:

1. Follow the directions. Don't exceed the recommended dosages.
2. Let your doctor know what you're taking. Some supplements can interfere with the effectiveness of prescription or over-the-counter medications or have other harmful effects. In addition to the type of supplement you're taking, let your doctor know which brand you're taking.
3. Keep track of what you take. Know what you take, how much you take and how it affects you.
4. Be cautious of products manufactured outside the United States. In general, European products are well regulated. However, toxic ingredients and prescription drugs have been found in some products that are manufactured elsewhere.

# Chapter 11

# Be proactive with your health care

Health care is a lot like anything else you may be involved in — the more you put into it, the more you get out of it.

Think of when you wash your hands after you've used the restroom or worked with raw meat in the kitchen. This simple step with soap and water — less than a minute of your time — limits the transfer of bacteria and viruses, greatly reducing your risk of illness. A little effort pays big dividends.

In the same way, if you see your doctor only when you're sick, there's a limit as to how much your doctor can help you fight disease and stay well. But if you see your doctor in good times and in bad — when you're feeling well in addition to when you're not — the opportunity for fending off disease increases

dramatically. This includes heart disease, cancer, diabetes and osteoporosis.

You and your doctor are a team. And it's up to you to work with your doctor to make sure that you receive recommended immunizations, screening tests and exams, and other care intended to prevent disease, or catch it early when it's most treatable. Although they may take some time and energy, preventive health measures are well worth the investment for your long-term health.

The bottom line: By becoming more actively involved in your own health care, you increase your odds of living a healthier, more productive life. In the pages that follow, you'll learn more about different ways that you can work with your doctor to stay healthy and active for many years to come.

# Developing a good relationship with your doctor

The best medical care results when you and your doctor share information and work together. Here are some ways you can help build and strengthen that relationship:

- **Be on time for office appointments.** If you must cancel, try to do so at least 24 hours in advance. You may arrive for your appointment only to find that your doctor is running late. You should be able to see your doctor within a reasonable amount of time. However, realize that he or she may be called away on occasion to address medical emergencies.

- **Be prepared for your appointments.** Before each visit, jot down a couple of main problems that are of concern to you. Also be ready to bring up relevant changes in your personal or family health history.

- **Answer all your doctor's questions truthfully and completely.** This helps your doctor better monitor your health, assess any health risks you may have and make a proper diagnosis, if one is needed. Even if the subject is a sensitive one, such as smoking, alcohol or drug use or sex, be truthful. Your doctor can only help you if he or she has an accurate picture of what's going on in your life.

- **Make sure you understand what has been said.** If you don't understand something, ask your doctor to clarify it for you until you do understand. You should know what your doctor is doing or recommending and why. If you think you're unlikely to remember, write it down.

- **Follow your doctor's treatment recommendations.** When your doctor prescribes a medication or another form of treatment, do what he or she recommends. Be patient — sometimes a treatment takes time to have an effect. However, if you experience any adverse effects or worsening symptoms, contact your doctor.

- **Consider bringing a friend or family member to your appointment.** He or she can provide moral support, remind you of questions you want to ask, and take notes to help you remember what was said. Having a friend or family member present is also helpful if you have difficulty driving or getting around on your own.

# How often to see your doctor

Throughout this chapter we mention that you should see your doctor on a regular basis for basic preventive care. What does "regular" mean?

The answer depends on your age, your health and your family medical history. In general, if you're fairly healthy and you have no symptoms of disease, it's a good idea to have a physical four to five times in your 50s and then annually once you turn 60. More-frequent visits may be advisable if you have certain health risks due to your personal or family health history.

Regular preventive exams are important because they help your doctor assess your overall health and identify possible risk factors for disease that —

## Need a new doctor?

The thought of switching to a different physician may seem overwhelming at first — especially if you've had a long relationship with your present doctor and he or she understands you and your health history. As you make the change, keep in mind that just as you're growing older and possibly contemplating retirement, so might be an older doctor. Whereas, if you switch to a younger doctor, that person will be around to see you through your 50s, 60s, 70s and beyond — to get to know you in your later years.

When looking for a new doctor, the most important thing is to find someone who will effectively partner with you in your care. Talk to friends and family about which doctors they recommend. You can also get recommendations from your current physician.

Once you have a short list of possible care providers, check to see if these people are part of your health insurance plan. If you need more information to make your decision, consider making an appointment with the individuals to see how well you communicate and get along.

with commitment and effort — you may be able to modify. And the payoff of these efforts is typically a longer, healthier life.

Many conditions, such as diabetes, high blood pressure or some forms of cancer, don't cause any noticeable signs or symptoms in their early stages —but they may still be detectable with screening. If your doctor identifies these conditions early, which can typically be done with standard screening tests, they can often be treated more effectively.

## When you shouldn't 'wait and see'

Oftentimes, when a particular sign or symptom develops, our natural response is to wait a day or two and see if it goes away. In many instances, such as if you develop a sore throat or experience back pain after a day of lifting, this approach is OK. But certain signs and symptoms demand an immediate response. Seek emergency medical care if you experience any of the following:

- Uncontrolled bleeding
- Difficulty breathing or shortness of breath
- Severe chest or upper abdominal pain or pressure
- Fainting, sudden dizziness or weakness
- Weakening or numbness of an arm or leg
- Sudden, marked change in vision
- Confusion or changes in mental state
- Any sudden or severe pain
- Severe or persistent vomiting or diarrhea
- Coughing or vomiting blood
- Suicidal or homicidal feelings

You may also have other warning signs to be aware of, based on your personal medical history.

# Recommended vaccinations

One of the best ways to prevent many diseases is to make sure you've received all of the recommended vaccinations. Vaccines work by stimulating your body's natural defense mechanisms to resist infectious disease, destroying the disease-causing microbes before you become sick.

Most vaccinations are given in childhood. But there are some vaccines that are recommended specifically for adults or may be recommended regularly throughout life. Or, it may be that you didn't receive a vaccination in childhood, which, if given now, still could be of benefit.

When in doubt, follow your doctor's advice on which vaccinations to receive and when to get them. He or she may recommend additional vaccinations depending on your occupation, hobbies or travel plans.

## If you travel internationally

If you're planning to travel out of the country, make sure you're up to date on routine vaccinations, such as those for tetanus, diphtheria, pertussis, flu (influenza), measles, mumps and rubella. Also, depending on your destination, length of stay and medical history, you may need additional vaccines.

The Centers for Disease Control and Prevention (CDC) recommends that international travelers consider the following additional vaccinations or booster vaccines:

- **Japanese encephalitis.** This vaccination is recommended if you will be traveling to rural areas in the Far East, Southeast Asia or the Asian subcontinent for four weeks or more.
- **Polio.** A single dose of this vaccine is recommended if you didn't have a polio booster as an adult and are traveling to Africa, Southeast Asia, the South Pacific islands, the Middle East, the Asian subcontinent, eastern Europe or one of the former republics of the Soviet Union.
- **Typhoid.** This vaccination is recommended if you're traveling to any area outside of the United States except Australia, New Zealand, western Europe or Canada. The vaccination is particularly important if you're traveling to developing countries, where typhoid fever is much more prevalent.

# Recommended vaccinations

| Disease | What it is |
| --- | --- |
| Chickenpox (varicella) | A viral disease that spreads easily from person to person. Chickenpox is much more serious in adults than in children. |
| Hepatitis A | A viral infection of the liver transmitted primarily through contaminated food or water or close personal contact. |
| Hepatitis B | A viral infection of the liver that's often transmitted through contaminated blood, sexual contact and prenatal exposure. |
| Influenza (flu) | A respiratory disease that spreads from person to person when you inhale infected droplets from the air. |
| Measles, mumps, rubella | Viral diseases that spread from person to person when you inhale infected droplets from the air. |
| Meningococcal disease | A disease caused by bacteria that can cause meningitis, an inflammation of the membranes surrounding the brain and spinal cord. |
| Pneumonia | An inflammation of the lungs, which can have various causes, such as bacteria or viruses. |
| Tetanus and diphtheria<br><br>or<br><br>Tetanus, diphtheria and pertussis | Tetanus is a bacterial infection that develops in deep wounds. Diphtheria is a bacterial infection spread when you inhale infected droplets from the air.<br><br>Whooping cough (pertussis) causes cold-like signs and symptoms and a persistent hacking cough. |
| Herpes zoster (shingles) | A viral infection that causes a painful rash. It's caused by the varicella-zoster virus — the same virus that causes chickenpox. |

| You're at increased risk if: | Doses for adults |
| --- | --- |
| You're a health care worker without immunity or an adult who has never been exposed to the disease or never been vaccinated. | Two-dose series given four to eight weeks apart. Avoid if you have weakened immunity or lymph node or bone marrow cancer or if you've had a serious allergic reaction to gelatin or the antibiotic neomycin. |
| You are traveling to a country without clean water or proper sewage, you have chronic liver disease or a blood-clotting disorder, use illegal drugs, or are male and homosexual. | Two-dose series with at least six months between doses. Avoid if you're hypersensitive to alum or 2-phenoxyethanol, a preservative. |
| Your occupation puts you at risk of exposure to blood and body fluids, you're on dialysis or have received blood products, or you're sexually active with multiple partners. | Three-dose series given during a six-month period can prevent this disease. Avoid if you're allergic to baker's yeast or if you've had a previous reaction. |
| You are age 50 or older, have a chronic disease or a weakened immune system, work in health care, or have close contact with people who are at high risk of the diease. | One dose every year for all adults. Avoid if you're allergic to eggs or if you've had a previous reaction to a flu shot. A high-dose version of this vaccine is available for adults age 65 and older. This vaccine contains four times as much flu virus antigen — the part of the vaccine that stimulates the immune system — as the standard flu vaccine. This is because older people produce 50 to 75 percent fewer antibodies than do younger adults. |
| You were born after 1956 and don't have proof of previous vaccination or immunity. | One or two doses. Avoid if you received blood products in the past 11 months, have weakened immunity or are allergic to the antibiotic neomycin. |
| You have a compromised immune system or you travel to certain foreign countries. | A single dose can prevent a bacterial form of the illness. |
| You're age 65 or older, you have a medical condition that increases your risk, such as chronic lung, liver or kidney disease, or you don't have a spleen or it's damaged. | One lifetime dose, but you may need a second dose if you're at higher risk or vaccination was before age 65. Need at least five years between doses. |
| You suffered a deep or dirty cut or wound. | Initial three-dose series (Td) with booster every 10 years. If your most recent booster was more than five years ago, get a booster within 48 hours after a wound. |
| You haven't received a previous pertussis vaccination— especially if you have close contact with an infant, for which pertussis is particularly risky. | Initial three-dose series (Tdap) if you didn't finish the Td series as a child. Otherwise, one dose of Tdap when you're due for a Td booster, followed by a Td booster every 10 years. |
| You're older than age 50 and have never had chickenpox. | A single dose. Avoid if you have a weakened immune system or are allergic to gelatin or the antibiotic neomycin. Also avoid if you're receiving treatment with steroids, radiation or chemotherapy. |

- **Yellow fever.** This vaccination is recommended if you're traveling to certain parts of Africa, the Caribbean, Central America or South America.

See your doctor at least four to six weeks before your departure to schedule the vaccinations you need. Some vaccinations require several injections spaced days or weeks apart. For more information on the vaccinations recommended for specific international destinations, visit the CDC's website at *www.cdc.gov/travel*.

# Recommended tests and those to consider

Preventive screening exams are the best way to catch potential problems in their early stages — when the odds for successful treatment are greatest. In the pages that follow, you'll find information on exams or tests generally recommended for people who don't have symptoms or risk factors for a particular medical condition. You'll also find information on additional screening tests you may want to consider.

Remember, these are general guidelines for screening. You and your doctor should determine what tests are best for you and the rightschedule for them. For example, if you're older than age 50 or you're at risk of a particular disease, your doctor may order additional tests or perform certain ones more frequently.

## Recommended tests

Following are tests that you should undergo on a regular basis.

# Preventive screening exams for women

Recommendations are based on average risk and normal results on prior testing.

| Test | Ages 50 to 59 | Ages 60 to 69 | Ages 70 to 79 | Age 80+ |
|---|---|---|---|---|
| Blood cholesterol | At least every 5 years | At least every 5 years | At least every 5 years | At least every 5 years |
| Blood pressure | At least every 2 years | At least every 2 years | At least every 2 years | At least every 2 years |
| Bone density | Ask your doctor | Screening at age 65 | Ask your doctor | Ask your doctor |
| Clinical breast exam and mammogram | Annually | Annually | Annually | Annually |
| Colon cancer | Every 5-10 years (depends on test) | Every 5-10 years (depends on test) | Every 5-10 years (depends on test) | Ask your doctor |
| Dental | Every 6 months to 1 year | Every 6 months to 1 year | Every 6 months to 1 year | Every 6 months to 1 year |
| Diabetes | Every 3 years | Every 3 years | Every 3 years | Every 3 years |
| Eye | Every 2-4 years; yearly if you wear glasses or contacts | Until age 65, every 2-4 years; beginning at age 65, every 1-2 years; yearly if you wear glasses or contacts | Every 1-2 years; yearly if you wear glasses or contacts | Every 1-2 years; yearly if you wear glasses or contacts |
| Pap test | Every 1-3 years | Every 1-3 years | Ask your doctor | Ask your doctor |

# Other tests women should consider

| Test | Ages 50 to 59 | Ages 60 to 69 | Ages 70 to 79 | Age 80+ |
|---|---|---|---|---|
| Hearing | Every 3 years | Every 3 years | Every 3 years | Every 3 years |
| Human papillomavirus (HPV) | Ask your doctor | Ask your doctor | Ask your doctor | Ask your doctor |
| Skin exam | Annually | Annually | Annually | Annually |
| Thyroid-stimulating hormone (TSH) | Ask your doctor | Ask your doctor | Ask your doctor | Ask your doctor |
| Transferrin saturation | Ask your doctor | Ask your doctor | Ask your doctor | Ask your doctor |

# Preventive screening exams for men

Recommendations are based on average risk and normal results on prior testing.

| Test | Ages 50 to 59 | Ages 60 to 69 | Ages 70 to 79 | Age 80+ |
|---|---|---|---|---|
| Blood cholesterol | At least every 5 years | At least every 5 years | At least every 5 years | At least every 5 years |
| Blood pressure | At least every 2 years | At least every 2 years | At least every 2 years | At least every 2 years |
| Colon cancer | Every 5-10 years (depends on test) | Every 5-10 years (depends on test) | Every 5-10 years (depends on test) | Ask your doctor |
| Dental | Every 6 months to 1 year | Every 6 months to 1 year | Every 6 months to 1 year | Every 6 months to 1 year |
| Diabetes | Every 3 years | Every 3 years | Every 3 years | Every 3 years |
| Eye | Every 2-4 years; yearly if you wear glasses or contacts | Until age 65, every 2-4 years; beginning at age 65, every 1-2 years; yearly if you wear glasses or contacts | Every 1-2 years; yearly if you wear glasses or contacts | Every 1-2 years; yearly if you wear glasses or contacts |
| Prostate-specific antigen (PSA) and digital rectal exam | Ask your doctor | Ask your doctor | Ask your doctor | Ask your doctor |

# Other tests men should consider

| Test | Ages 50 to 59 | Ages 60 to 69 | Ages 70 to 79 | Age 80+ |
|---|---|---|---|---|
| Hearing | Every 3 years | Every 3 years | Every 3 years | Every 3 years |
| Skin exam | Annually | Annually | Annually | Annually |
| Thyroid-stimulating hormone (TSH) | Ask your doctor | Ask your doctor | Ask your doctor | Ask your doctor |
| Transferrin saturation | Ask your doctor | Ask your doctor | Ask your doctor | Ask your doctor |

# Blood cholesterol numbers

| Total cholesterol level | Total cholesterol category |
|---|---|
| Less than 200* | Desirable |
| 200 to 239 | Borderline high |
| 240 and above | High |

| LDL** cholesterol level | LDL cholesterol category |
|---|---|
| Less than 100 | Optimal |
| 100 to 129 | Near optimal |
| 130 to 159 | Borderline high |
| 160 to 189 | High |
| 190 and above | Very high |

| HDL*** cholesterol level | HDL cholesterol category |
|---|---|
| Less than 40 for men, less than 50 for women | A major risk factor for heart disease |
| 40 to 59 for men, 50 to 59 for women | The higher, the better |
| 60 and above | Protective against heart disease |

Triglycerides also can raise your risk of heart disease. Levels that are borderline high (150 to 199 mg/dL) or high (200 mg/dL or more) may require treatment.

Source: National Cholesterol Education Program, 2004
*Numbers are expressed in levels of milligrams of cholesterol per deciliter of blood (mg/dL).
**LDL means low-density lipoprotein.***HDL means high-density lipoprotein.

## Blood cholesterol test

A blood cholesterol test is actually several blood tests (serum lipids). It measures total cholesterol in your blood, as well as the levels of low-density lipoprotein (LDL, or "bad") cholesterol, high-density lipoprotein (HDL, or "good") cholesterol and other blood fats called triglycerides.

**What's the test for?** To measure the levels of cholesterol and triglycerides (lipids) in your blood. Undesirable lipid levels raise your risk of heart attack and stroke. Problems occur when your LDL cholesterol forms too many fatty deposits (plaques) on your artery walls or when your HDL cholesterol carries away too few.

**When and how often should you have it?** Have a cholesterol evaluation at least every five years if the levels are within normal ranges. If the readings are abnormal, have your cholesterol checked more often. Cholesterol testing is especially important if you have a family history of high cholesterol or heart disease, are overweight, are physically inactive, or have diabetes. These risk factors put you at increased risk of developing high cholesterol and heart disease.

**What do the numbers mean?** The National Cholesterol Education Program has established guidelines to help determine which numbers are acceptable and which carry increased risk. However, desirable ranges vary, depending on your individual health conditions, habits and family history. Talk with your doctor about what cholesterol levels are best for you and what you can do to maintain or achieve them.

**Blood pressure measurement**
This test — using an inflatable cuff around your arm — measures the peak pressure your heart generates when pumping blood out through your arteries (systolic pressure) and

## Blood pressure numbers

| Top number (systolic) | Bottom number (diastolic) | Category |
| --- | --- | --- |
| lower than 120* and | lower than 80 | Normal** blood pressure |
| 120 to 129 and | lower than 80 | Elevated |
| 130 to 139 or | 80 to 89 | Stage 1 hypertension |
| 140 or higher or | 90 or higher | Stage 2 hypertension |
| higher than 180 and/or | higher than 120 | Hypertensive crisis |

*Numbers are expressed in millimeters of mercury (mm Hg).

**Normal means the preferred range in terms of cardiovascular risk.

Source: Whelten PK, et al. 2017 Guideline for the Prevention, Detection, Evaluation, and Management of High Blood Pressure in Adults.

the amount of pressure in your arteries when your heart is at rest between beats (diastolic pressure).

**What's the test for?** This test is used to detect high blood pressure. If you have high blood pressure, the longer it goes undetected and untreated, the higher your risk of a number of diseases, including heart attack, stroke, heart failure and kidney damage.

**When and how often should you have it?** Have your blood pressure checked at least every two years. However, you'll probably have it checked every time you see a doctor. If your blood pressure is elevated, your doctor may recommend more frequent testing. Testing is especially important if you're black, overweight, inactive or have a family history of the condition. These factors put you at increased risk of high blood pressure.

**What do the numbers mean?** An ideal or normal blood pressure for an adult of any age is 119 millimeters of mercury (mm Hg) over 79 mm Hg or lower. This is commonly written as 119/79 mm Hg.

## Bone density measurement
Bone density is measured by way of a specialized X-ray scan of your lower back and hip region, wrist, or heel.

**What's the test for?** To detect osteoporosis — a disease most common to women that involves gradual loss of bone mass, making your bones more fragile and likely to fracture. Osteoporosis most often increases the risk of fractures of the hip, spine and wrist.

There are several different types of scans available. They include dual energy X-ray absorptiometry (DXA) and computerized tomography (CT).

**When and how often should you have it?** Women should have a baseline exam after menopause. However, if you have a family history of osteoporosis or other risk factors, earlier testing is a good idea.

Risk factors for osteoporosis include early menopause, frequent or extended use of steroid medications, smoking, low body weight, and a history of fractures. Talk with your doctor about a bone density testing schedule that's right for you.

**What do the numbers mean?** The T-score is a number that describes how much your bone density varies from what's considered normal.

"Normal" is based on the typical bone mass of people in their 30s — the period in life when bone mass is at its peak. Peak bone mass varies from one person to another and is influenced by many factors, including heredity, sex and race. Men tend to have higher bone mass than do women, and whites and Asians generally have lower bone density than do blacks and Hispanics.

- T-scores ranging from +1 or higher to -1 mean that your bone density is considered normal, and you're at low risk of bone fractures.
- T-scores ranging from -1 to -2.5 indicate you have relatively low bone mass.

- T-scores of -2.5 and lower indicate you have osteoporosis and are at greater risk of bone fractures.

## Clinical breast exam and mammogram

These two tests are generally done in conjunction with one another.

### Clinical breast exam

A clinical breast exam is a physical check of a woman's breasts and armpits that's typically part of a routine physical.

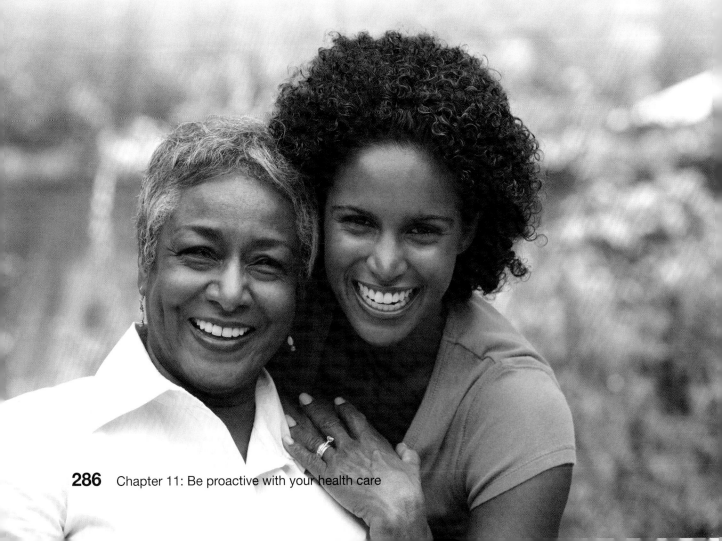

**What's the test for?** To detect cancer and precancerous changes in the breasts. Your doctor examines your breasts, looking for lumps, color changes, skin irregularities and changes in your nipples. He or she then feels for swollen lymph nodes in the armpits.

**When and how often should you have it?** Before age 40, women should have a clinical breast exam at least every three years. For women age 40 and older, the exam is best done every year. Having regular breast exams is particularly important if you have a family history of breast cancer or other factors, including advancing age, which put you at increased risk of breast cancer.

### Mammogram

In this screening test, X-rays are taken of your breast tissue while your breasts are compressed between plates.

**What's the test for?** To help detect cancer and precancerous changes in female breasts. Some small breast lumps and calcifications, which can be the first indication of early-stage breast cancer, are too small to be detected on a physical examination.

**When and how often should you have it?** There's been disagreement in recent years over the best screening schedule for mammograms. In 2009, the U.S. Preventive Services Task Force issued revised mammogram guidelines. They said that screening mammograms should be done every two years beginning at age 50 for women at average risk of breast cancer and that screening mammograms before age 50 should not be done routinely.

These guidelines differ from those of the American Cancer Society (ACS). The ACS mammogram guidelines call for yearly mammogram screening beginning at age 40 for women at average risk of breast cancer.

At Mayo Clinic, the current practice is to continue to recommend an annual screening mammogram beginning at age 40 — this aligns with the ACS recommendation. Screening mammography is not a perfect exam, but it's the best available tool to detect breast cancer early.

Talk with your doctor about a schedule that's right for you. Regular mammograms are particularly important if you have a family history of breast cancer or have had prior abnormal breast biopsies.

If your breasts are sensitive, taking a pain reliever an hour or two before the test may help ease your discomfort.

Avoid using underarm deodorant on the day of your mammogram. It affects the accuracy of the results.

## Colon cancer screening

For this screening exam, a variety of screening tests may be used. You may have just one or a combination.

- **Colonoscopy.** With this exam, a long, flexible tube (colonoscope) is inserted into the rectum, which allows the doctor to examine the entire length of your colon.
- **Virtual colonoscopy.** For this exam, a computerized tomography machine is used to produce cross-sectional images of your abdominal organs, including your colon.
- **Fecal occult blood test.** With this, a stool sample is tested in a lab for hidden (occult) blood.
- **Flexible sigmoidoscopy.** Similar to a colonoscopy, a thin tube is inserted into your rectum. However, this test only evaluates the lower part of the colon (sigmoid colon).
- **Barium enema.** For this test, an X-ray is taken of your colon after you have an enema with a white, chalky substance that outlines the colon (barium X-ray).

**What's the test for?** To detect cancer and precancerous growths (polyps) on the inside wall of the colon that could become cancerous. Many people are afraid to have colon cancer screening because of fear of embarrassment or worry of discomfort. However, this screening could save your life by detecting precancerous polyps that can be removed, preventing this common cancer from occurring. Early detection of cancer can also be lifesaving.

**When and how often should you have it?** If you're at average risk of developing colon cancer, have a screening test every five to 10 years, beginning at age 50. The frequency of screening will depend on the type of test you have.

Talk with your doctor about which screening approach and frequency are best for you, given your particular health issues. If you're at increased risk of developing colon cancer, your doctor may recommend beginning screenings at an earlier age.

## Dental checkup

Your dentist examines your teeth and checks your tongue, lips, mouth and soft tissues.

**What's the test for?** A dental exam is done to detect tooth decay, problems such as tooth grinding and diseases such as periodontal disease. Your

# Prostate-specific antigen (PSA) numbers

| Age | Upper limit | Age | Upper limit |
|---|---|---|---|
| 40 or under | 2.0* | 62 | 4.1 |
| 41 | 2.1 | 63 | 4.2 |
| 42 | 2.2 | 64 | 4.4 |
| 43 | 2.3 | 65 | 4.5 |
| 44 | 2.3 | 66 | 4.6 |
| 45 | 2.4 | 67 | 4.8 |
| 46 | 2.5 | 68 | 4.9 |
| 47 | 2.6 | 69 | 5.1 |
| 48 | 2.6 | 70 | 5.3 |
| 49 | 2.7 | 71 | 5.4 |
| 50 | 2.8 | 72 | 5.6 |
| 51 | 2.9 | 73 | 5.8 |
| 52 | 3.0 | 74 | 6.0 |
| 53 | 3.1 | 75 | 6.2 |
| 54 | 3.2 | 76 | 6.4 |
| 55 | 3.3 | 77 | 6.6 |
| 56 | 3.4 | 78 | 6.8 |
| 57 | 3.5 | 79 | 7.0 |
| 58 | 3.6 | 80 or older | 7.2 |
| 59 | 3.7 | | |
| 60 | 3.8 | | |
| 61 | 4.0 | | |

*Numbers are expressed in nanograms per milliliter (ng/mL).
Source: Mayo Clinic

Beginning at age 65, have an eye exam every year or two. Regular eye exams are especially important if you have diabetes, high blood pressure, or a family history of glaucoma, cataracts or age-related macular degeneration.

## Pap test
In this test, a doctor inserts a plastic or metal speculum into a woman's vagina to observe the cervix. Then, using a soft brush, he or she gently scrapes a few cells from the cervix, places the cells on

# PSA: To test or not?

Use this chart to help you prepare for a conversation with your doctor about prostate-specific antigen (PSA) testing.

| Pros of PSA testing | Cons of PSA testing |
| --- | --- |
| PSA screening may help you detect prostate cancer early. | Some prostate cancers are slow growing and never spread beyond the prostate gland. |
| Cancer is easier to treat and is more likely to be cured if it's diagnosed in the early stages of the disease. | Not all prostate cancers need treatment. Treatment for prostate cancer may have risk and side effects, including urinary incontinence, erectile dysfunction or bowel dysfunction. |
| PSA testing can be done with a simple, widely available blood test. | PSA tests aren't foolproof. It's possible for your PSA levels to be elevated when cancer isn't present and not to be elevated when cancer is present. |
| For some men, knowing is better than not knowing. Having the test can provide you with a certain amount of reassurance — either that you probably don't have prostate cancer or that you do have it and can now have it treated. | A diagnosis of prostate cancer can provoke anxiety and confusion. Concern that the cancer may not be life-threatening can make decision making more complicated. |
| The number of deaths from prostate cancer has gone down since PSA testing became available. | It's not yet clear whether the decrease in deaths from prostate cancer is due to early detection and treatment based on PSA testing or if it's due to other factors. |

a glass slide or in a bottle, and sends the sample to a laboratory for analysis.

**What's the test for?** The Pap test detects cancer and precancerous changes in the cervix.

**When and how often should you have it?** Women should have a Pap test every one to three years. If you've had normal Pap test results for three years in a row, you and your doctor may opt for a longer interval.

For women who've had a total hysterectomy for a noncancerous condition, routine Pap tests aren't necessary. They're also not necessary if you're age 70 or older, you've had normal test results over the past 10 years (including the last three tests), and you aren't at high risk of developing cervical cancer.

When in doubt, ask your doctor what's appropriate for you.

Getting regular Pap tests is especially important if you smoke or have had a sexually transmitted infection or multiple sex partners or if you have a history of cervical, vaginal or vulvar cancer.

### Prostate-specific antigen test and digital rectal exam

The prostate-specific antigen (PSA) test is a blood test that measures the amount of a specific protein secreted by the male prostate gland. A digital rectal exam is a physical exam done by a doctor in which he or she inserts a lubricated, gloved finger into the male rectum and feels the prostate gland for enlargement, tenderness, lumps or hard spots.

**What are the tests for?** The digital rectal exam can detect prostate enlargement or prostate cancer. Don't be alarmed if your doctor tells you that your prostate gland is enlarged. More than half of men older than age 50 have an enlarged prostate caused by a noncancerous condition called benign prostatic hyperplasia (BPH).

With the PSA test, increased PSA levels may indicate prostate cancer. However, other noncancerous conditions can elevate PSA.

**When and how often should you have them?** Professional organizations vary in their recommendations about who should — and who shouldn't — get a PSA screening text. Organizations that do recommend PSA screening generally encourage the test annually in men between the ages of 40 and 75, and in younger men with an increased risk of prostate cancer due to their race or family history. Talk with your doctor about what's right for you.

**What do the numbers mean?** The age-adjusted PSA scale (see page 291) shows the normal upper PSA limits, based on the PSA test used at Mayo Clinic. Upper limits increase almost every year as you age. If your PSA level is above the normal upper limit for your age, talk with your doctor about what your next step should be. Even if your PSA is normal but it has increased substantially, further testing may be warranted.

## Tests to consider

The screening exams that follow are recommended for some individuals, depending on their health and personal risk factors. Talk with your doctor to see if any of these tests may be appropriate for you.

## Full-body skin examination

In this exam your doctor examines your skin from head to toe, looking for moles and spots that are irregularly shaped, have varied colors, are asymmetrical, are greater than the size of a pencil eraser, bleed or have changed since the previous visit.

**What's the test for?** To check for signs of skin cancer, or other skin changes that may put you at increased risk of skin cancer.

**When and how often should you have it?** Have a full-body skin exam every three years in your 20s and 30s. Once you turn 40, have the exam every two years. Once you turn 50, have it every year.

Regular screening for skin cancer is especially important if you have many moles, fair skin, sun-damaged skin, a family history of skin cancer or if you've had two or more blistering sunburns in childhood or adolescence. These factors put you at increased risk of developing skin cancer.

## Hearing test

During a hearing test, a doctor checks how well you recognize speech and sounds at various volumes and frequencies.

**What's the test for?** To check for hearing loss, which becomes more common with increased age.

**When and how often should you have it?** Have your hearing checked every 10 years until age 50. Starting at age 50, have it checked every three years.

Hearing tests are especially important if you've been exposed to loud noises through your job or recreational activities, have had frequent ear infections, or are older than age 60. These factors increase your risk of hearing loss.

## Hepatitis screening

This is a simple blood test.

**What's the test for?** The test is used to screen for chronic hepatitis B or C. Hepatitis is an inflammation of the liver. People with chronic hepatitis B or C, caused by a viral infection, are at greater risk of liver disease and liver cancer.

**When and how often should you have it?** Have a baseline test if you have one or more risk factors for hepatitis B or C. Risk factors include being exposed to human blood or body fluids, having had multiple sex partners, having received a blood transfusion before 1993, and living or traveling in an area where hepatitis B is common.

## Human papillomavirus screening

This test is an additional screening option for cervical cancer that typically accompanies a Pap test.

**What's the test for?** It's done to check for the presence of a high-risk strain of the human papillomavirus (HPV). Almost all cervical cancers are linked to infection with a high-risk strain of this virus.

**When and how often should you have it?** The HPV test involves the same method used to collect cervical cells during a Pap test. In fact, the test can be done at the same time as a Pap test.

If your Pap test indicates the presence of abnormal cells and you didn't have an accompanying HPV test, you should request one. Although there's no known cure for HPV infection, the cervical changes that result from it can be treated.

## Thyroid-stimulating hormone test

This is a simple blood test.

What's the test for? This test measures the level of thyroid-stimulating hormone (TSH) in your blood, helping to determine whether your thyroid gland is functioning properly. TSH, made by the brain's pituitary gland, stimu-lates the thyroid gland to produce the hormone thyroxine. Sometimes, the thyroid produces too little thyroxine (possible hypothyroidism) or too much (possible hyperthyroidism).

**When and how often should you have it?** Experts disagree about who can benefit from screening and at what age to begin. Talk with your doctor about a screening schedule that's right for you. If you have high cholesterol, a family history of thyroid problems or symp-toms of a thyroid condition, such as in-creased irritability or sluggishness, you may need more-frequent testing than do others in the general population.

## Transferrin saturation test

This is a simple blood test that mea-sures the amount of iron bound to an iron-carrying protein (transferrin) in your bloodstream.

**What's the test for?** It can detect hemo-chromatosis, also called iron overload disease, a condition in which your body stores too much iron. Excessive iron can damage your organs and lead to diabe-tes, heart disease and liver disease. He-mochromatosis is an underrecognized but treatable hereditary disease.

**When and how often should you have it?** Doctors don't regularly test for hemochromatosis, but talk with your doctor about testing if you have a family history of the disease or you have a condition that can be caused by hemochromatosis. They include joint disease, severe and continuing fatigue, heart disease, elevated liver enzymes, erectile dysfunction, and diabetes. Some experts recommend a baseline test around age 30, with periodic repeat testing.

# Managing your medications

If you're fortunate, you don't have to take any medications. But the fact is, as you get older, the odds that you'll need to take a medication at some point increase.

Medications serve a vital role in maintaining good health, and taking a drug doesn't mean that your health is poor. When used with care, medications can mean improved quality of life — and sometimes the difference between life and death. But almost anything with the power to heal also carries the power to harm, when used incorrectly.

If you take medication regularly, remember these important tips:

- **Be sure your doctor knows about all the medications you're taking, including over-the-counter medicines, vitamins and supplements.** Before your appointments, list all the medications, vitamins and supplements you take, or bring the bottles with you. This allows your doctor to make sure the products aren't causing symptoms or interacting with each other.
- **For each medication you take, you should know what it is, why you're taking it, how to take it and for how long to take it.** If you don't have this information, ask your doctor to provide it. It may be helpful to create a medication log and carry it with you.
- **If possible, use one pharmacy for filling all of your prescriptions.** This will help your pharmacist detect whether there are duplications or adverse interactions with your medications.
- **Use your pharmacist as a resource.** If any instructions on a medication label are unclear, ask your pharmacist to clarify. If your prescription looks different from what you expected, ask your pharmacist why.
- **Develop a routine so that you remember to take your medications at the right time.** Use reminders if you need to, such as pillbox com-

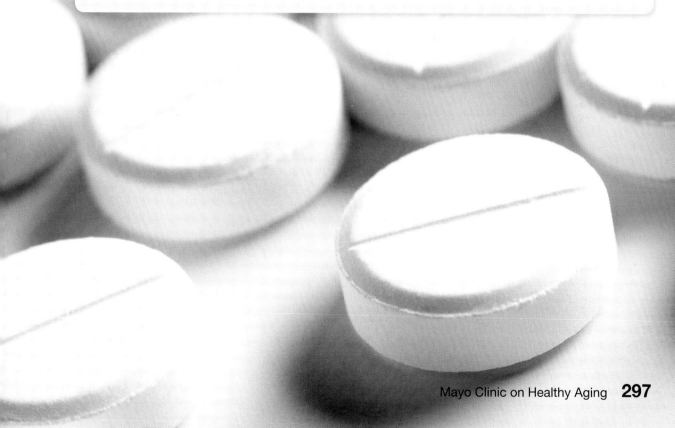

## Disposing of unused medications

According to the Food and Drug Administration (FDA), it's important to take certain precautions before tossing out unused drugs. Here are the guidelines for disposing of them safely.

- Follow any specific disposal instructions listed on the drug label or on information that accompanies the medication. Or you can ask your pharmacist. Don't flush prescription drugs down the toilet unless specifically instructed to do so.
- Take advantage of community drug take-back programs. These programs allow you to bring in unused medications to a central location for proper disposal.
- If no instructions are available and no take-back program is offered in your area, put your unused drugs in the trash. But first, take them out of their original containers and mix them with an undesirable substance, such as used coffee grounds or kitty litter. This way, the drug will be less appealing to children and pets, and unrecognizable to anyone who may come upon it.

partments, medication containers with alarms, reminder watches, charts or calendars.

- **Always take your medication as directed.** Don't stop taking it just because you're feeling better, unless your doctor instructs you to do so.
- **Don't take medications with alcohol, hot drinks, or vitamin or mineral supplements.** These combinations can all cause drug interactions. Also, don't stir drugs into food unless the label says to do so.
- **Don't take medication prescribed for another person, and never give your medicine to anyone else.** What helps you might harm others and vice versa.
- **Store your medications in their original labeled containers.** Otherwise, you may forget what the drug is and when it expires.
- **Don't store your medications in the bathroom, near the kitchen sink, on a windowsill or in your car.** Moisture, heat and direct light can change a medication's strength. Better storage options are a high kitchen cabinet or bedroom dresser drawer, out of the reach of children and pets.
- **Periodically get rid of unused, unlabeled or outdated drugs.** Medication deteriorates over time. If a medication has changed from its original form or has an unusual odor, dispose of it and replace as needed. See "Disposing of unused medications" on page 297 for tips on getting rid of old drugs safely.

Remember that while medications can be a marvel, they can also be dangerous and even deadly when used improperly. Even nonprescription medications can cause side effects and be dangerous if misused. Follow the same safety precautions for over-the-counter products as you do for prescription medications.

# Part 3

# Other important issues

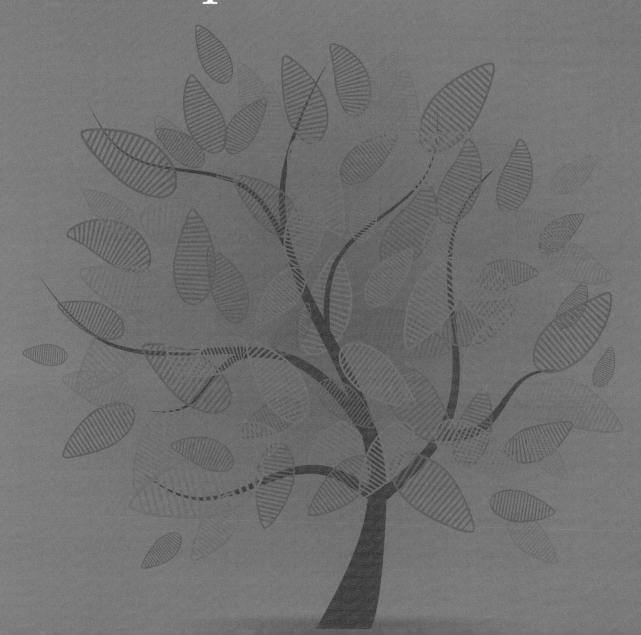

# Chapter 12

# Insurance issues

Reading about topics such as health insurance and long-term care insurance isn't exactly exciting or intellectually stimulating. But these are very important matters, especially within the context of aging. As you enter your second 50 years — the time in your life when you're most likely to need medical care — it's important that you have appropriate health insurance.

Making sure you have adequate health insurance is more than just a smart financial move. Good insurance also can affect your health. How so? You're more likely to see a doctor for preventive care and when a problem arises if you know that your insurance will help cover the cost. This results in earlier diagnosis and treatment of illness, which is typically when the chances of a cure are greatest.

A good health insurance plan also reduces stress. Instead of worrying how you'll pay your latest bill, you can concentrate on other more enjoyable — and less stressful — matters, and hopethis will fully allow you to enjoy some of your financial resources. Ultimately, it's reassuring to know that you're covered if a health problem or incident were to occur.

This chapter aims to give you an overview of health insurance, including specifics on Medicare and other plans. We also talk about long-term care insurance and who might benefit most from this type of insurance. Where possible, you'll be pointed toward additional resources that offer more-detailed information, which can help you make appropriate decisions based on your particular needs.

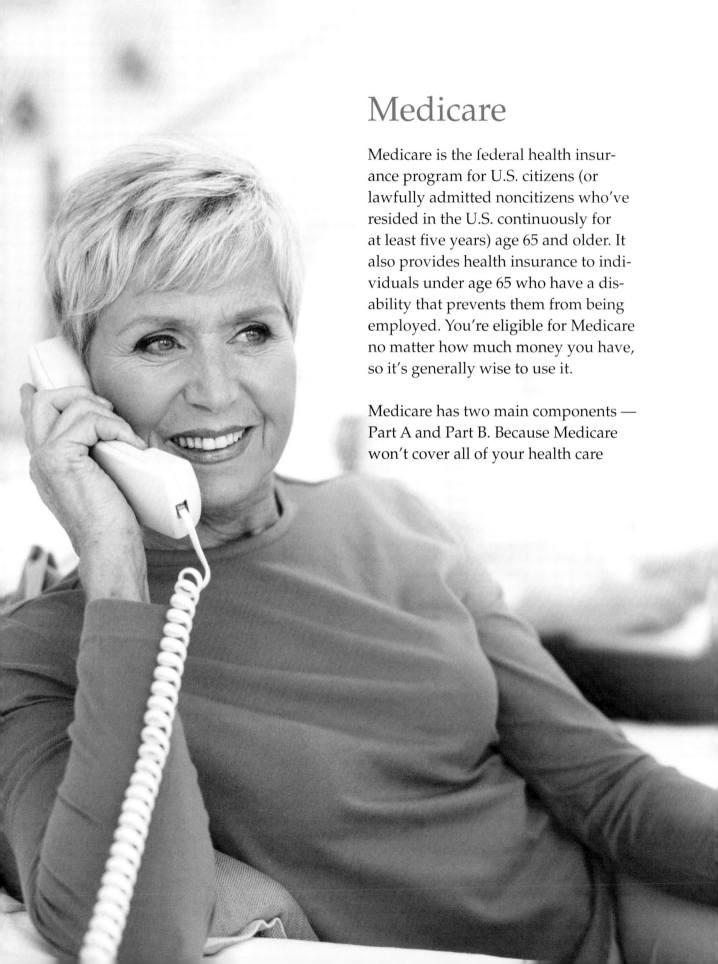

# Medicare

Medicare is the federal health insurance program for U.S. citizens (or lawfully admitted noncitizens who've resided in the U.S. continuously for at least five years) age 65 and older. It also provides health insurance to individuals under age 65 who have a disability that prevents them from being employed. You're eligible for Medicare no matter how much money you have, so it's generally wise to use it.

Medicare has two main components — Part A and Part B. Because Medicare won't cover all of your health care expenses, you have a number of options to supplement your basic Medicare insurance.

## Medicare Part A

If you're already receiving Social Security benefits, you're automatically enrolled in Medicare Part A.

Even if your Social Security benefits don't begin until a later age or you don't plan on retiring until later, you're still eligible for Medicare at age 65.

Part A pays for most of these services:

- Hospital stays in a semiprivate room, including mental health care
- Post-hospitalization skilled nursing care, including rehabilitative services, for a limited time
- Home health care visits from a nurse or therapist and durable medical equipment such as a wheelchair or hospital bed
- Hospice care, including drugs for pain relief and symptom control

As long as you or your spouse paid Medicare taxes while working, you don't pay premiums for Part A, but you do pay deductibles — $1,184 for one- to 60-day hospital stays in 2013 — and

you do pay copays. Copay amounts are subject to annual changes by Congress.

## Medicare Part B

You can enroll in Part B, which is optional, during the seven-month period that begins three months before the month of your 65th birthday and ends three months after the month of your 65th birthday. If you miss this enrollment period, you can join during any general enrollment period, held every year from Jan. 1 through March 31. Be aware that the cost of Part B increases the longer you wait to enroll.

If you're working past your 65th birthday and you're receiving health insurance coverage from your employer, you can delay enrollment in Part B until this coverage ends or your employment ends — or join anytime you're still covered through your current employment — without paying extra. Talk with an insurance adviser to learn more about this special enrollment period if it may apply to you.

Medicare Part B pays for some or most of these services:

- Visits to your health care provider. This includes a one-time "Welcome to Medicare" preventive visit within the first year of obtaining Part B, and a yearly "wellness visit" to assess your health and risk factors once you've had Part B for more than 12 months.

- Outpatient hospital care, including outpatient physical or speech therapy
- Flu and pneumoccal vaccinations, and hepatitis B vaccinations for people considered at high risk.
- Second opinions for nonemergency surgery
- Home health care
- Laboratory services
- Some medical equipment and supplies
- Preventive screenings, including mammograms and colonoscopies
- Adult care, mental health treatment and some counseling
- Alzheimer's-related therapy
- Weight-loss therapy
- Tobacco cessation counseling

Part B does not cover:

- Treatment that isn't deemed medically necessary, such as cosmetic surgery or alternative therapies
- Other vaccinations
- Most medications, with the exception of some administered by a medical professional, such as some

immunosuppressant, anti-cancer and dialysis drugs
- Hearing and routine eye exams
- General dental work or dentures
- Acupuncture

You pay a monthly premium for Part B. In 2013, the standard monthly premium was approximately $105, which is deducted automatically from your Social Security check if you receive one. This premium usually increases every January.

In addition, you pay an annual deductible, currently $147. After you've paid the deductible for the year, you pay 20 percent of the amount Medicare has agreed to pay your health care provider. For example, if Medicare allows $100 for your doctor visit, you pay $20 (20 percent of $100). Some services are covered 100 percent, such as home health care visits, laboratory services, and flu and pneumonia shots. Other services, such as outpatient mental health treatment, are covered at only 50 percent of the approved amount. You pay the other 50 percent.

You may have heard the expression "accepting Medicare assignment." Doctors who accept assignment have agreed to charge you no more than what Medicare is willing to pay. You

# Finding out more about Medicare

Navigating through the ins and outs of Medicare and all of its plans can be an overwhelming task, but there are a number of resources to help you:

**Medicare's website.** Medicare has an interactive online tool called the Medicare Plan Finder that lists Medigap and Medicare Advantage and other supplemental policies in your ZIP code area. The organization also has a number of helpful publications. You can get free copies of these publications by visiting Medicare's website, *www.medicare.gov*, or by calling (800) 633-4227. There's an additional portal within the Medicare site that provides free access to personalized information about your current Medicare benefits and services. To access this, register at *www.mymedicare.gov.*

**State health insurance department.** Every state has a program — often called the state health insurance assistance program (SHIP) — to help people sort out Medicare issues, Medigap policies and managed care plans. SHIP staff not only can assist you with information regarding Medicare but also may often be able to help you sift through various policies and help you find the pros and cons of each. Check your local phone directory for the toll-free number, or visit *www.shiptalk.org.*

**Insurance agent.** An insurance agent can help you find a supplemental health insurance policy, but agents generally work with certain companies. To get a broad selection, talk to more than one insurance agent.

**Medical personnel.** Medical social workers at many hospitals and clinics can help you understand your choices and navigate the system.

**Friends and family.** Ask around. Your friends and extended family members may be able to give you valuable firsthand reports on how well different Medicare plans fit their needs.

still pay the copay and deductible, but you don't pay anything beyond that. Ask your doctor in advance if he or she accepts Medicare assignment. If not, your expenses may be higher.

# Getting medicare coverage

Medicare offers several types of health plans, with varying amounts of coverages and varying costs. No matter which you pick, you're still in the Medicare program.

## Original Medicare

This is the traditional basic plan you're automatically enrolled in unless you choose another privately funded option. Most people stay with Original Medicare. It pays Medicare's share of your costs under Parts A and B. You pay the balance. You receive all services Medicare covers, but no extra benefits.

## Medigap policies

Since Original Medicare isn't designed to cover all of your medical expenses,

you may wish to consider buying a supplemental insurance policy. More than half of Medicare recipients age 65 or older purchase private insurance to supplement their Original Medicare. These are commonly called Medigap policies because they pay for gaps in coverage — things that Original Medicare doesn't pay for.

All private insurance companies that sell Medigap policies offer Plan A. Other options available — including Plans B, C, D, F, G, K, L, M and N — vary depending on your insurance company and state laws. All Medigap plans are required to offer basic benefits including coverage of:

- Medicare Part A copayment during a hospital stay plus an additional 365 days after Medicare's coverage ends
- Medicare Part B copayments
- The first three pints of blood each year for blood transfusions

Some levels help pay limited amounts for prescription drugs, but policies sold after Jan. 1, 2006, aren't allowed to include prescription drug coverage. Instead, you're eligible to participate in the Medicare Prescription Drug Plan — otherwise known as Medicare Part D (see page 310).

Currently, Medigap policies on the market don't cover:

- Long-term care
- Routine eye or dental care
- Hearing aids
- Private-duty nursing

Insurance companies must enroll you in the Medigap plan of your choice if you apply within six months in which you're both age 65 and enrolled in Part B. During this time, insurance companies can't deny you coverage, place conditions on your policy or charge you more because of pre-existing health conditions. They must also shorten the waiting period for pre-existing conditions based on your previous health care coverage.

This open enrollment period is offered only once for an individual. If you miss it, you may not be able to purchase the policy you want later or you may have to pay more for it. One significant advantage is that your Medigap insurer must renew your policy for life provided you pay your premiums. You can switch to a different Medigap policy, but certain rules apply.

You will need only one Medigap policy to supplement your Original Medicare plan. In fact, it's illegal for an insur-ance company to sell you a policy that duplicates coverage you already have. However, your Medigap policy applies only to you. You and your spouse must purchase separate Medigap policies.

## Medicare Advantage (Medicare Part C)

The Medicare Advantage Plan, commonly known as Medicare Part C, is designed to cover gaps in Original Medicare, as well. But with this choice of Medicare, you receive your health care entirely through a managed care plan. This plan might be a health maintenance organization (HMO) or a preferred provider organization (PPO).

Managed care plans are based on the same idea: A limited network of doctors and hospitals provides care for you, often at a lower out-of-pocket cost to you than if you were insured by Original Medicare.

To join Medicare Part C, you need to have both Medicare Part A and Part B. You'll need to pay the premium for Part B to Medicare, and you may need to pay an additional premium to the managed care plan. However, these premiums are generally less expensive than are premiums for Medigap policies.

Some managed care plans charge no premium at all. You don't need a separate Medigap policy if you join a Medicare managed care plan. That's because the managed care plan agrees to cover some of the same services Medigap plans do.

When you enroll in a managed care plan, Medicare pays the plan a fixed amount no matter how many services you need. That means the health plan has a financial incentive to restrict services. For example, you may only be able to see the doctors and hospitals that are in the managed care plan's network. For that reason, managed care plans may not be a good choice if you travel frequently or live in another country for part of the year.

Managed care plans might save you money if you follow plan rules and get only the care your plan approves. In some cases you might also get additional benefits, such as prescription drug coverage and vision or dental care. However, these plans may not cover hospice care.

These plans offer the best benefits in states that receive higher Medicare reimbursements from the federal government — often but not always the more populated states.

## Private Fee-for-Service (PFFS) Plans

In this type of Medicare Advantage Plan, you choose a private insurance plan that accepts Medicare beneficiaries. Private fee-for-service plans offer more flexibility than managed care plans in that you're not restricted to particular networks of health care providers — you can see any doctor or go to any hospital in the country that accepts the plan's payment terms. However, in return for this flexibility, you typically pay higher premiums and out-of-pocket expenses.

To enroll, you must have Medicare Part A and Part B. You don't need a Medigap policy if you have this type of Medicare plan.

The private insurance company, not Medicare, decides how much it will pay for services and how much you will pay. You get all the services covered in Medicare Parts A and B. You may also get additional benefits not offered by Original Medicare.

With a PFFS plan, you still pay the Part B premium to Medicare and usually an additional monthly premium to the insurance company. You'll likely have a copay for each visit or service provided, as well.

# Bridging the 'donut hole'

Most Medicare drug plans have a coverage gap (also called the "donut hole"). This means that there's a temporary limit on what the drug plan will cover for drugs. Not everyone will enter the coverage gap — it begins after you and your drug plan have spent a certain amount for covered drugs.

Currently, once you enter the coverage gap, you get more than a 50 percent discount on covered brand-name drugs and more than 20 percent off generic drugs. And although you'll only pay a percentage of the price for that drug, the entire price will count as out-of-pocket spending, which will help you get out of the coverage gap.

Here are some ways to lower your costs while in the donut hole:
- **Generics or other lower cost drugs.** Talk to your doctor to find out if there are generic or less-expensive brand-name drugs that would work just as well as the ones you're taking now.
- **Pharmaceutical Assistance Programs.** Some drug companies offer help for people enrolled in Medicare Part D. Find out whether there's a pharmaceutical assistance program for the drug you take by visiting *www.medicare.gov/pharmaceutical-assistance-program/index.aspx.*
- **State Pharmaceutical Assistance Programs.** Many states also offer help paying drug plan premiums and other drug costs. Find out if your state has a program by visiting *www.medicare.gov/pharmaceutical-assistance-program/state-programs.aspx.*
- **Social Security assistance.** Medicare and Social Security have a program for people with limited income that helps you with prescription drug costs. You can learn more at *www.ssa.gov/prescriptionhelp* or by calling 800-772-1213.
- **National and Community-Based Charitable Programs.** There are charitable groups that offer programs to help with drug costs. Learn about the programs available in your area by visiting *www.benefits-checkup.org.*

### Special needs plans (SNP)

This type of Medicare Advantage Plan is designed to focus on specific groups of people, such as individuals in long-term care facilities or people with a particular chronic disease like cancer or dementia. These plans seek to provide more-targeted health care to meet the special needs of a covered group in a more efficient and effective manner. To find out if any specialty plans are available in your area, call Medicare or log on to its website (see page 305).

## Medicare Prescription Drug Plan (Medicare Part D)

Separate from the other plans listed, Medicare also offers plans through private companies to cover some prescription drug costs. This is known as Medicare Part D. Participation is voluntary. To enroll, you must have Medicare Part A or Part B. The drug coverage may come as part of a Medicare Advantage (Part C) plan or as a stand-alone plan that works with Original Medicare.

In general, this is how the standard Medicare drug benefit works as of 2013. After you pay a $325 deductible for the year, your plan will pay 75 percent of the next $2,610 you spend on prescriptions. Once your total prescription expenses for the year reach $2,970 (including the deductible), you enter the no-coverage zone — sometimes called the donut hole. While in this coverage gap, you pay 47.5 percent of the plan's cost for covered brand-name prescription drugs and 79 percent of the plan's cost for covered generic drugs. (See page 309 for more information.) These costs apply until your total out-of-pocket expenses have reached $4,750. After this, you will pay a small amount for each covered drug — $2.65 for generic or preferred drugs and $6.60 for all other drugs (or 5 percent, whichever is greater) — for the rest of the year.

Other options — including prescription drug plans with smaller premiums and lower deductibles — are also available.

# Making a decision

When choosing a Medicare plan that's right for you, keep the following points in mind:

## Coverage away from home

If you travel often or you live in another part of the country for part of the year, make sure that your plan covers you while you're away from home. Managed care plans offer only limited coverage while you're away from home.

In addition, Medicare doesn't cover care received in a foreign country, although some private health insurance plans may provide this benefit.

If you're taking a trip outside of the country, you may wish to purchase a temporary, one-time health insurance policy that will cover you while you're away. These are often available through your travel agent.

## Specialists when you want them

Medigap and fee-for-service plans let you see any specialist whenever you want to. Most managed care plans require you to see specialists who are part of the plan's network. Often you must get a referral from your regular doctor first. Make sure the specialists you desire are part of your plan's network. If they aren't, you'll pay much more out of pocket when you see them.

## Limited budget

Medicaid is a government program that helps people with low incomes pay medical bills. To qualify for Medicaid, you and your spouse must have a low income and only a few assets. If you're eligible for Medicaid, it acts like a Medigap policy. The lower your income and assets are, the more Medicaid helps

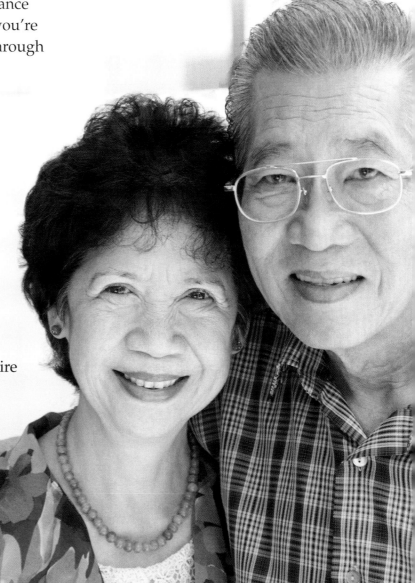

pay for your Medicare out-of-pocket expenses. Medicaid also pays for nursing homes and other long-term care.

Each state has different Medicaid rules. To find out if you qualify in your state, call your state's department of social or human services.

## Employer-based coverage

Not everyone retires at age 65, so you may still be receiving health insurance coverage from your employer when you become eligible for Medicare. Usually, employers require that you sign up for basic Medicare when you become eligible but offer their group health insurance benefits in conjunction with Medicare.

If you work for a company with more than 20 employees, your work health insurance remains the primary payer for your health care bills even after you join Medicare. As a result, you may wish to delay enrolling in Medicare Part B. Otherwise, you're paying a premium for services that are likely already covered under your work health insurance. If you work for a smaller company (fewer than 20 employees), Medicare is the primary payer. In this case, talk to your health benefits ad-

ministrator at work before making a decision about enrollment.

Some companies offer health insurance benefits as part of a retirement package. Even if you're eligible for work-related health insurance, it may be worth your while to compare plans offered through your current or former employer with Medicare plans to see which offers the best value.

# Long-term care insurance

Long-term care insurance may provide some financial protection if you're unable to care for yourself because of a chronic illness, disability or mental impairment, such as Alzheimer's disease.

Long-term care insurance is designed to help pay the cost of long-term medical care, protecting your savings and other assets. This type of insurance generally covers a wide variety of services, from the cost of home health care to monthly nursing home payments.

Long-term care is often very expensive and generally isn't covered by Medicare or involves substantial copayments. According to the latest figures from the National Center for Health Statistics, average charges for residing in a nursing home run close to $4,000 a month, or $48,000 a year. Other figures estimate double that amount.

When thinking about long-term care insurance, it's important to consider all the pros and cons.

## Do you need it?

Some of the reasons why people buy long-term care insurance include:

- Protecting assets you plan to leave to heirs
- Preventing the need for your family to take care of you or pay your bills
- Avoiding being dependent on the government for long-term care

Most of all, people buy long-term care insurance for peace of mind. But did you know that most people never end up staying in nursing homes, and of those who do, the majority are there for only a short period of time?

Family and friends remain the primary caregivers, not institutions. However, this could change as families become more spread out and fragmented.

Consider the following statistics:

- There were 39.6 million people age 65 and older in the U.S. in 2009. Of these, 2.8 million — or 7.1 percent — had a nursing home stay. Of those age 85 and older, 21.5 percent had a nursing home stay.
- Of the people who stay in a nursing home, 60 percent are there only temporarily, usually for less than a year.
- The average stay for permanent nursing home residents is two and a half years.
- Most people who need long-term care — about 80 percent — live at home or in a community setting such as assisted living.
- The average stay in an assisted living residence is more than two years.
- Of older adults who don't live in a nursing home and need long-term care, about two-thirds depend on family and friends alone for help, 28 percent use a combination of family help and paid help, and 8 percent use paid help alone.

As you can see, your chances of an extended stay in a nursing home are fairly low. This is not to say that long-term care insurance can't be useful. Such insurance may help for other types of care, especially home health care or assisted living. However, long-

## Need some help?

Long-term care insurance can be complicated. It's a good idea to talk to an expert before you buy. Financial advisers and attorneys who specialize in long-term care insurance can help you decide if you need a policy. They can also help you understand the fine print.

All states offer free health insurance counseling. Contact your local Area Agency on Aging, or you can call the Eldercare Locator service, which offers a free directory of aging services in every state. The phone number is (800) 677-1116, or you enter your location into their website at *www.eldercare.gov.*

The following organizations also can provide more information:

- AARP, formerly known as the American Association of Retired Persons *(www.aarp.org)*
- Centers for Medicare & Medicaid Services *(www.cms.gov)*
- Consumer Reports *(www.consumerreports.org)*
- Insure.com *(www.insure.com)*

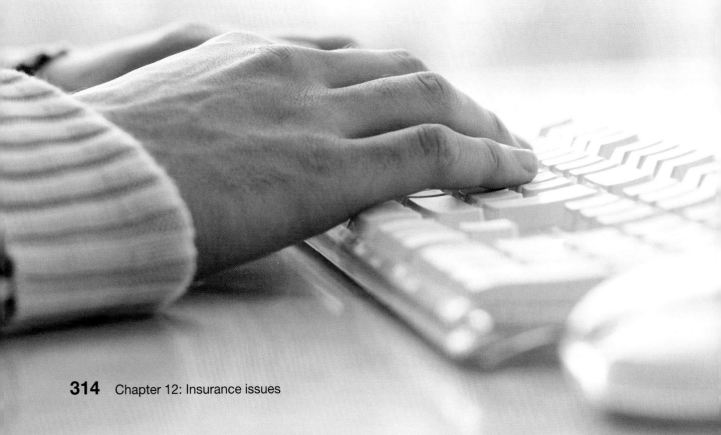

term care isn't the best choice for everyone, and knowing the facts may help you in your purchase decisions.

## Who should buy it?

A long-term care insurance policy is most appropriate for people whose income is in the middle-class range and who have a limited amount of assets they want to protect. *Consumer Reports*, for example, puts the middle-class income range at a net worth — all of your assets minus any debt or liabilities — between $200,000 and $1.5 million.

If you do purchase long-term care insurance — or are considering it — keep these points in mind: As a general rule, don't use more than 5 to 7 percent of your annual income to pay for premiums. Also, don't purchase a policy if paying the premium forces you to change your lifestyle or if you can't afford premium increases of 20 to 30 percent during the policy's lifetime.

If your net worth is less than $200,000, your smartest choice will probably be to rely on Medicaid to pay for any long-term care that becomes necessary, once you have paid what you can. If your net worth is more than $1.5 million, you can most likely pay for any long

term care yourself without exhausting your funds. In fact, some authorities recommend forgoing long-term care insurance if your net worth is more than $500,000.

If you have questions about whether long-term care insurance is for you, you may wish to consult a financial adviser. He or she can help you sort through the pros and cons of purchasing a policy based on your finances.

## At what age should you buy it?

In general, the younger you are when you buy a long-term care insurance policy, the lower your premiums will be. But if you buy it too young, you may pay many years of unnecessary premiums. You might not use your policy until you're in your late 70s or 80s. In addition, new types of care may be developed that aren't covered by current policies.

Decide when to buy based on your health, family medical history and finances. Many experts agree that a good time for most healthy adults to buy is when they're in their 60s. Other experts recommend buying a policy within 10 years of expected use.

Insurance company representatives may tell you that your premiums will generally stay the same once you lock in at a certain age. However, premiums can be — and often are — increased to cover inflation and other costs.

# What to look for

Buying insurance is always somewhat of a gamble because you never know exactly what kind of coverage you'll need. Here are some things to be aware of that may help you get the best policy for your money.

One caution: Be sure that the policy you choose explains your benefits very specifically so that later you're not stuck in a dispute with your insurance company over the interpretation of the benefits listed. In addition, look for a policy that allows you a 30-day free look. A free look gives you the option of returning the policy for a full premium refund if you aren't satisfied with the coverage.

### Company reputation
Choose an insurance company that will be able to back your claims when it becomes necessary. You don't want a company that's going to go under after years of receiving your premiums.

It's generally wise to select a company that's been around for at least 10 years. You can also check company ratings with rating agencies. Look for a rating of AAA or A+.

### Range of services
It's a good idea to buy a policy that's fairly flexible in terms of its coverage. Ideally, a policy would cover at-home care — including adult care, hospice services and respite care — and care in an assisted living facility as well as in a nursing home. Some policies also cover home modifications, such as ramps and railings.

Look for a policy that covers at-home services at the same rate as nursing home services.

### Maximum daily benefit
The maximum daily benefit is how many dollars a day a policy pays for care. This may vary according to the type of care received. For example, benefit payments for home care are usually less than payments for nursing home care.

Many companies today offer policies with pooled benefits, which means they pay a fixed amount a day, month or year regardless of the type of care you use. As a general rule, you should buy enough coverage to pay for at least two-thirds to three-fourths of the daily nursing home costs in your area.

### Duration of benefit

Most people buy long-term care policies that pay for two to six years of coverage. Remember that the average nursing home stay for permanent residents is 2½ years, so a policy that pays for three to four years should be adequate for most people.

A four-year policy doesn't mean that you get benefits for only four years. It means your benefits last until four years' worth of the maximum daily benefit has been used.

### Inflation protection

You'll pay more for a policy with inflation protection, but it's usually worth it in the long run.

The costs of long-term care are rising steadily. It could be many years before you use your policy. Inflation protection increases your benefit amounts so that they keep pace with rising costs.

### One-time elimination period

An elimination period is the number of days you agree to pay for your care out of pocket before the policy starts paying.

For example, if you choose a policy with a 90-day elimination period — which is common — and need nursing home care at $100 a day, you must pay the first $9,000. Shorter elimination periods cost more. Avoid policies that require you to meet the elimination period each time you need care.

### Premium waiver

If you have a premium waiver in your policy, you're not required to pay premiums once you or your spouse enters a nursing home or is receiving home care. You will start paying premiums again when you're no longer receiving these services.

Read the policy carefully to make sure you don't have to be receiving care for a certain length of time before you can stop paying your premiums.

### Nonforfeiture benefits

Some policies allow holders, for an added fee, to reclaim some of their investment if they decide to drop coverage. This can be in the form of cash, typically a percentage of the premiums you paid, or in the form of a shortened benefit period.

For example, you may still receive some long-term care benefits after you drop the coverage but at the expense of a reduced benefit period. But make sure you can afford the premiums for the life of the policy before you think about adding on this potentially expensive rider.

### Benefit triggers

Benefit triggers are requirements that you must meet before the policy begins to pay for the services provided:

- **Pre-existing conditions.** Policies often require a period of time to pass before they pay for care related to a problem you had when you became insured.
- **Activities of daily living (ADLs).** These include things such as bathing, eating, dressing and using the bathroom. Many policies start to pay when you can no longer perform two ADLs. It's a good idea to make sure bathing is one of the trigger ADLs because that's often the first activity people need help with.
- **Household chores.** If you buy a policy that pays for home care, decide if you want to have benefits trigger once you need people to help cook and clean.
- **Doctor approval.** Look for a policy that allows your doctor to give approval for when you're eligible to receive benefits.

# Chapter 13

# Future health planning issues

Decisions regarding your health continue throughout your life. Even at the end of life, there are important decisions to be made. That doesn't mean, though, that you should wait until your final days to make these crucial decisions or to let your wishes be known to others.

One of the most important steps that you can take in the prime of your life — when you're healthy and able to have a discussion with your family — is to let your thoughts be known regarding your final days — how you'd like to spend them and whether you'd like measures to be taken to extend your life, if possible.

It may be difficult to think about such things, but it's important that you do. Letting your wishes be known helps ensure that if you're incapacitated or dying, matters will be taken care of in the manner you prefer. And it also benefits your family by providing guidance in medical and ethical issues that are potentially divisive and costly.

## Advance directives

With the advent of modern medications, surgical techniques and life-sustaining technologies, medicine has become increasingly capable of prolonging the life and easing the pain of seriously ill people. Sometimes, death due to natural failure of the heart, lungs or other organs can be postponed with life-prolonging measures.

One of the most important things that you can do with your doctor and your family is to have a frank discussion about how you wish to be treated when you don't have the capacity to make decisions for yourself, such as when you're unconscious or too sick to communicate.

Under these circumstances, an advance directive can guide your family and caretakers. An advance directive is a legal document that spells out the types of medical treatments and life-sustaining measures you do or do not want. It may also specify an individual that you've appointed to make medical decisions on your behalf.

In some states this type of document may be known by a different name, such as a health care directive or health care declaration.

If you're older than age 18 and are being admitted to a hospital, nursing home, hospice or home health care agency that receives Medicare funds, the institution is required by federal law to ask whether you have an advance directive. That information is documented in your record. In the absence of an advance directive, a doctor will rely on your next of kin for guidance.

The institution must also give you written information about your right, under

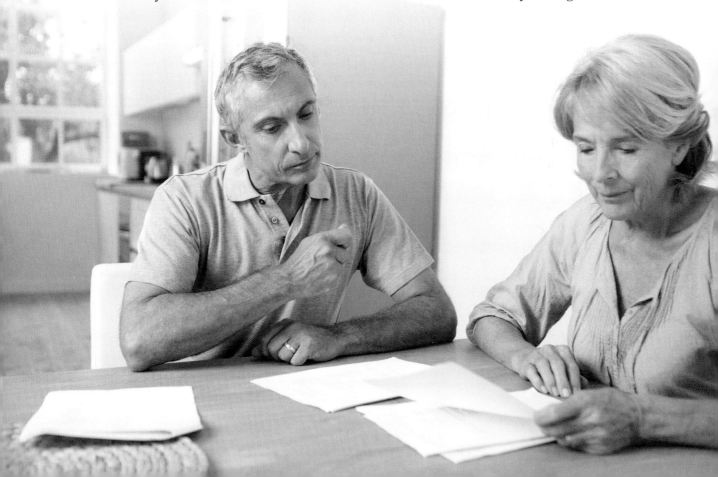

state law, to accept or reject medical treatment. Whether or not you have an advance directive, federal law requires the institution to provide all individuals the same treatment options.

The most common types of advance directives are a durable power of attorney for health care (a person) and a living will (a document). A combination of the two provides maximum personal participation in the face of medical situations that require difficult decisions.

## A durable power of attorney for health care

One of the most important actions you can take is appointing someone you trust to make health-related decisions for you should you become unable or unwilling to do so, giving this person legal authority to act on your behalf. A durable power of attorney for health care identifies this person, also called a proxy, in writing.

Your proxy helps ensure that your wishes aren't misinterpreted or ignored. When selecting someone to serve as your proxy, choose a person you're comfortable with acting as your representative. He or she should fully understand your medical care phi-

losophy and wishes and agree to serve in representing them. It may also be helpful, but not necessary, if this person lives close to you.

The reason it's so important to have a proxy is because it's impossible to predict all of the things that might require a decision in the future, or what the circumstances will be when those decisions need to be made.

Your proxy can respond specifically to possible questions and decisions that your condition may create. For example, you may say you don't want a feeding tube. But what many people mean is that they don't want a feeding tube if death is near and inevitable. There are circumstances in which a temporary feeding tube could be very helpful to recovery.

The only way to tease out these nuances is to have a conversation with your proxy about your overall goals for health care. For example, your overall goal may be to avoid medical interventions that will prolong your life unnecessarily if there is no reasonable chance of recovery.

Don't confuse a durable power of attorney for health care with a financial power of attorney. A financial power of attorney allows a person you authorize to manage your money and property if you aren't able to do so.

## A living will

A living will is a document you create to specify which medical treatments you want or don't want at the end of your life. Because no one can anticipate all of the possible circumstances surrounding his or her death, it's hard to be specific in living wills. For example, you may state that you don't want heroic procedures to extend your life when death is imminent, but then your doctor has to make certain distinctions as necessary: Is the use of a respirator a heroic measure? What about a blood transfusion?

The question becomes increasingly complicated as new technologies develop and yesterday's heroic treatments become routine. For doctors, one of the biggest challenges is keeping patients and family members informed of ever-changing life-sustaining technologies and the personal impact of those treatments.

Nonetheless, a living will is a place where you can record your overall health care goals and intentions.

In determining your wishes, think about your values and core beliefs. When would you consider it appropriate to refuse life-sustaining measures? Would it matter what stage of an illness or injury you were in? Would it matter what your prognosis was or if your condition was improving?

To help you get started in planning your living will, here are the main potential life-sustaining treatments to consider:

- **Resuscitation.** Resuscitation restarts the heart when it has stopped beating (cardiac death). Determine if and when you would want to be resuscitated by cardiopulmonary resuscitation (CPR) or by a device that delivers an electric shock to stimulate the heart.
- **Mechanical ventilation.** Mechanical ventilation takes over your breathing if you're unable to do so. Consider if, when and for how long you would want to be placed on a mechanical ventilator.
- **Nutritional and hydration assistance.** These steps supply the body with nutrients and fluids intravenously or via a tube in the stomach. Decide if, when and for how long you would want to be maintained in this manner.

- **Hemodialysis.** Hemodialysis removes waste from your blood and manages fluid levels if your kidneys no longer function. Determine if, when and for how long you would want to receive this treatment.
- **Treatments in the end stages of life.** Examples include, but are not limited to, antibiotics, pain medication and mechanical ventilation. Would you want to receive these as a form of comfort (palliative) care if your prognosis was that they would only delay imminent death?

Also decide if you would like to donate your organs for possible transplantation or your body for scientific study.

A living will by itself carries only moral force in stating your preferences. To give legal authority to living wills, most states have passed statutes, often called natural death acts. In these states, the statutes interpret the extent of the authority and the legal force of the living will.

The statutes aren't uniform among states. To ensure that your living will conforms to your state's requirements and will be followed, be familiar with the appropriate laws in your state before you prepare your living will or let an attorney help you.

## Do not resuscitate order

A do not resuscitate (DNR) order is a request to not have cardiopulmonary resuscitation if your heart stops or if you stop breathing. Your resuscitation requests may be included in your living will, or a DNR order can stand on its own — your doctor can put a DNR order in your medical chart.

# Preparing your directives

You may want to enlist the help of an attorney to help you prepare an advance directive, although this isn't necessary. Your doctor or hospital staff can give you the necessary forms and provide resources explaining the relevant state laws. You can also obtain state-appropriate forms on a variety of websites, such as the National Hospice and Palliative Care Organization.

Other possible sources include your local library or state medical, hospice or bar association.

The forms should come with directions for filling them out. If you have any questions, ask your doctor or attorney.

Before naming someone to make health care decisions on your behalf, discuss your decision with that person. He or she may be required to sign an acceptance form to act as your proxy. Usually, you'll need to have witnesses or a notary sign the forms.

Once you've filled out the necessary forms, make sure that your proxy and other important people in your life — your spouse, adult children, doctor, lawyer — have copies of the forms or know how to get them. Also let them know who is your designated proxy. At home, keep a copy in a place where it's easily accessible by others. Some people also keep a copy in a safe-deposit box.

## Changing your directives

You can update your advance directive at any time. In fact, it's probably wise to take a look at your advance directive on a periodic basis, especially if your health status changes.

To change an advance directive, a witness, notary or both may be required. Check the requirements in your state. If you move to another state, you may want to update your directive, even though most states will honor directives from other states. Be sure to discuss major changes with your proxy and to give updated copies to your proxy and other copy holders.

# Chapter 14

# Independence issues

If you're like many people, independence is the bedrock upon which you've built your life. More than virtually anything else, you treasure your freedom from the control of others — the opportunity to act according to your will and to make decisions for yourself as you see fit.

Your later years, however, can present a significant challenge to the self-reliance that you've enjoyed from young adulthood onward. As the years go by, your body and mind may change in ways that can affect both your safety and security.

Perhaps you're not at the point in your life in which you need to be concerned about these issues yet. But you may be caring for older parents and you're confronted with aspects of independence from the opposite side. The information here can help you make suggestions or decisions regarding their care and daily living.

Fortunately, options for ensuring independence grow more numerous every day. Whole industries have evolved to give older adults additional choices in their lives, while decreasing infringements on their independence. And increasing technology allows them to interact with the world like never before, opening up numerous new opportunities for information, communication and growth.

In this chapter, we explore many of the tools and resources that can help older adults retain their valuable independence and "live smarter" in their golden years.

# Tools for living smarter

You may have heard the phrase "Work smarter, not harder." If you swap *live* for *work*, you'll begin to understand the idea behind assistive devices.

These tools can help you with everyday tasks, such as writing a check or buttoning your shirt. Some are simple handle extensions that provide more leverage, while others are specially designed devices backed by high-tech engineering.

Now, you might be thinking that the use of assistive devices really signals old age, and you'd like to stay away from them for as long as possible. But before you relegate assistive devices to forms of weakness or physical surrender, consider how many of them you already rely on to make your life easier and more enjoyable.

For example, it's unlikely that you hesitate before climbing into an automobile for that short drive to the grocery store. A car is an assistive device. The vehicle helps you to accomplish your goal: getting from point A to point B with greater speed and comfort.

All assistive devices play that same role, to one degree or another. Whether it's something you do every day, such as reaching down to pick up the newspaper, or something you do less often, such as moving heavy objects around the garden, these aids can help.

Medical supply stores, websites, catalogs, your hospital's physical therapy department and even your local hardware store are full of specifically designed items and materials that can help you with daily tasks. By using these tools, you can ease pain, add comfort, increase safety, bolster confidence, enhance ability and sustain your independence.

## Daily needs devices

Assistive devices are most often used to accomplish simple daily tasks. Using the right tool can facilitate almost everything you need or want to do at home.

In the bathroom, one of the most dangerous rooms in the home, there are a number of options to help you move around safely and reduce strain on your wrists and back. Examples include folding shower seats, grab bars, elevated toilet seats, adjustable shower

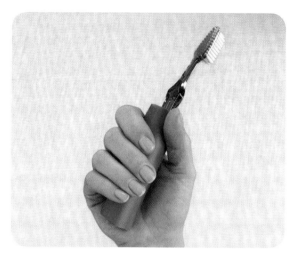

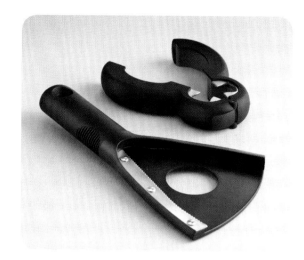

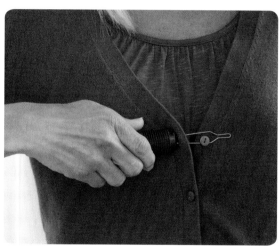

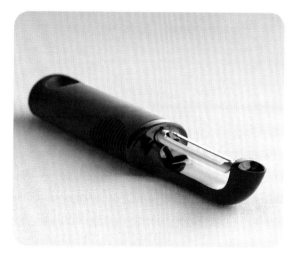

## Common daily assistive devices

A foam tube that slides onto objects such as a toothbrush can make them easier to grip (top left). Different types of opening devices can make a stubborn jar lid or bottle cap easier to tackle (top right). A buttonhook can help you grasp and fasten buttons on your clothes (middle left). Many kitchen tools, such as vegetable peelers, can be purchased with larger handles (middle right). A lever attachment makes it easier to work a doorknob (bottom).

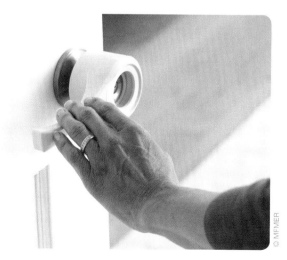

heads and single-lever faucets. You can also buy long-handled brushes, combs and sponges so that you don't have to reach over or behind your head as much. Several manufacturers now make toothbrushes and hand mirrors with foam rubber grips for an easier grasp.

In the kitchen, a wheeled cart can help you transport many items at once, which saves time and energy. Electric can openers do all the maneuvering for you, and many can be installed under a kitchen cabinet for easy access. Look for vegetable peelers, ladles, knives and other utensils with larger, preferably rubberized, grips. Holding on to something that has a large handle eases the strain on your hand and wrist; the rubber will help maintain your grip.

On your chairs and sofas, try some extra cushioning. Seating that's higher and firmer is easier to get out of than is seating that's lower and softer. To make it easier to slide in and out of your car, place a silky pillowcase or brown paper bag on your car seat.

And don't forget one of the greatest tools of all — proper lighting. Use the highest wattage bulbs allowed on your light fixtures to illuminate work and leisure areas.

## Health and fitness devices

Mountaineers often use ski poles while hiking through rough terrain. You can do the same for a walk around your neighborhood. Stationary bicycles, stair steppers and treadmills make great assistive additions to any home gym. They give you better stability and a way to regulate your workout routines. If you have access to a swimming pool, look at the variety of flotation equipment that water-trained runners and water aerobics enthusiasts commonly use.

For working in the garden, look for tools with wider handles and a better grip. Spring-loaded clippers and pruners eliminate the need to open the tools and reduce the pressure needed to close them. Rakes, hoes and other tools with long handles let you do your work with less bending.

## Electronic devices

Yes, they can often seem intimidating. But the wide variety of electronic "gadgets" on the market aren't just for the young. These devices can open up a new world of convenience and opportunity if you take the time to learn the basics.

# When is it time to give up the keys?

You may reach a point when retiring your car keys is in everyone's best interest. Or, perhaps, you're worried about a parent who's still driving. Knowing when to give up — or take away — the keys can be a tough call.

Some signs that it's time to quit driving are more obvious: being involved in preventable accidents or receiving an increased number of traffic tickets or warnings. But sometimes the signs may be more subtle. Consider giving up the keys if you or someone else notices that you're consistently:

- Moving too slowly on the highway
- Failing to come to a full stop at stop signs
- Being inattentive
- Making erratic moves
- Reacting too slowly
- Being honked at by other drivers
- Missing traffic signs or signals or being uncertain of what they mean
- Getting anxious at busy intersections, being unsure what to do or being afraid to drive
- Upsetting your passengers, who may refuse to ride with you

By understanding your limitations as a driver, you can better prepare for driving or perhaps giving up driving altogether. Listen to your friends and family. If they suggest you cut back on your time behind the wheel, they're only doing it with your best interests in mind. Talk to your doctor about how your health may affect your driving.

You may have family and friends to rely on for occasional rides. Most communities have options available to help you get around, as well. Mass transit services, including city buses and subways, may provide discounted fares to seniors. Senior transit may be available, often in the form of shuttle services. Taxis and delivery services also can help in a pinch.

## Internet devices

"Knowledge itself is power," said Sir Francis Bacon. And, he might have added, power means independence. One of the most useful devices at your disposal is the computer and the access it gives you to the Internet — the most rapidly growing communication medium in history.

If you've embraced this technology, good for you. But if you're resistant to it, you're missing out on a tool that can bring the world to your door. The Internet can transport you to just about anywhere, from the Smithsonian Institution to your own local library. You can also access almost any news source online.

You can use the Internet to purchase gifts and have them delivered, order groceries, send or receive emails and family photos, do your banking and pay bills, or video chat in real time with a friend or family member who lives across the country. The Internet's wealth of information and contacts can help you no matter what you want to accomplish, whether it be facing new medical challenges or finding a good plumber. And don't forget about all the websites mentioned in this book.

If you haven't ventured into cyber-space yet, consider taking a computer class as a way to get started. Classes are fun, and you can meet people with the same interests.

Along with standard stationary computers, laptops, netbooks and tablets have become increasingly popular in recent years. These devices can perform most of the same tasks as a standard computer with the added convenience of portability.

## Basic and 'smart' cellphones

More and more older adults are leaping into the cellphone market, drawn by the convenience of being able to make and take calls on the go.

Choose a cellphone that's comfortable for you. While a device with all the bells and whistles may be all the rage, you may never need all of those features. For example, if you don't think you'd ever text or access the Internet from your phone — or you don't wish to pay extra for these services — stick with a "talk" plan with a basic phone instead of a smartphone.

Additionally, there are cellphones designed with aging needs in mind. Some phones come with larger buttons and screens. Some also include an SOS button that can be used to connect with an emergency phone number.

### E-readers

Why would you want to read a book on a screen rather than in paper? There are numerous reasons to enjoy a good, tangible book. But the recent explosion of e-books and e-readers is for good reason, too.

The biggest convenience of an e-reading device is that you can carry multiple books, magazines and newspapers with you within a small, portable device. An e-reader will also save your place and allow you to highlight any passages you'd like to remember.

Older adults especially may discover advantages of e-readers. They tend to be lighter weight and easier to hold than traditional books. Most e-readers also have features that allow you to adjust the book to your needs, such as changing to a larger type-size or turning on audio capabilities.

Many public libraries offer classes on using e-readers, as well as a wide selection of e-books to check out.

### Navigation devices

Driving around in unfamiliar territory can be a challenge for anyone. But Global Positioning System (GPS) technology can make navigation significantly easier.

GPS navigation devices use satellites to pinpoint your location and the destination that you enter. They can then provide you maps and step-by-step driving instructions. Some devices also provide traffic and road construction updates, giving you a better idea of what to expect on the road ahead.

## Movement and mobility devices

A cane or walker can dramatically extend or increase your independence. Although these devices may seem awkward and hard to use at first, they can help you get around on your own without relying on someone else for help.

Awkwardness with any device is natural. Remember the first time you tried riding a bike or casting a fishing rod? Ease will come with practice.

Walking aids come in a variety of sizes, weights and designs, so it's best to have a health care professional recommend one that would be most appropriate for you. Ask the same person to help you determine the proper size and fit, as well as the best ways to use it.

It's a common mistake, for example, to choose a cane that's too long. The extra

# Choosing and using canes

Generally, choosing a grip is a matter of personal preference. Consider a foam grip or a grip that's shaped to fit your hand. The candy-cane-style cane (left) and swan-neck handle (right) are common choices. But other styles also are available.

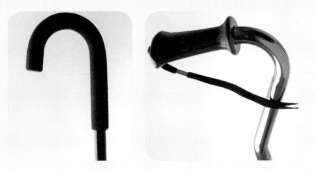

To make sure your cane fits you properly:

- **Check your elbow bend.** With the cane in your hand, your elbow should bend at a comfortable angle, about 15 to 20 degrees. You might bend your elbow slightly more if you're primarily using the cane for balance.
- **Check your wrist height.** With your arm hanging straight down at your side, the top of your cane should line up with the crease in your wrist.

If you use a cane for stability, you may grip it in either hand — whichever feels the most comfortable. Pick up and move your cane in unison with the opposite leg. Don't place your cane too far ahead of you. If you have an injury or disability affecting your hip, knee or ankle, your doctor or physical therapist might recommend a specific walking pattern.

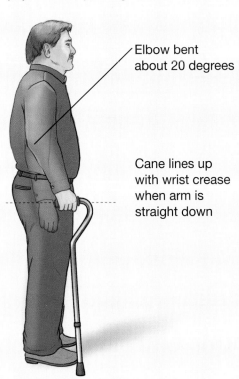

Elbow bent about 20 degrees

Cane lines up with wrist crease when arm is straight down

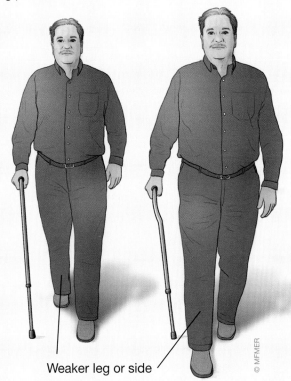

Weaker leg or side

© MFMER

length pushes up one arm and shoulder, causing strain to those muscles and your back. The candy-cane-style cane (with a hooked handle) probably won't be the most comfortable if you use a cane daily. Instead, one with a swan-neck handle will put your weight directly over the cane's shaft.

Another mobility aid you may wish to look into is a mobility scooter. If you live in an urban setting and are close to a grocery store, for example, a scooter can help you make the trip there and back with minimal effort and allow you to bring your purchases back home with you.

Technology also offers a wide variety of assistive devices to make driving easier. For example, hand controls can be mounted on a steering column. Wheelchair loaders and van lifts improve access. The cost of more advanced equipment can be high, but the mobility it provides may make the expense worthwhile. You may also be able to get financial help from Medicare or Medicaid for certain assistive devices.

## Keeping an open mind

Assistive devices can't do all things for all people. But your attitude toward them is just as important as the devices themselves. If you look at assistive devices as anchors that will drag you down the path of frailty and disability, you may fulfill your own prophecies. But if you view them as tools that enable you to exercise your independence and personal freedom, they can prove very useful in helping you overcome physical limitations.

# Housing options

It's no surprise that, according to an AARP survey, more than 80 percent of older Americans prefer to live and die in their own homes. Most people fear that someday they'll be helplessly trapped in a nursing home, but U.S. Census Bureau and other national survey figures show that less than 5 percent of Americans older than age 65 live in these facilities. By contrast, more than 90 percent of older adults between the ages of 65 and 84 live in traditional residential homes.

Staying in your present dwelling is just one of many housing options. Broadly speaking, your choices will fall under four categories: independent living, shared living, shared assisted living and fully supported living arrangements.

Ultimately, where you live and how much support you choose will depend on your physical and mental conditions, personal preferences, interests, financial resources, family and your willingness to adapt to change.

## Independent living

Your home is the place you feel most comfortable, safe and secure. Maybe you've already paid off your mortgage, so except for taxes and maintenance you're virtually home-free. Perhaps you've rented an apartment for years, but it's home and you really can't see moving out of the city.

At the same time, however, take an objective look at your present residence to be sure it makes sense long term. Most homes in the United States are designed for able-bodied occupants and may not accommodate the needs of someone older than age 65.

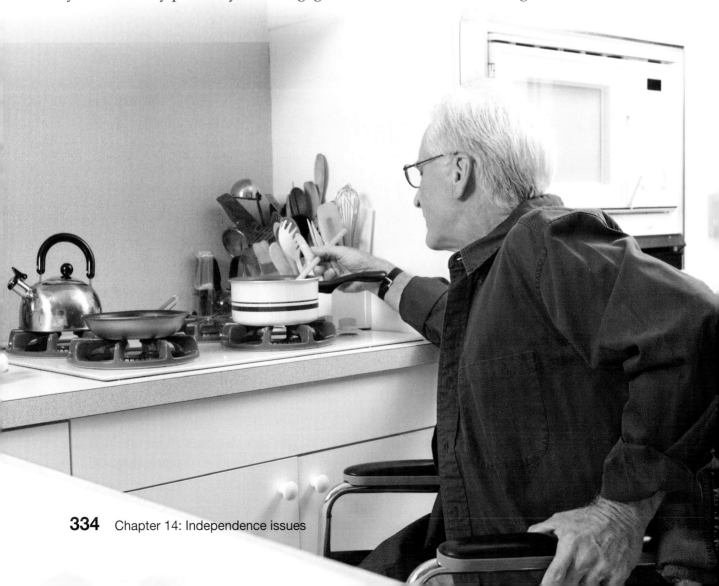

For example, will the stairs of your two-story home eventually present a problem? Is the only bathroom on the second floor? Is the laundry in the basement? Does the big backyard still hold some appeal, or is the upkeep becoming more of a burden? Major repairs may also become more common as plumbing and heating systems age and wear out.

### Home modification

If you really want to stay in your home, you may need to make some modifications to make it more convenient and accessible. Whether it's replacing doorknobs with more easily operated lever handles, installing grab bars in the bathroom or lowering countertops for better access, well-thought-out remodeling plans can build new life into your home.

Research suggests that 30 to 50 percent of home accidents can be prevented through home modification and repair.

### Moving to a different home

A cold, hard look at your house might convince you that it's time to move while you're still in good physical condition. Maybe a single-story ranch makes more sense or maybe all you really need is a two-bedroom home. Downscaling could also ease your expenses. Standard apartments, condominiums and townhouses can provide the living space you need without the worries of exterior upkeep. Nearby neighbors can offer both social and safety advantages as well.

### Retirement communities

Retirement communities provide a variety of options for independence. Often, they're multi-unit complexes of condos, townhouses or apartments.

One of the major benefits of a retirement community is reduced hassles of home ownership. Such a facility also draws like-minded older adults together and delivers the community services that residents most want and need.

Continuing care retirement communities go even further. These facilities offer multiple services on an a la carte basis so that as residents' needs change, they can receive additional care within the same setting. A retirement community may provide the independent living setting that you want now and the assisted living setting you may need in the future.

## Shared living

Despite the freedom it offers, living alone isn't for everyone. You can gain some real advantages, both for your

## Resources for independent living

Part of living independently means recognizing limitations that present themselves and seeking help in managing them. Numerous resources exist that can help you continue to live independently and stay productive for many years to come.

- **Home health care.** Some health care services can be provided at home by trained professionals, such as home health nurses.
- **Household maintenance.** While staying in your house may be appealing, there may be certain tasks that become difficult with time. Look for people or resources in your community that can help with housekeeping, shopping or handyman services.
- **Personal care.** This involves help with daily living, such as dressing, bathing or meal preparation. You might hire a personal care aide or home health aide.
- **Social interaction.** Feelings of isolation may crop up from time to time. Your local senior center and community education are both excellent resources for recreational and educational activities that can keep you socially involved. Some areas may also have adult day care options for adults with greater health care and social needs.

A great place to start searching for resources in your area is the Eldercare Locator, provided by the U.S. Administration on Aging. You can access this information at *www.eldercare.gov* or by calling 800-677-1116.

emotional well-being and your physical safety, by sharing your residence, moving in with another person or family, or finding a group of like-minded individuals to share living arrangements with.

### House sharing

Sharing your home with one or more people or joining someone else in his or her home can be a joy, a disaster or something in between. Consider any arrangement on a trial basis to start and have open discussions beforehand about issues such as rent, cooking, cleaning, repairs and maintenance, and personal space.

### Family connections

Moving in with family used to be the way most older adults transitioned out of their own homes. But with today's far-flung families, that's not always an option.

If you want to live with your children or they're urging you to move in with them, have frank discussions about each other's expectations. Consider everything from spousal relationships and finances to living space allocations and child care before you start unpacking.

### Cohousing

Unrelated people often enjoy the advantages of living as a family unit. Organizations throughout the country offer a collection of privately or cooperatively owned small-group residences.

These arrangements usually include a live-in manager and at least some staff, but they're primarily for residents in at least relatively good health.

### Senior housing

The federal government and most states have programs that help pay for housing for older adults with minimal income and assets. Rent is based on a percentage of your income. Usually, you live in your own apartment in a multiunit housing development.

Some programs also offer help with meals, housekeeping, shopping and laundry. The federal government also offers housing vouchers that allow qualified individuals to lease or purchase a house or apartment.

## Shared assisted living

If you need some assistance with bathing, dressing, meal preparation and housekeeping, then assisted living could be a valid alternative to hiring private help in your own home.

Continuing care retirement communities, board-and-care homes, retirement centers, congregate housing and senior residential housing all offer varying levels of support staff, depending on the operator and the needs of their residents.

These assisted living centers usually offer a menu of options, allowing you to tailor your services and costs to your specific needs. Facilities that provide fewer services usually allow outside specialists to give you private help if you need it.

Many assisted living arrangements charge a monthly rental fee for an apartment with utilities, meals, housekeeping, laundry and an emergency call system provided. Additional services generally include extra fees.

These supervised living arrangements work well for residents who have moderate functional impairment. Condition-specific facilities, such as Alzheimer's centers, also have opened. None of these replaces nursing homes, which offer fully supported care, but they are a reasonable alternative for people who require some degree of assistance with daily living.

## Fully supported living

As more living options become available for older adults, nursing home use is declining. These days, nursing homes — now often referred to as skilled nursing facilities — are most suited for rehabilitative care and care in which 24-hour services are required.

For many people, a stay in a nursing home is temporary while they recover from a hip fracture or some other mishap. Once rehabilitated, the individual is often able to return to independent living. This type of arrangement is often referred to as temporary rehabilitation or skilled nursing home care. Other people enter a nursing home because they need full care for a condition that may not improve.

The average nursing home resident has several chronic illnesses that require medical attention. More than half have Alzheimer's disease or some other mental impairment.

When independent living, assisted living or care by family members isn't feasible or threatens to destroy the fabric of a family, a nursing home should be considered. If you're physically able to visit prospective nursing homes and psychologically fit enough to help make the decision, you should participate in the selection process.

In terms of your independence, you would undoubtedly experience some feelings of compromise should you eventually need to move to a fully supported care facility. But you still have the power to choose how you think about those challenges and how they shape your outlook on life.

# Part 4

# Quick guide

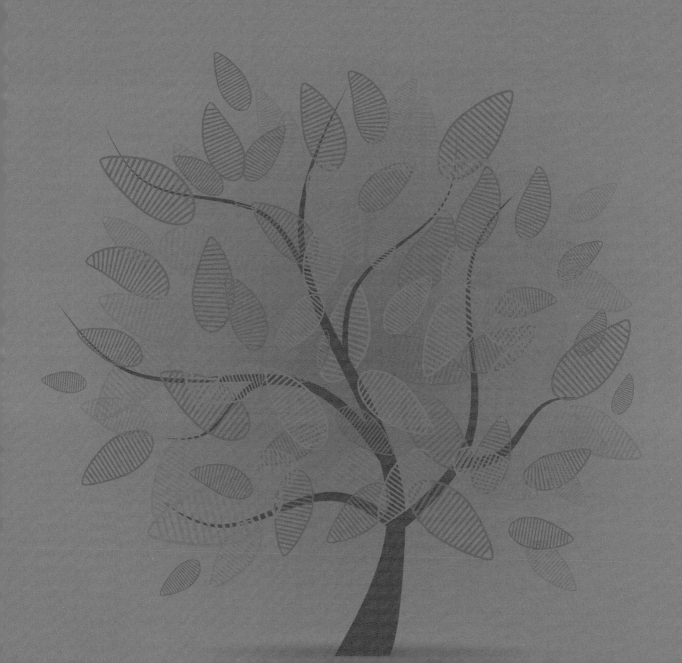

# Quick guide

Americans are living longer than ever before. And increasingly, people's later years are relatively healthy ones. Still, the physical processes of aging are inevitable. Perhaps you've already been diagnosed with a particular condition or illness, or maybe you're hoping to avoid one — or more than one!

This Quick Guide describes some of the diseases and disorders that become more common with age. That's not to say, though, that these conditions are inevitable. As explained earlier in this book, some of the diseases and disorders often blamed on aging are more a result of inactivity, a poor diet and other unhealthy lifestyle choices than they are age. Fortunately, that means there are often actions you can take to lower your risk.

If you or a loved one has a specific medical condition, use this section to read up on current treatment options, as well as self-care tips for managing the disease or disorder.

If you don't have any serious health problems, it's not a bad idea to take a few minutes to review the risk factors for some of the conditions listed. By identifying potential risk factors, you may be able to make changes in your lifestyle to avoid developing a particular disease or disorder down the road and keep your body operating at its best possible level.

Not all diseases and conditions are avoidable, but many of the most serious ones can be prevented with good lifestyle habits, including having regular medical checkups.

# Alzheimer's disease

Alzheimer's disease primarily affects adults over the age of 60. But this doesn't mean that Alzheimer's disease is an inevitable illness as you get older, or that all older adults will eventually display its signs and symptoms. Many older adults remain mentally alert and active and as intelligent as they ever were.

## The basics

Everyone has occasional lapses in memory. It's quite normal, for example, to forget the names of people whom you rarely see. The kinds of problems with memory and thinking that interfere with a person's daily functioning are known as dementia. The difficulties with memory and thinking that occur with the dementia of Alzheimer's disease go beyond simple forgetfulness. It may start with slight memory loss and confusion, but it eventually destroys your ability to remember, reason, learn and plan for the future. Because Alzheimer's disease is the most common cause of dementia, people sometimes forget that

there are other causes, such as strokes and the brain disease that also causes Parkinson's disease.

With Alzheimer's disease, healthy brain tissue progressively degenerates, leading to irreversible mental impairment. Most people with Alzheimer's disease share certain signs and symptoms. These may include:

- A gradual loss of memory for recent events and an inability to process new information
- A progressive tendency to repeat oneself, misplace objects, become confused and get lost
- A gradual disintegration of personality and judgment
- Increasing irritability, anxiety, depression, confusion and restlessness

These changes generally happen very gradually. As the disease progresses, its signs and symptoms become more serious and more noticeable.

The causes of Alzheimer's disease aren't well understood. However, researchers have found that in people with the condition, nerve cells in the brain (neurons) slowly die. The two hallmarks of Alzheimer's are clumps of protein called amyloid-beta, that form what are called neuritic plaques, and twisted threads of a protein called tau, known as neurofibrillary tangles. Researchers continue to study these abnormal structures to better understand why the disease causes neuron death.

Although there's no cure or surefire way to prevent Alzheimer's disease, scientists continue to make great progress in understanding the disease. Doctors are now able to diagnose the condition at much earlier stages, but there are no definitive treatments. Some treatments are available that can help improve the quality of life for people with Alzheimer's disease.

New drugs also are being studied, and scientists have discovered several genes associated with Alzheimer's disease, which may lead to new treatments to block the progression of the disease.

## Risk factors

Scientists have identified several risk factors that may increase your likelihood of developing Alzheimer's disease. They include:

- **Age.** Alzheimer's disease becomes more common with age, doubling in frequency every five years after age 65.

- **Heredity.** Your risk of developing Alzheimer's disease appears to be slightly higher if a parent or sibling has or had the disease. Certain, rare forms of early-onset Alzheimer's (occurring before age 65) are caused by specific genetic mutations. In addition, one form of the apolipoprotein E gene (APOE) increases your chance of developing late-onset Alzheimer's disease.
- **Sex.** Women are more likely than men are to develop the disease, mainly because they live longer.
- **Unhealthy lifestyle.** The same factors that put you at risk of heart disease, such as high blood pressure and diabetes, may also increase your risk of developing Alzheimer's.
- **Head injury.** The fact that some ex-boxers eventually develop dementia begs the question of whether serious head injury may be a risk factor for Alzheimer's. Studies have produced conflicting results, but one theory is that head injury may interact with a form of the APOE gene, leading to a higher risk of Alzheimer's disease.

## Treatment

Medications are the primary treatment for Alzheimer's disease. These drugs can't stop or reverse the underlying disease process, but they may slow it down, lessening its signs and symptoms. Medications that may be prescribed include:

- **Cholinesterase inhibitors.** These medications are commonly recommended for people with mild to moderate Alzheimer's. They work by improving the levels of acetylcholine in the brain, a chemical messenger that plays an important role in attention and memory skills. Around 50 percent of people taking cholinesterase inhibitors, such as donepezil (Aricept), rivastigmine (Exelon) and galantamine (Razadyne) have some improvement in their signs and symptoms.
- **Memantine.** This drug, which works by protecting brain cells from damage caused by the chemical messenger glutamate, is the only medication specifically indicated for treating moderate to severe Alzheimer's. Memantine (Namenda) seems to slow the loss of daily living skills, such as dressing and managing personal hygiene.

Doctors also sometimes prescribe mild sedatives, antidepressants or antipsychotic medications to improve behavioral symptoms that often accompany Alzheimer's. These drugs, often used in low doses, can improve a person's quality of life and assist family members in caring for their loved one.

Aside from medications, using memory aids also may help an individual with Alzheimer's disease supplement cognitive losses and maintain a degree of independence and dignity. Nonmedication strategies include writing down all important information, such as appointments and social events, and keeping it in visible places, along with clocks and calendars.

## What you can do

There's currently no way to prevent the onset of Alzheimer's disease. But researchers have some hopeful — if preliminary — leads on how to possibly reduce your risk or at least slow the progression of the disease.

- **Adopt a healthy lifestyle.** Taking steps to improve your cardiovascular health, such as losing weight, exercising, and controlling high blood pressure and cholesterol, also may help prevent Alzheimer's disease. Some studies have also suggested that eating a low-fat diet as well as consuming foods rich in omega-3 fatty acids, such as fatty fish, may be helpful.

- **Take steps to maintain your mental fitness.** Some researchers believe that lifelong mental exercise and learning may promote the growth of additional connections between neurons, giving you a greater reserve as you age and possibly delaying the onset of dementia.

# Arthritis

Arthritis is one of the most common health problems in the world. And it's the No. 1 cause of disability in the United States. An estimated 50 million Americans have arthritis.

## The basics

Osteoarthritis — often known simply as arthritis — results when the slippery, lubricated substance that normally cushions the ends of bones, called cartilage, breaks down. This breakdown causes the lining in a joint (synovium) to become inflamed, further damaging the cartilage. As the ends of the bones become exposed, they thicken and form bony growths, and bone rubs against bone, causing pain.

Arthritis can affect any joint in your body. It may initially strike only one joint, such as a knee or a hip. Or it may involve multiple joints, such as the joints of the fingers. Wear and tear on cartilage in a joint, affecting its mobility, is a principal feature of the disease.

If you have swelling or stiffness in your joints that lasts more than two weeks, seek medical advice. If you have arthritis, your doctor can work with you to develop a pain management and treatment plan.

## Risk factors

The exact causes of arthritis are unclear, but these factors increase your risk:

- **Age.** More than half of people older than age 65 have osteoarthritis in varying degrees of severity.
- **Sex.** Of people older than age 65 who have osteoarthritis, 75 percent are women.
- **Certain hereditary conditions.** Some people are born with defective cartilage or with slight defects in the way their joints fit together. With age, these defects can cause early cartilage breakdown.
- **Joint injury.** If you've injured a joint due to sports, work-related activity

or an accident, you may be at increased risk of developing osteoarthritis — especially of the knees.

- **Obesity.** Excess weight puts unnecessary pressure on your spine, knees and hips and can lead to osteoarthritis.
- **Other medical conditions.** Diseases that change the normal structure and function of cartilage, such as rheumatoid arthritis, gout or pseudogout, can increase your risk of developing osteoarthritis.

## Treatment

There's no known cure for osteoarthritis, but treatments can help reduce pain and maintain joint movement. Your doctor may recommend a combination of medication, self-care and exercise. In some cases, surgery may be necessary.

For pain without inflammation, analgesics may be recommended. Acetaminophen (Tylenol, others) is often the first choice. Other analgesics include tramadol (Ultram) and narcotics containing oxycodone or hydrocodone.

Nonsteroidal anti-inflammatory drugs (NSAIDs) reduce both pain and inflammation. Nonprescription NSAIDs include ibuprofen (Advil, Motrin IB, others) and naproxen (Aleve). Some NSAIDS are available only by prescription, such as the COX-2 inhibitor celecoxib (Cele-

### Rheumatoid arthritis

There are more than 100 forms of arthritis. Rheumatoid arthritis is among the most debilitating, causing joint pain, swelling and stiffness. Unlike osteoarthritis, rheumatoid arthritis is an autoimmune disorder. It's thought to result from your immune system attacking your body's synovium — the tissue that lines your joints. Rheumatoid arthritis is often more debilitating than is osteoarthritis.

There's no cure for rheumatoid arthritis. But with proper treatment — medication, rest, exercise and self-care — you can live a long, productive life with this condition.

brex). This drug blocks the production of an enzyme called cyclooxygenase (COX), which produces hormone-like substances that trigger inflammation and pain. Unlike traditional NSAIDs, it doesn't cause stomach bleeding and ulcers, but it may pose cardiovascular and gastrointestinal risks.

Sometimes, a doctor may suggest injecting an arthritic joint with a derivative of hyaluronic acid, a substance found naturally in joint fluid. Preparations of hyaluronic acid include hyaluronate (Hyalgan) and Hylan G-F 20 (Synvisc). A series of injections of one of these medications may provide pain relief for osteoarthritis of the knee. Your doctor may also recommend an injection of a corticosteroid medication into a joint that's inflamed and not responding to other treatments.

Some studies suggest that the dietary supplements glucosamine and chondroitin sulfate can help ease the symptoms of arthritis by maintaining existing cartilage and stimulating new cartilage growth. For more information on these products, see page 267.

If you have long-term deterioration, your doctor may recommend replacing your damaged joint with an artificial one. Replacement surgery is most often performed on hip and knee joints. If the joints in your hands have deteriorated significantly, an operation may help relieve pain and increase finger mobility.

Other surgical techniques are designed to remove loose fragments of bone or cartilage that may cause pain or mechanical problems such as "locking."

## What you can do

You can relieve much of the discomfort of osteoarthritis by adopting a healthy lifestyle and using simple self-care techniques.

- **Control your weight.** Excess weight puts added stress on joints in your back, hips, knees and feet. Excess weight can also make joint replacement surgery more difficult.
- **Develop an exercise program.** Appropriate exercise helps keep joints flexible and builds muscle strength. Work with your doctor.
- **Apply heat, especially before exercising.** It will ease your pain, relax tense, painful muscles and increase blood flow in the area.
- **Apply cold for occasional flare-ups.** Cold may dull the sensation of pain the first day or two. It can also decrease muscle spasms.

- **Wear comfortable shoes that properly support your weight.** This is especially important if you have arthritis in your weight-bearing joints or back.
- **Maintain good posture.** Poor posture causes uneven weight distribution and may strain your ligaments and muscles. Walking can improve your posture.
- **Practice relaxation techniques.** Hypnosis, guided imagery, deep breathing and muscle relaxation can all be used to control pain.
- **If you're tired, rest.** Prioritize your energy. Arthritis can make you prone to a deep exhaustion.

# Cancer

Cancer affects the basic units of life — your cells. Normally, human cells grow and divide in an orderly fashion. But sometimes this growth gets out of control — cells continue dividing without restraint, crowding out neighboring normal cells. In addition, these abnormal cells affect the function and growth of normal cells by competing with them for essential nutrients.

Uncontrolled cell growth typically results in a mass of tissue, called a tumor. Tumors may be either noncancerous (benign) or cancerous (malignant). Cells from cancerous tumors can invade and damage nearby tissues and organs. They can also spread to other parts of your body.

What causes cancer? That's a question that doctors and scientists are still trying to fully answer. However, they are learning more about what happens within some cells to cause normal cells to become cancerous.

You may fear cancer, perhaps because you view it as an incurable disease. The truth is that although cancer remains a serious illness, it's no longer the inevitable death sentence it once was. Instead, it's increasingly becoming a tale of survivorship. An estimated 12 million Americans living today have a history of cancer.

The following pages contain information on three of the most common cancers among Americans: breast cancer, lung cancer and prostate cancer.

## Breast cancer

The National Cancer Institute estimates that about 1 in 8 women in the United States will develop breast cancer at some point during her lifetime. Your risk of breast cancer increases with age. Most breast cancers occur in women older than age 50, and the average age at diagnosis is 61.

## The basics

Breast cancer most commonly develops in breast ducts, small tubes designed to carry milk from the small sacs that produce milk (lobules) to the nipple. But cancer may also occur in the lobules or in other breast tissue.

The most common sign of breast cancer is a lump or thickening in the breast. Often, the lump is painless. Other signs of breast cancer include:

- Clear or bloody discharge from your nipple
- An inverted nipple — if it isn't normally inverted
- A change in the size or contours of your breast
- Any dimpling or puckering of the skin over your breast
- Redness or pitting of the skin over your breast, looking similar to the skin of an orange

Although most breast changes aren't cancerous, it's important to have any change evaluated promptly. If breast cancer is detected and treated early —

while the tumor is small and before cancerous cells have spread to neighboring lymph nodes — odds are it'll be successfully treated.

## Risk factors

Scientists don't know what causes most breast cancer. However, they do know that the following factors may increase your risk:

- **Sex.** Although men can develop breast cancer, it's 100 times as common in women.
- **Age.** Your risk of breast cancer increases as you get older.
- **A personal history of breast cancer.** Having cancer in one breast increases your chances of developing it in the other.
- **Family history.** Women who have a mother or sister with breast cancer have a greater chance of developing breast cancer themselves.
- **Genetic predisposition.** Defects in one of several genes, such as BRCA1 or BRCA2, put you at greater risk of developing the disease.
- **Excess weight.** Obesity increases your breast cancer risk, especially after menopause.
- **Exposure to estrogen.** Much of this is related to your reproductive system. If you reach menopause late (after age 55) or you began men-

struating before age 12, you have a higher risk of developing breast cancer. The same is true if you've never given birth or if your first pregnancy occurred after age 30.

- **Race.** Caucasian women are more likely to develop breast cancer than are black or Hispanic women.
- **Smoking.** A Mayo Clinic study found that smoking significantly increases the risk of breast cancer in women with a strong family history of breast and ovarian cancers.
- **Excessive use of alcohol.** Women who consume more than one alcoholic drink a day have a slightly greater risk of breast cancer than do women who don't drink.
- **Hormone therapy.** Women who take combination hormone therapy (estrogen plus progestin) have a slightly higher risk of breast cancer.

## Treatment

Treatment for breast cancer depends on several factors, but it usually involves some combination of surgery, radiation therapy, hormone therapy or chemotherapy.

When discovered at its earliest stages, breast cancer is highly curable with surgery. At one time, the only type of breast cancer surgery was radical mastectomy, which removed the entire breast, along with chest muscles beneath the breast and all the lymph nodes under the arm. Today, this operation is rarely performed. Instead, the majority of women are candidates for breast-saving operations in which only a portion of the breast is removed, or surgery in which all of the breast is removed but the chest muscles are left intact.

Many times, surgery is followed by chemotherapy, radiation or both. Radiation to your chest wall or underarm area can kill cancer cells that may have escaped surgical removal. Chemotherapy drugs are also taken to destroy cancer cells that might have spread to other parts of your body.

Hormone therapy is another common form of treatment. The hormones estrogen or progesterone might encourage the growth of breast cancer cells in your body. Drugs such as tamoxifen bind to hormone receptors in your breast and at other locations, preventing estrogen from attaching to them and feeding the cancer.

Medications called aromatase inhibitors work by keeping an enzyme called aromatase from converting testosterone (yes, women have some testosterone) to estrogen. The aromatase inhibitors currently used for breast cancer treatment are anastrozole (Arimidex), exemestane (Aromasin) and letrozole (Femara).

For women who have breast tumors that produce excessive amounts of a protein called HER2, the drug trastuzumab (Herceptin) may be an important part of treatment. Trastuzumab attaches to HER2 receptors on cancer cells, cutting the cells off from chemical signals they need to function and maintain themselves. This inhibits the growth of HER2 positive cancer cells and, in many cases, is able to shrink the cancer.

## What you can do

These suggestions may help reduce your risk of breast cancer:

- **Stay physically active.** How exercise may affect breast cancer is a fairly new area of research. Many studies indicate that an inactive lifestyle may increase breast cancer risk, whereas one large, long-term study found that women who exercised for 30 minutes a day reduced their breast cancer risk by 10 percent. Exercise may influence hormone levels and it also promotes a healthy weight.
- **Maintain a healthy weight.** There's a clear link between obesity and

breast cancer, especially having excess weight after menopause.

- **Limit your intake of dietary fat.** Some observational studies have reported a correlation between a high dietary fat intake and breast cancer risk. However, not all studies support this.
- **Eat plenty of fruits and vegetables.** They contain vitamins, minerals and antioxidants that may help protect you from cancer.
- **Drink less than one alcoholic drink a day or avoid alcohol completely.** Compared with nondrinkers, women who consume one alcoholic drink a day have a very small increase in breast cancer risk, while women who consume more than three drinks a day have about 1.5 times the risk.
- **If you're taking hormone therapy, discuss your options with your doctor.** You may be able to manage your menopausal symptoms with exercise, dietary changes or nonhormonal therapies.
- **Ask your doctor about aspirin and other drugs.** Studies suggest drugs such as acetaminophen (Tylenol, others), ibruprofen (Advil, Motrin IB, others) or aspirin may help protect against breast cancer. However, regular NSAID use can produce side effects. Talk with your doctor.

# Lung cancer

Lung cancer is the leading cause of cancer deaths in the United States, among both men and women. Each year, it claims more lives than prostate, breast and colon cancers do combined. The good news is that most lung cancer deaths are highly preventable. That's because smoking accounts for about 80 to 90 percent of lung cancers.

## The basics

The two main types of lung cancer are small cell and non-small cell carcinomas. Small cell lung cancer spreads aggressively and is best treated with chemotherapy and radiation. It occurs almost exclusively in smokers and accounts for about 15 percent of lung cancers in the United States. Non-small cell lung cancer is much more common. If caught early, when confined to a small area, it may be removed surgically.

Lung cancer usually doesn't cause signs or symptoms until the disease is advanced. When symptoms do appear, they may include:

- Coughing — either a dry cough or one that produces sputum, which may contain blood
- Shortness of breath
- Chest pain
- Hoarseness
- Fever

Lung cancer also may cause fatigue, loss of appetite and weight loss. Al-

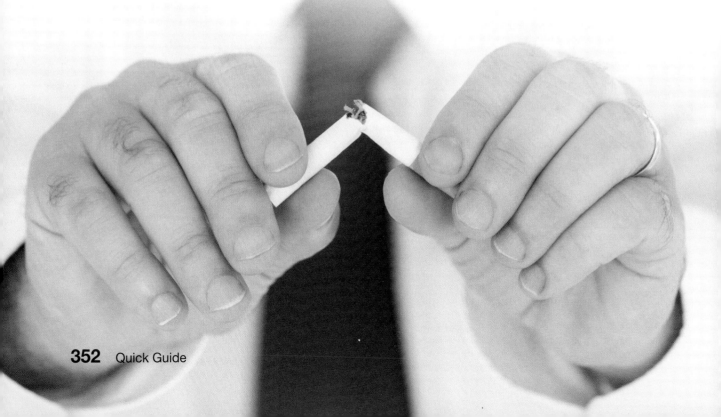

though many of these symptoms might be attributed to other causes, talk to your doctor if you experience such problems. The earlier you discover and treat lung cancer, the better chance you have of lengthening your life and reducing symptoms.

## Risk factors

Smoking is the greatest risk factor for lung cancer. Your risk increases with the number of cigarettes you smoke each day and the number of years you've smoked. Your risk is also greater if you start smoking early in life. Quitting smoking, on the other hand, even after many years of smoking, can greatly reduce your risk of developing lung cancer.

Other known risk factors for lung cancer include:

- **Sex.** Women who smoke or once smoked are at greater risk of lung cancer than are men who've smoked an equal amount. Women may be more susceptible to the cancer-causing substances found in tobacco, or estrogen may play a role.
- **Race.** Black men are slightly more likely to develop lung cancer than are white men. They also develop the disease at an earlier age and are less likely to survive.

- **Exposure to radon gas.** This is second only to smoking as a cause of lung cancer. Radon comes from the natural (radioactive) breakdown of uranium in soil, rock and water. Radon eventually may become part of the air you breathe.
- **Exposure to secondhand smoke.** Daily exposure to secondhand smoke may increase your chances of developing lung cancer by as much as 30 percent.
- **Exposure to carcinogens.** Workplace exposure to substances such as asbestos, vinyl chloride, nickel chromates and coal products also can increase your risk of developing lung cancer, especially if you're a smoker.

## Treatment

Treatment of lung cancer depends on the size, location and type of cancer, as well as on your overall health.

Because most small cell lung cancers have spread beyond the lungs by the time they're discovered, surgery usually isn't a treatment option. Instead, the most effective treatment is chemotherapy, either alone or in combination with radiation therapy.

Radiation therapy uses X-rays to kill cancer cells. Unfortunately, small cell lung cancer often spreads to the brain. For that reason, your doctor may recommend brain radiation therapy to prevent cancer from spreading to that part of the body or to eliminate small areas of cancer spread (micrometastases) that aren't yet detectable with imaging studies.

For early-stage non-small cell lung cancer, surgery is usually the treatment of choice. In some cases, only the portion of the lung that contains the tumor is removed (wedge resection). In others, one lobe (lobectomy) or even the entire lung (pneumonectomy) may be taken. Because pneumonectomy can decrease lung function considerably as well as lead to other complications, it's performed only when absolutely necessary. More advanced non-small cell lung cancers are generally treated with chemotherapy, radiation or a combination of the two.

### What you can do

The best known way to prevent lung cancer is to not smoke. Still, there's hope for current smokers. If you smoke, quitting now can significantly reduce your cancer risk — even if you've smoked for years.

These measures also can help prevent lung cancer:

- **Avoid secondhand smoke.** The less your exposure to these harmful chemicals, the better
- **Have the radon levels in your home checked.** This is especially important if you live in an area where radon is known to be a problem. The best tests are those that take three to six months.
- **Avoid carcinogens.** Take precautions to protect yourself from toxic chemicals such as vinyl chloride, nickel chromates and coal products.
- **Eat a healthy diet.** A diet high in fruits and vegetables appears to offer protection against some cancers. Certain chemicals in cruciferous vegetables such as broccoli, cabbage and bok choy may be especially protective against lung cancer. Other chemicals called flavonoids, found in all fruits and vegetables, also appear to help protect against lung cancer.
- Consider screening. If you're at high risk of lung cancer due to current or past smoking, you may want to consider early detection with CT screening. Talk to your doctor.

## Prostate cancer

Prostate cancer is the most commonly diagnosed life-threatening cancer in men in the United States. As you age, your risk of prostate cancer increases. Almost 2 out of 3 prostate cancers are found in men older than age 65.

## The basics

Prostate cancer is cancer that affects the prostate gland — the small, walnut-shaped gland that surrounds the bottom portion of a man's bladder and about the first inch of the urinary tube (urethra).

Typically, prostate cancer grows slowly and remains confined to the prostate gland, where it usually doesn't cause serious harm. But not all cancers act the same. Some forms of prostate cancer are aggressive and can spread quickly.

Prostate cancer often doesn't produce any symptoms in its early stages. That's why many cases of prostate cancer aren't detected until they've spread beyond the prostate. When signs and symptoms do occur, they may include:

- Dull pain in your lower pelvic area
- Urgency of urination
- Difficulty starting urination
- Pain during urination
- Weak urine flow and dribbling
- Intermittent urine flow
- A sensation that the bladder isn't empty after urination

- Frequent urination at night
- Blood in your urine
- Painful ejaculation

A digital rectal exam and a blood test called the prostate-specific antigen (PSA) test may be used to screen for prostate cancer. The PSA test isn't foolproof, but it can identify increases in a specific substance often associated with prostate cancer. If you're a man older than age 50 and you haven't been screened for prostate cancer, talk with your doctor about whether screening is right for you. If you're black or you have a family history of the disease, you may want to have this discussion earlier.

## Risk factors

Factors that put you at increased risk of prostate cancer include:

- **Age.** As you get older, your risk of prostate cancer increases.
- **Ethnic background.** For reasons not well understood, black men are more likely to get and die of prostate cancer than are men of any other ethnic group. Black men also are more likely to get prostate cancer at a younger age, and to get an aggressive form.
- **Family history.** If your father or brother has or had prostate cancer, your risk of developing the disease

is at least twice that of the average American man.

- **Diet.** A high-fat diet and obesity may increase your risk of prostate cancer. Researchers theorize that fat increases production of the hormone testosterone, which may promote the development of prostate cancer cells.
- **Sexual activity.** Men with a history of sexually transmitted infections (STIs) may be at higher risk of prostate cancer.
- **Tobacco.** Cigarette smoking may increase the risk of prostate cancer in younger men.
- **Supplemental hormones.** Large doses of the nutritional supplement dehydroepiandrosterone (DHEA) may promote the development of prostate cancer.

## Treatment

Prostate cancer can be treated in a number of ways. For some men, a combination of treatments works best. The treatment you and your doctor choose will depend on how fast the cancer is growing, whether it has spread beyond the prostate, and your age and overall health. In some cases, immediate treatment may not be necessary.

Surgical removal of the prostate gland is the most effective way to treat cancer that's confined to the gland. During this procedure, a surgeon uses special techniques to completely remove the prostate gland, while trying to spare muscles and nerves that control urination and sexual function.

If you're older or in poor health and might have trouble withstanding surgery, radiation therapy is generally the preferred treatment for prostate cancer. For cancer confined to the prostate, radiation is often as effective as surgery for up to 10 years. The two forms of radiation therapy for prostate cancer are external beam and radioactive seed implants. External beam radiation is delivered by beams from a large machine that's placed over your body. Radioactive seed implants are generally used in men with smaller or moderate-sized prostates with small and lower grade cancers.

Cryotherapy is a treatment option that involves inserting thin metal rods into the prostate and freezing the tissue around the rods. The formation of ice crystals within cancer cells causes them to rupture and die.

Hormone therapy uses certain medications to stop the body from producing most male sex hormones or to block the hormones from entering cancer cells. This is effective because male sex hormones have been found to make cancer cells in the prostate gland grow more quickly. Hormone therapy is the most common treatment for advanced prostate cancer. It's also used in some early-stage cancers.

Chemotherapy is generally used in situations when the cancer has continued to grow and spread despite other forms of treatment.

**What you can do**

To reduce your risk of developing prostate cancer or possibly slow the disease's progression:

- **Eat well.** Diets high in fat have been linked to prostate cancer. Instead, emphasize plenty of fruits and vegetables each day. Studies show that frequent consumption of tomato products and other lycopene-rich foods may be associated with lower risk of prostate cancer. Lycopene is the chemical that gives food its red color.
- **Get regular exercise.** Studies indicate that regular exercise may reduce your cancer risk, including your risk of prostate cancer.
- **Get screened.** Ask your doctor when you should begin screening and how long to have it.

# Coronary artery disease

Coronary artery disease is the most common type of heart disease, affecting over 16 million Americans. It's also the leading cause of death in both men and women.

Coronary artery disease may exhibit no warning signs, or it can produce very noticeable symptoms such as chest pain or shortness of breath. Some people aren't even aware that they have coronary artery disease until they experience a heart attack or they develop signs and symptoms of heart failure — extreme fatigue with exertion, shortness of breath, and swelling in their feet and ankles.

## The basics

Your coronary arteries encircle your heart like a crown and branch off into your heart muscle, supplying it with blood. When they're healthy, these arteries are clean, smooth and slick. The artery walls are flexible and can expand to let more blood through when necessary. If these arteries are unhealthy, you're at risk of heart failure or a heart attack.

# Signs and symptoms of a heart attack

Not all people who have heart attacks experience the same signs and symptoms or experience them to the same degree. For example, heart attack symptoms in women, older adults and people with diabetes tend to be less pronounced. Some people have no symptoms at all. Still, there are warnings that a heart attack may be occurring:

- Pressure, fullness or a squeezing pain in the center of your chest that lasts for more than a few minutes
- Pain extending beyond your chest to your shoulder, arm, back or even to your teeth and jaw
- Increasing episodes of chest pain
- Prolonged pain in the upper abdomen
- Shortness of breath
- Sweating
- Impending sense of doom
- Lightheadedness
- Fainting
- Nausea and vomiting

Most people who experience a heart attack have mild warning signs and symptoms for hours, days or weeks in advance. The earliest predictor of an attack may be recurrent chest pain (angina) that's triggered by exertion and relieved by rest.

An injury to the lining of the coronary arteries is thought to trigger the disease. This injury makes them susceptible to atherosclerosis — the slow, progressive buildup of deposits (plaques) on the inner artery walls. Over time, these plaques — deposits of fat, cholesterol, calcium and other cellular sludge from your blood — can narrow your coronary arteries, so less blood flows to your heart muscle. Reduced blood flow to your heart can cause chest pain (angina). The deposits can also become fragile and rupture, forming blood clots that can block blood flow to your heart or other organs. Complete blockage of blood flow to your heart is what causes a heart attack.

You can prevent or slow coronary artery disease by taking steps to improve the health of your heart and blood vessels. Drugs and surgical techniques also can repair narrowed coronary arteries. The best long-term solution, however, is a healthy lifestyle to control risk factors for the disease.

## Risk factors

Several factors place you at added risk of coronary artery disease. Some you can control, and others you can't. Uncontrollable risk factors include:

- **Sex.** Men are generally at greater risk of heart disease than are women. However, after menopause, the risk of heart disease increases in women.
- **Heredity.** If your siblings, parents or grandparents have coronary artery disease, you may be at risk, too. Your family may have a genetic condition that contributes to higher blood cholesterol levels or high blood pressure.
- **Race.** Blacks, Hispanics, American Indians and native Hawaiians have a higher risk of heart disease and high blood pressure than do whites.
- **Age.** Most people who die of coronary artery disease are older than 65.

Controllable risk factors for coronary artery disease include:

- **Smoking.** Exposure to cigarette smoke combined with other factors greatly increases your risk of coronary artery disease by damaging blood vessels.
- **High blood pressure.** Over time, high blood pressure can damage your coronary arteries by accelerating atherosclerosis.
- **High blood cholesterol.** The risk of coronary artery disease increases as your blood cholesterol level rises. When your level of low-density

lipoprotein (LDL, or "bad") cholesterol is high, there's a greater chance that you will develop coronary artery disease.

- **Diabetes.** People with diabetes have an increased risk of coronary artery disease. That risk is even higher if your blood sugar level isn't well controlled.
- **Obesity.** Excess weight increases strain on your heart, raises your blood pressure, increases your blood cholesterol levels and increases your risk of diabetes.
- **Physical inactivity.** Regular physical activity is important in preventing heart disease.
- **Stress and anger.** Stress and anger may increase your risk of coronary artery disease. This is especially true if they cause you to engage in other risk factors, such as overeating or smoking.
- **Excessive alcohol consumption.** Drinking too much alcohol can raise your blood pressure and your triglyceride level. Triglycerides are another form of blood fat.

Risk factors often occur in clusters and may feed one another. For example, obesity commonly leads to diabetes and high blood pressure. Even a small increase in one factor becomes more critical when combined with others.

## Treatment

Changing your habits is the single most effective way to treat underlying atherosclerosis and prevent progression of coronary artery disease. A diet low in cholesterol and saturated fat helps reduce high blood cholesterol, a primary cause of atherosclerosis. Eating a diet rich in fruits and vegetables and having at least one or two servings of fish a week also can reduce your risk of a heart attack. Quitting smoking and getting regular exercise dramatically lowers your risk of complications from atherosclerosis.

If lifestyle changes alone aren't enough, your doctor may recommend drug therapy. Medications to prevent or treat coronary artery disease include:

- **Cholesterol-lowering drugs.** These medications help lower the level of "bad" cholesterol in your blood while raising the level of "good" cholesterol.
- **Aspirin and other blood thinners.** They can reduce the tendency of your blood to clot, which may help prevent obstruction of your coronary arteries.
- **Blood pressure medications.** Blood pressure medications relax and open up your blood vessels and

allow blood to flow from your heart more easily, decreasing your heart's workload.

- **Nitroglycerin.** Nitroglycerin tablets, spray and patches help control chest pain (angina) by both opening up your coronary arteries and reducing your heart's demand for blood.

In some cases, medications don't provide adequate relief, and the blocked artery must be widened to allow adequate blood flow. This is done with a procedure called coronary angioplasty. In this procedure, a balloon-tipped catheter is inserted into an artery in your groin or arm and threaded to the narrowed artery. When the catheter reaches the blockage, the balloon is inflated to widen the artery and improve blood flow. Often small metallic mesh tubes (stents) are placed into the area where the blockage occurred to keep the artery from narrowing again.

If angioplasty doesn't widen the artery or if complications occur, you may need coronary bypass surgery. This procedure creates an alternate route for blood to flow around a blocked stretch of artery. A blood vessel, usually taken from your leg or chest, is grafted directly onto a narrowed artery, bypassing the blocked area. If more than one artery is blocked, a bypass can be done on each.

## What you can do

The following steps can help prevent coronary artery disease, as well as a heart attack and congestive heart failure. If you have coronary artery disease, these steps can also prevent your condition from becoming worse.

- **Don't smoke and avoid secondhand smoke.** Nicotine constricts blood vessels and forces your heart to work harder. Carbon monoxide reduces oxygen in blood and damages the lining of blood vessels.
- **Get regular checkups.** Some of the main risk factors for coronary artery disease — high blood cholesterol, high blood pressure and diabetes — have no symptoms in their early stages. But your doctor can check for these conditions. If a problem is found, you and your doctor can manage it early to prevent complications.
- **Get ample physical activity.** Exercise helps prevent coronary artery disease by helping you to achieve and maintain a healthy weight and control diabetes, elevated cholesterol and high blood pressure.
- **Maintain a healthy weight.** Being overweight increases your risk of coronary artery disease. Losing weight can reduce that risk.

- **Eat a heart-healthy diet.** Too much saturated fat and cholesterol in your diet can narrow the arteries leading to your heart. Too much salt can also raise blood pressure in some people. Focus on fruits and vegetables. They contain antioxidants — vitamins and minerals that help prevent wear and tear on your coronary arteries. Fish also is part of a heart-healthy diet because it contains omega-3 fatty acids, which help improve blood cholesterol levels and prevent blood clots.
- **Minimize or manage stress.** Stress can increase your risk of a cardiac event, such as a heart attack.

# Depression

Depression is a medical disorder that influences your thoughts, moods, feelings, behavior and physical health. It affects an estimated 1 in 10 adults at any given time.

## The basics

Depression is an illness with a biological basis that's often influenced by psychological and social stress. A complex interplay of factors involving genetics, stress, and changes in brain and body function is thought to play a role in its development.

Depression can take many forms. The most common is major depression. Its hallmark symptoms are:

- Depressed mood
- Loss of interest in activities once enjoyed

Other signs and symptoms of depression may include:

- Sleep disturbances, such as early awakening, sleeping too much or having trouble falling asleep
- Decreased concentration, attention and memory
- Increased or decreased appetite and unexplained weight gain or loss
- Restlessness, agitation, irritability, annoyance or ambivalence
- Fatigue and loss of energy
- Feelings of helplessness, hopelessness, worthlessness or guilt
- Continuous pessimism
- Neglect of personal responsibilities or personal care
- Decreased interest in sex
- Thoughts of death or suicide

Depression can also cause a wide variety of physical complaints, such as headache, digestive problems and chronic pain.

There's no single cause for depression. But experts believe a genetic vulnerability to the disease combined with environmental factors, such as stress or physical illness, may trigger an imbalance in brain chemicals called neurotransmitters, resulting in depression. Imbalances in three neurotransmitters — serotonin, norepinephrine and dopamine — seem to be linked to depression.

If you have signs and symptoms of depression, see your doctor. With proper treatment, most people improve — often within weeks — and return to normal activities.

## Risk factors

Scientists have identified a number of risk factors — events and conditions that appear to increase your likelihood of becoming depressed. They include:

- **Family history.** If your parent, sibling or child is depressed, you're at increased risk. The increase in risk may be due to genetics, family environment or both. However, not everyone with a family history of depression develops the disorder.

- **Stressful situations.** Major life events, particularly a loss or threatened loss of a loved one through death or divorce, can trigger depression. Other losses, such as a job layoff, also can lead to the illness.
- **Past experiences.** People who've survived deeply upsetting events in the past, such as childhood abuse, wartime combat or witnessing a serious crime, are at increased risk of developing depression.
- **Dependence on alcohol or drugs.** About 30 percent of people who abuse alcohol meet the medical criteria for depression. Of those who abuse drugs, approximately 20 percent are depressed or have experienced depression in the past.
- **Psychological issues.** Certain personality traits, such as having low self-esteem and being overly self-critical, pessimistic or easily overwhelmed by stress, can make a person more vulnerable to depression.
- **Other mental illnesses.** Up to half the people with an anxiety disorder also experience depression. Depression is also common among people with eating disorders.
- **Medical conditions.** Having a chronic illness, such as heart disease, stroke, diabetes, cancer or chronic pain, puts you at higher risk

## St. John's wort

Some studies suggest that the herbal preparation St. John's wort may work as well as antidepressants in treating mild depression and with fewer side effects. But studies suggest that it's of minimal benefit in treating major depression.

A concern about St. John's wort is that it can interfere with the effectiveness of prescription medications, including antidepressants, drugs to treat human immunodeficiency virus (HIV) infections and AIDS, and drugs to prevent organ rejection in people who've had transplants. It can also increase the risk of a rare but potentially life-threatening side effect called serotonin syndrome if you take it with a serotonin-active antidepressant.

For more on St. John's wort, see page 270.

of developing depression. Having an underactive thyroid (hypothyroidism) also can cause depression.

In many cases, depression results from not just one risk factor but a combination of them.

## Treatment

Antidepressant medications, which affect the levels of or availability of neurotransmitters in your brain, are often the first line of treatment for depression. They can relieve symptoms and generally have few side effects. Many types of antidepressants are available. Your doctor will determine what type may be best for you based on your symptoms, family history and the match between your symptoms and the medication's effects.

Once your signs and symptoms have eased, your doctor may recommend continuing the medication for up to 12 months to prevent relapse. If you've had recurrent depression, your doctor may recommend that you continue taking medication longer — perhaps for years.

Another common treatment for depression is psychotherapy, also called talk therapy or counseling. Psychotherapy involves meeting with a mental health professional who can help you understand the source of your feelings and find better ways of coping with problems and conflicts that may be triggering them. The most effective treatment for depression is often the combination of antidepressant medication and psychotherapy.

In case of severe depression that doesn't respond to medication or psychotherapy, electroconvulsive therapy (ECT) may be used. This form of treatment involves passing an electrical current through your brain for one to three seconds while you're under light general anesthesia. The stimulus causes a controlled seizure, which typically lasts for 20 to 90 seconds. Experts aren't sure how this therapy helps treat depression, but they theorize that when administered on a regular basis over several weeks, it produces chemical changes in the brain that build upon one another, somehow reducing depression. The most common side effect of electroconvulsive therapy is confusion that may last a few minutes to several hours. ECT may also affect short-term memory, at least temporarily.

An alternative treatment similar to ECT under study is called transcranial magnetic stimulation. Instead of an electrical current, it relies on a strong magnetic pulse to produce chemical changes in the brain.

## What you can do

There are several things you can do to meet life's challenges while managing depression and to experience greater joy and pleasure in life.

- **Don't isolate yourself.** Instead, participate in activities that make you feel good or feel like you've achieved something.
- **Eat well, exercise and get adequate sleep.** This helps you maintain your strength and energy. Exercise can also help treat some forms of depression, ease stress, and help you relax and sleep better.
- **Avoid alcohol and recreational drugs.** Abuse of alcohol and drugs will slow or prevent your recovery.
- **Learn healthy ways to manage anger and sadness.** This can help preserve your emotional well-being.
- **If someone has wronged you, try to forgive.** Holding on to anger may harm your emotional health.
- **If you've suffered a loss, let yourself feel it.** Don't be afraid to ask for help from friends and family as you cope with your grief.

- **Keep a journal.** Writing down your thoughts and feelings can help relieve stress.
- **Slow down.** If your busy lifestyle seems to be a source of stress, perhaps you need to cut out some activities or delegate some tasks to others.
- **Take your medications as prescribed and see your doctor regularly.** Your doctor can monitor your progress, provide support and encouragement, and adjust your medication if necessary.

# Diabetes

More Americans have diabetes than ever before. The disease affects almost 26 million adults and children, yet a large number of them may not know they have it. That's because diabetes can develop gradually over many years, often with no symptoms. In addition, there are approximately 79 million Americans with prediabetes.

## The basics

Diabetes is a condition that affects the way your body uses blood sugar (glucose), your main source of energy.

Normally, glucose is able to enter your cells with the aid of insulin, a hormone secreted by your pancreas. But in diabetes, this process goes awry. Instead of being transported into your cells, glucose accumulates in your bloodstream and eventually is excreted in your urine. The accumulation of glucose in your blood can damage almost every major organ in your body.

Diabetes mainly occurs in two forms. Type 1 diabetes develops when your pancreas makes little or no insulin. Type 2 diabetes occurs when your body is resistant to the effects of insulin or your pancreas produces some, but not enough, to maintain a normal glucose level. Type 2 diabetes is far more common, affecting up to 95 percent of people with diabetes older than age 20.

Often, diabetes produces signs and symptoms that are easily dismissed. This is most common with type 2 diabetes. Other times, signs and symptoms can develop rather suddenly. They may include:

- Increased thirst
- Frequent urination
- Hunger
- A flu-like feeling, including weakness and fatigue
- Unexplained weight loss

- Blurred vision
- Irritability
- Slow healing of cuts and bruises
- Tingling or numbness in your hands or feet
- Recurring infections of the gums, skin, vagina or bladder

If you experience any of these signs and symptoms, especially increased thirst and urination, see your doctor.

## Risk factors

Although researchers don't fully understand why some people develop diabetes and others don't, it's clear that certain factors increase your risk. These factors include:

- **Family history.** Your chance of developing type 1 or type 2 diabetes increases if you have a parent, sibling or child with the disease.
- **Being overweight.** The more fatty tissue in your body, the more resistant your cells become to your own insulin.
- **Inactivity.** The less active you are, the greater your risk of diabetes.
- **Age.** Your risk of type 2 diabetes increases as you get older — especially past the age of 45. But diabetes is also increasing dramatically

among people in their 30s and 40s, and even teens.
- **Race.** More than 8 percent of the general population has received a diagnosis of diabetes, but that rate is significantly higher for blacks and Hispanics and nearly doubles for American Indians. Type 1 diabetes is more common among whites.

## Treatment

Some people are able to control their diabetes with diet, exercise and weight loss. But if these lifestyle changes aren't enough, you may need the help of medication. Medications used to treat diabetes include:

- **Insulin.** Everyone with type 1 diabetes and some people with type 2 diabetes must take insulin every day to replace what their pancreas is unable to produce. Insulin can only be administered by injection with a syringe or insulin pen or through constant infusion with an insulin pump. It isn't available in pill form because its chemical structure is destroyed during digestion, making the hormone ineffective by the time it gets to your bloodstream. There are many types of insulin. They differ in how long it takes them to begin working and how long they last. The type and dosage of insulin your doctor recommends will depend on your specific needs.

- **Oral medications.** In addition to insulin, there are six different families of oral medications available for treating diabetes. Each has its own method for lowering blood sugar. To effectively control your blood sugar, you may need a combination of oral medications or an oral medication plus insulin.
- **Other injectable medications.** The drugs pramlintide (Symlin), exenatide (Byetta) and liraglutide (Victoza) are all synthetic forms of natural hormones found in the body. They are typically helpful for people unable to reach their A1C goals (a common measurement of how well you're managing your diabetes) with other treatments.

Pancreas transplantation may be an option for some people, but it's uncommon and it isn't always successful. Islet cell transplantation is another possible option. In this experimental procedure, doctors infuse insulin-producing pancreas cells into your liver. The cells spread throughout the liver and begin to produce insulin. This approach is undergoing further research and isn't readily available.

Whatever treatment your doctor recommends, monitoring your blood sugar is an essential part of it. People who take insulin for diabetes test their blood sugar frequently. If you don't take insulin, you may not have to test your blood sugar as often.

## What you can do

These steps can help reduce your risk of diabetes, or prevent complications if you already have it.

- **Don't smoke.** People with diabetes who smoke are three times as likely to die of cardiovascular disease as are nonsmokers.
- **Maintain a healthy weight.** For some people with type 2 diabetes, weight loss is all that's needed to restore blood sugar to normal levels. In fact, losing 5 to 10 percent of your current weight also can help prevent diabetes.
- **Eat well.** Eat more fruits, vegetables and whole grains and fewer foods high in fat and sugar.
- **Get at least 30 minutes of exercise most days of the week.** Physical activity helps you control your weight, uses up glucose, makes your cells more sensitive to insulin and improves circulation.

- **Monitor your glucose levels.** If you have diabetes, testing is crucial because it tells you whether you're keeping your glucose levels in a safe range.
- **Have a yearly physical.** This is an opportunity to check for complications of diabetes.
- **Take care of your feet.** Diabetes can damage nerves in your feet, and reduce blood flow to your feet. As a result, you may develop a cut or other injury without realizing it. To help prevent foot problems, check your feet every day. See your doctor if any sores don't start to heal in a few days.
- **Get a yearly flu shot.** Diabetes can weaken your immune system, increasing your risk of influenza or making its symptoms more severe. Also make sure you're up to date on your pneumonia vaccine.

# Upper gastrointestinal disorders

Your digestive, or gastrointestinal, tract runs from your mouth to your anus. Conditions affecting the upper portion of this tract, including the esophagus and stomach, are often referred to as upper gastrointestinal (GI) disorders. Conditions affecting the lower part of the gastrointestinal tract, including the intestines and rectum, are known as lower GI disorders.

A few common disorders of the upper gastrointestinal tract, which are discussed here, include gastroesophageal reflux disease (GERD), ulcers and a condition called nonulcer dyspepsia.

## Gastroesophageal reflux disease

Nearly everyone has experienced heartburn, that burning sensation in your chest or throat from stomach acid that washes back into your esophagus.

An occasional episode of heartburn generally isn't anything to worry about. Frequent heartburn, however, can be a serious problem, and it deserves medical attention. Most often, it's a symptom of GERD.

### The basics
When you swallow, food travels down your esophagus through a muscular valve called the lower esophageal sphincter, which opens to allow food

to pass into your stomach and then closes again. Sometimes, though, this valve relaxes abnormally or weakens, allowing stomach acid to wash back into your lower esophagus, causing frequent heartburn. Over time, this constant backwash of acid can irritate the lining of the esophagus, causing it to inflame (esophagitis). GERD is the name for chronic acid reflux that causes esophageal irritation or inflammation.

Most people with GERD have acid reflux and heartburn. But you may also experience the following:

- Regurgitation of fluid or food in the back of the throat
- Chest pain, especially after a heavy meal or at night while lying down
- Difficulty swallowing (dysphagia)
- Coughing, wheezing, asthma, hoarseness or sore throat
- Regurgitated blood
- Black stool, which may mean it contains partially digested blood

If you experience heartburn at least twice a week for several weeks or your symptoms seem to be getting worse, see your doctor.

### Risk factors
Several factors can significantly increase your risk of GERD.

- **Hiatal hernia.** In this condition, part of your stomach protrudes into your lower chest. If the protrusion is large, it can worsen heartburn by further weakening the lower esophageal sphincter.
- **Certain foods.** Caffeinated beverages, fatty or spicy foods, chocolate, onions, mint and chewing gum all may contribute to or aggravate GERD by causing the valve to become weaker.
- **Being overweight.** Excess weight puts extra pressure on your stomach and diaphragm, forcing open the lower esophageal sphincter. Eating very large or fatty meals may cause similar effects.
- **Excessive alcohol.** Alcohol reduces pressure on the lower esophageal sphincter, allowing it to relax and open. Alcohol may also irritate the lining of the esophagus.
- **Smoking.** It may increase acid production and aggravate reflux. Smoking also lowers the pressure in the lower esophageal sphincter.
- **Family history.** If your parents or siblings have or had GERD, your chances of having the condition are increased.
- **Other medical conditions.** Asthma, diabetes, peptic ulcer and connective tissue disorders can aggravate or precipitate symptoms of GERD.

## Treatment

The first step in treating GERD is making healthy lifestyle changes, such as cutting back on fatty foods, eating smaller meals, losing weight and going to bed on an empty stomach. For people with more-severe symptoms, medication is generally the main treatment. Drugs used to treat GERD include:

- **Antacids.** Available over-the-counter, antacids (Maalox, Rolaids, others) neutralize gastric acid and provide quick, temporary relief. But they won't cure the cause of your reflux. Antacids are generally safe, but if taken regularly they can cause side effects such as diarrhea or constipation. Some antacids can also interfere with other medications taken for kidney or heart disease.

- **Acid blockers.** Also known as histamine (H-2) blockers, these medications — including nizatidine (Axid), famotidine (Pepcid), cimetidine (Tagamet) and ranitidine (Zantac) — are available over-the-counter and by prescription. Instead of neutralizing acid, they reduce acid secretion, so they can prevent acid reflux and heartburn, not just relieve it. These medications are generally safe, but some may interact with other drugs. Check with your doctor or pharmacist for possible drug interactions.

- **Proton pump inhibitors.** These medications, most often prescribed for severe symptoms, are the most effective treatment for GERD. Proton pump inhibitors — including omeprazole (Prilosec), esomeprazole (Nexium), lansoprazole (Prevacid) and pantoprazole (Protonix) — inhibit acid production and allow time for damaged esophageal tissue to heal.

## GERD

Because of the effectiveness of medications, surgery for GERD is uncommon. However, it may be an option. The most common type of surgery involves tightening the lower esophageal sphincter to prevent reflux by wrapping the very top portion of the stomach around the outside of the lower esophagus. Other procedures to treat GERD include:

- **Surgery to create a barrier that prevents the backup of stomach acid.** A device is inserted in order to fold the tissue at the base of the stomach into a replacement for the sphincter valve.

- **A procedure that uses electrode energy to form scar tissue in the esophagus.** This scar tissue helps to strengthen the muscles.

- **Surgery to strengthen the lower esophageal sphincter.** A magnetic ring is wrapped around the junction of the stomach and esophagus. The magnetic pull is strong enough to keep the opening between the two closed to refluxing acid, but weak enough so that food can pass through it.

### What you can do

Lifestyle changes are a big part of preventing or managing GERD.

- **Don't smoke.** Smoking increases acid reflux and can dry up saliva, which helps protect your esophagus from stomach acid.
- **Eat smaller meals.** This reduces pressure on the lower esophageal sphincter, reducing acid reflux.
- **Limit fatty foods.** They relax the lower esophageal sphincter and slow stomach emptying, both of which contribute to acid reflux.
- **Avoid problem foods and beverages.** Everyone has different triggers, but common ones include caffeinated drinks, chocolate, onions, spicy foods, citrus fruits, tomato-based foods and mint.
- **Limit or avoid alcohol.** Alcohol relaxes the lower esophageal sphincter and may irritate the esophagus, worsening symptoms.

- **Lose excess weight.** Excess pounds put pressure on your abdomen, pushing up your stomach and causing acid to back up into your esophagus.
- **Don't exercise immediately after a meal.** Wait two or three hours before engaging in strenuous physical activity.
- **Don't lie down after eating.** Wait at least three hours after eating before going to bed or taking a nap. By then, most of the food in your stomach will have emptied from your stomach into your small intestine.
- **Raise the head of your bed.** This helps prevent acid from flowing back into your esophagus as you sleep. You can do so by placing 4- to 6-inch blocks under the legs at the head of your bed. Or place a foam wedge between your mattress and box spring.
- **Take time to relax.** When you're under stress, digestion slows, worsening GERD symptoms.

## Peptic ulcer

A peptic ulcer is an open sore that develops on the inner lining of your stomach, upper small intestine or esophagus. Peptic ulcers are fairly common. Statistics suggest that about

1 of every 10 people will experience a peptic ulcer at some point in life.

## The basics

Depending on their location, ulcers have different names. A peptic ulcer that occurs in your stomach is called a gastric ulcer. If the ulcer develops in your upper small intestine (duodenum), it's called a duodenal ulcer. An esophageal ulcer is usually located in the lower portion of your esophagus.

The most common symptom of a peptic ulcer is a gnawing pain in your upper abdomen between your navel and breastbone (sternum). The pain is often worse when your stomach is empty, and therefore eating, drinking or taking an antacid often temporarily relieves the pain. Other signs and symptoms of a peptic ulcer may include:

- Black-colored or even bloody stools
- A bloated feeling after meals
- Nausea or vomiting
- Vomiting blood, which may appear bright red or black like coffee grounds
- Unexplained weight loss
- Pain in the midback

Not long ago, the belief was that peptic ulcers were the result of stress or too much spicy food. Doctors now know that many ulcers are caused by the bacterium *Helicobacter pylori*, which lives and multiplies within the mucous layer that covers and protects the lining of your stomach and small intestine.

Often, *H. pylori* causes no problems. But sometimes it can disrupt the mucous layer and inflame and erode digestive tissues, producing an ulcer. Regular use of nonsteroidal anti-inflammatory drugs (NSAIDs), such as naproxen (Aleve), ibuprofen (Advil, Motrin IB, others) or celecoxib (Celebrex) also can irritate or inflame the lining of your stomach and small intestine and lead to an ulcer.

## Risk factors

It's not clear exactly how *H. pylori* spreads. It may be transmitted from person to person by close contact, such as kissing. People may also contract *H. pylori* through food and water. Factors that increase your risk of *H. pylori* infection, and therefore increase your risk of developing a peptic ulcer, include:

- Being born in a developing country
- Low socioeconomic status
- Living in a large family or crowded conditions
- Having an infant in the home
- Exposure to vomit from an infected person

Other risk factors for peptic ulcer, not related to *H. pylori* infection, include:

- **Regular use of NSAIDs.** These drugs inhibit production of the enzyme cyclooxygenase, which produces hormone-like substances called prostaglandins. Prostaglandins help protect your stomach lining from injury.
- **Smoking.** Nicotine in tobacco increases the volume and concentration of stomach acid, increasing your risk of an ulcer.
- **Excessive alcohol consumption.** Alcohol can irritate and erode the mucous lining of your stomach, and it increases the amount of stomach acid that's produced. It's uncertain, however, whether this alone can progress into an ulcer or whether other contributing factors also must be present.

## Treatment

An ulcer isn't something you should treat on your own. Over-the-counter antacids and acid blockers may relieve the gnawing pain, but the relief is short-lived. With a doctor's help, you can find prompt relief from ulcer pain as well as a lifelong cure from the disease.

Because many ulcers stem from *H. pylori* bacteria, treatment is usually aimed at achieving two objectives. The first is to kill the bacteria. The second objective is to reduce the level of acid in your digestive system to relieve pain and encourage healing.

Accomplishing these two steps requires using at least two, and sometimes three or four, of the following types of medications:

- **Antibiotics.** Several combinations of antibiotics kill *H. pylori*. Some pharmaceutical companies package a combination of two antibiotics together, with an acid suppressor or other agent specifically for treating *H. pylori* infection. You'll likely take antibiotics for about two weeks.
- **Acid blockers.** Acid blockers — including nizatidine (Axid), famotidine (Pepcid), cimetidine (Tagamet) and ranitidine (Zantac) — may be available with or without a prescription. These drugs reduce the amount of hydrochloric acid released into your digestive tract, which relieves ulcer pain and encourages healing.
- **Proton pump inhibitors.** These medications — including esomeprazole (Nexium), lansoprazole (Prevacid) and omeprazole (Prilosec) — reduce stomach acid by shutting down the tiny "pumps" within acid-secreting

cells. Proton pump inhibitors also appear to inhibit *H. pylori*. Some of these drugs may be available without a prescription.

- **Antacids.** Your doctor may recommend taking an antacid (Maalox, Rolaids, others) in addition to an acid blocker or in place of one. Instead of reducing acid secretion, antacids neutralize existing stomach acid and can provide rapid pain relief.
- **Cytoprotective agents.** These medications help protect the tissues that line your stomach and small intestine. Bismuth subsalicylate (Pepto-Bismol) is an over-the-counter cytoprotective agent. Bismuth preparations also appear to inhibit *H. pylori* activity.

Surgery may be an option in cases where the peptic ulcer doesn't respond to drug treatment. Surgery may also be used in the case where serious complications arise, such as a hemorrhage, obstruction or perforation. However, with the advent of newer medications and a better understanding of what causes most ulcers, surgical treatment of peptic ulcer is now uncommon.

To ensure that the *H. pylori* bacteria are eradicated, testing is generally recommended approximately three months after the completion of treatment.

## What you can do

While an ulcer is healing, watch what you eat and control stress. Acidic or spicy foods may increase ulcer pain. The same is true for stress. Stress slows digestion, allowing food and digestive acid to remain in your stomach and intestines for a longer period.

Other steps to aid in healing or help prevent ulcers include:

- **Don't smoke.** Smoking may interfere with the protective lining of the stomach, making your stomach more susceptible to the development of an ulcer. Smoking also increases stomach acid.
- **Limit or avoid alcohol.** Excessive use of alcohol can irritate and erode the mucous lining in your stomach and intestines, causing inflammation and bleeding.
- **Avoid NSAIDs.** If you use pain relievers regularly, talk to your doctor about which medication is the best for you to take.
- **If you have a history of ulcers, mention it when you receive a new medication.** If an ulcer-provoking medication is absolutely necessary to treat another condition, your doctor can prescribe a second medication to reduce the risk of a recurrent ulcer.

# Nonulcer dyspepsia

Sometimes, people will see their doctors for what they think is an ulcer, but isn't. Although they may have gnawing upper abdominal pain, diagnostic tests don't reveal an ulcer or other digestive problem. Many of these people have nonulcer dyspepsia, which may also be called functional dyspepsia.

## The basics

Nonulcer dyspepsia is a disorder of the upper gastrointestinal tract. Its most common symptom is pain, or an uncomfortable feeling in your upper abdomen. Other signs and symptoms may include bloating, belching, gas, nausea and an early feeling of fullness with meals.

The exact cause of nonulcer dyspepsia is unknown. In some cases, the culprit may be a temporary problem, such as eating too quickly, overeating or dealing with a stressful event. Nonulcer dyspepsia may be a chronic condition, but for many people its symptoms are often short-lived and preventable.

## Risk factors

Certain lifestyle factors may increase your risk of this condition:

- Eating too quickly, sometimes with air swallowing

- Overeating
- Drinking carbonated beverages
- Eating spicy foods
- Eating greasy or fatty foods
- Consuming too much caffeine or alcohol
- Smoking
- Taking certain medications, especially antibiotics and nonsteroidal anti-inflammatory drugs (NSAIDs)
- Stress

## Treatment

Nonulcer dyspepsia is most often treated by changing your daily habits. This may include avoiding foods that seem to worsen symptoms and controlling stress. Some people find that eating smaller, more frequent meals and low-fat foods also improves symptoms.

If these practices don't help, your doctor may recommend drug therapy. Many of the same drugs used to treat ulcers, including acid blockers and proton pump inhibitors, are recommended for nonulcer dyspepsia.

If your doctor believes your condition may be related to stress, he or she may recommend that you see a health care professional who can help you develop ways to control stress or deal with matters that may be contributing to your symptoms.

likely cause, it's important to identify the disorder and then begin treatment.

For diarrhea from malabsorption issues, such as gluten sensitivity or lactose intolerance, a special diet may be recommended.

### What you can do

To help prevent or reduce the signs and symptoms of chronic diarrhea:

- **Limit caffeine and alcohol.** These stimulants may be triggering your diarrhea or worsening symptoms.
- **Don't take antacids containing magnesium.** Magnesium can cause diarrhea. Check the label.
- **Ask about your medications.** Ask your doctor or pharmacist if it may be a medication side effect.
- **Ask about over-the-counter products.** Nonprescription products

## Preventing traveler's diarrhea

People who travel to developing countries commonly experience diarrhea. Often, the condition results from inadequate sanitation and contaminated food and water. To reduce your risk:

- Eat hot, well-cooked foods.
- Drink bottled water, soda, beer or wine served in its original container. Beverages from boiled water, such as coffee and tea, also are usually safe. Remember that alcohol and caffeine can aggravate diarrhea and dehydration.
- Use bottled water even for brushing your teeth. Don't use ice cubes in your beverages. Keep your mouth closed while you shower.
- Avoid raw fruits and vegetables, unless they can be peeled and you peel them yourself. Also avoid raw or undercooked meats, raw vegetables, dairy foods, tap water and ice cubes.

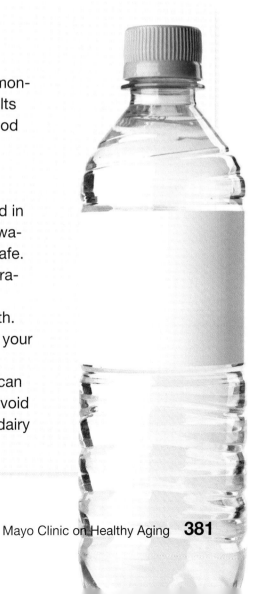

such as Imodium, Pepto-Bismol and Kaopectate may slow diarrhea, but they may not speed your recovery. Ask your doctor if they may be appropriate for you.

- **Reduce stress.** For some forms of chronic diarrhea, such as IBS, therapies to reduce stress can help reduce diarrhea symptoms.

## Constipation

The normal frequency of a person's bowel movements varies widely — from three a day to three a week. What's normal for you may not be normal for someone else.

However, if you have bowel movements just once or twice a week, or you have to strain to pass stool, chances are you're constipated. In some cases, you may also feel bloated or sluggish or experience discomfort or pain.

### The basics
Constipation can occur for many reasons, and it tends to become more common with age. Many medications, including many narcotics, antacids containing aluminum and drugs used to treat Parkinson's disease, high blood pressure and depression, can cause constipation.

In rare cases, constipation may be a sign of a more serious medical condition, such as colorectal cancer or a hormonal or electrolyte disturbance. See your doctor if you experience a recent, unexplained onset of constipation or change in bowel habits, or any of the following signs or symptoms:

- Intense abdominal pain
- Blood in your stool
- Rectal pain
- Thin, pencil-like stools
- Unexplained weight loss

### Risk factors
You're more likely to have problems with constipation if you're inactive, eat a low-fiber diet or don't drink enough fluids. You're also at increased risk if you take certain medications or you're having chemotherapy to treat cancer.

### Treatment
Changes in your lifestyle are the safest way to manage constipation. A few common-sense lifestyle changes, such as getting more exercise, eating high-fiber foods and drinking plenty of water, can help prevent or alleviate many cases of constipation.

Laxatives also relieve constipation, but talk to your doctor before taking any laxative other than fiber supplements.

If you overuse stimulant laxatives (Dulcolax, Ex-Lax, others), you may develop lazy bowel syndrome, a condition in which your bowels become dependent on laxatives to function properly. In fact, overuse of laxatives can cause a number of problems, including poor absorption of vitamins and other nutrients, damage to your intestinal tract and worsening constipation.

Your doctor may recommend a stool softener, such as docusate (Colace, Surfak). These drugs soften fecal matter so that it passes through your intestines more easily.

## What you can do

Take these steps to help prevent or relieve constipation:

- **Drink plenty of liquid every day.** Liquid helps keep your stool soft. Aim for eight 8-ounce glasses a day. Water is preferable.
- **Gradually add more high-fiber foods to your diet.** Fiber helps bulk up and soften stool so that it passes smoothly through your digestive tract. If you're a woman older than age 50, try for 21 grams a day. For men older than age 50, the goal is 30 grams. Fruits, vegetables, beans and whole-grain cereals and breads, are your best fiber sources.

- **Limit problem foods.** Foods that are high in fat and sugar and those low in fiber may cause or aggravate constipation.
- **Enjoy regular meals.** Eating on a regular schedule promotes normal bowel function.
- **Exercise regularly.** Physical activity stimulates the digestive muscles, hastening the passage of food through your digestive tract. Getting at least 150 minutes of moderate exercise a week is recommended. Try to exercise most, if not all, days of the week.
- **Heed nature's call.** The longer you delay going to the bathroom once you feel the urge, the more water that's absorbed from stool and the harder it becomes.
- **Try using a fiber supplement.** These natural supplements (Metamucil, Citrucel, others) help make stools softer and are safe to use every day. Be sure, though, to drink plenty of fluids. Otherwise, fiber supplements can worsen constipation. Be sure to add fiber to your diet slowly to avoid problems with gas.
- **Reduce stress.** Stress can slow the digestion process. For some forms of chronic constipation, relaxation practices such as yoga, massage, acupressure or aromatherapy may reduce symptoms.

# High blood pressure

Because it's so common, many people think that having high blood pressure (hypertension) isn't a big deal. It is. High blood pressure is a leading cause of stroke, heart attack, heart failure, kidney failure and dementia.

## The basics

Your blood pressure is determined by measuring the pressure within your arteries. Two numbers are involved in a blood pressure reading — both are equally important. The first, or top, number is your systolic blood pressure. Systolic blood pressure is the amount of pressure in your arteries when your heart contracts. The second, or bottom, number — your diastolic blood pressure — tells how much pressure remains in your arteries between beats, when your heart is relaxing.

An ideal blood pressure for an adult of any age is 115/75 millimeters of mercury (mm Hg) or less. Once your blood pressure rises above that threshold, your risk of cardiovascular disease may begin to increase. Your blood pressure is still considered to be normal if it's less than 120/80 mm Hg. It's considered high if your systolic pressure averages 140 mm Hg or higher or your diastolic pressure averages 90 mm Hg or higher. Systolic blood pressure readings from 120 to 139 mm Hg and diastolic readings from 80 to 89 mm Hg are generally referred to as prehypertensive.

Fortunately, high blood pressure can be easily detected and once you know you have it, you can work with your doctor to control it.

## Risk factors

There are four major risk factors for high blood pressure that you can't control.

- **Age.** Your risk of high blood pressure increases as you get older, particularly after age 65.
- **Race.** High blood pressure occurs far more frequently in blacks than in any other racial group in the United States.
- **Sex.** In young adulthood and early middle age, men are more likely to have high blood pressure than women are. After about age 50, the opposite is true — women are more at risk after menopause.
- **Family history.** High blood pressure tends to run in families.

Risk factors that you can control or manage include:

- **Obesity.** The more you weigh, the more blood you need to supply oxygen and nutrients to your tissues. More blood flowing through your blood vessels creates extra force on your artery walls.
- **Inactivity.** If you're inactive, you tend to have a higher heart rate. Your heart has to work harder with each contraction, increasing the force on your arteries. Lack of physical activity also increases your risk of being overweight.
- **Tobacco use.** The chemicals in tobacco can damage the lining of your artery walls, causing fatty deposits that contain cholesterol (plaques) to form in the arteries. Nicotine also constricts your blood vessels and forces your heart to work harder.
- **Sodium sensitivity.** People who are sodium sensitive retain sodium more easily, leading to fluid retention and increased blood pressure.
- **Low potassium intake.** Potassium helps balance the amount of sodium in your cells. If you don't consume or retain enough potassium, you

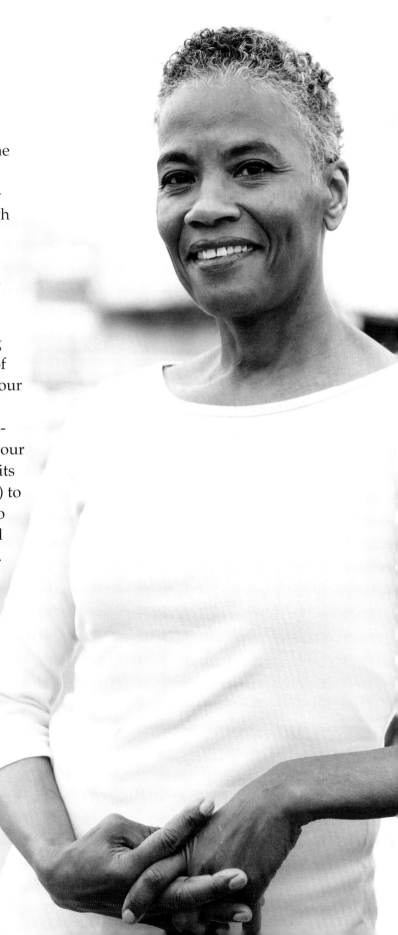

can accumulate too much sodium. This increases your risk of high blood pressure.

- **Excessive alcohol.** Exactly how or why alcohol increases blood pressure isn't understood. In addition, over time, heavy drinking can damage your heart muscle.
- **Stress.** Stress doesn't cause persistent high blood pressure, but a high level of stress can cause a temporary but dramatic increase in blood pressure. If this happens often enough, it can eventually damage your blood vessels, heart and kidneys in the same manner as persistent high blood pressure.

You may also be at increased risk of high blood pressure if you have certain chronic conditions, such as atherosclerosis, diabetes, chronic kidney disease, sleep apnea or heart failure.

## Treatment

The safest way to control your blood pressure is to change your lifestyle. This means by eating well, exercising and adopting other healthy habits.

Sometimes lifestyle changes alone can't reduce your blood pressure enough. In this case, you may need medication.

Taking medication for high blood pressure doesn't mean, though, that you can abandon your healthy habits. Maintaining a healthy lifestyle may improve the effectiveness of your medications and may mean you'll need fewer drugs or lower dosages.

There are a number of medications used to control high blood pressure:

- **Diuretics.** These medications help your body eliminate sodium and water, reducing blood volume. Diuretics often are a first choice in treatment because they're often the most effective.
- **Beta blockers.** These medications — including propranolol (Inderal LA, Innopran XL, others) and metoprolol (Lopressor) block the effects of certain adrenaline-related chemicals, causing your heart to beat more slowly and less forcefully.
- **Angiotensin-converting enzyme (ACE) inhibitors.** These medications — including enalapril (Vasotec) and benazepril (Lotensin) — help relax blood vessels. They do so by blocking the formation of a naturally occurring chemical that narrows blood vessels.
- **Angiotensin II receptor blockers.** These medications — including candesartan (Atacand) and eprosartan

— help relax blood vessels by blocking the action, not the formation, of a naturally occurring chemical that narrows blood vessels.

- **Calcium antagonists, also known as calcium channel blockers.** These medications — including diltiazem (Cardizem, Tiazac, others) and amlodipine (Norvasc) — help relax the muscles of blood vessels. Some slow your heart rate.
- **Renin inhibitors.** Aliskiren (Tekturna) slows the production of renin, an enzyme produced by your kidneys that starts a chain of chemical steps that increases blood pressure.

To achieve your blood pressure goal, your doctor may recommend using multiple drugs. In fact, combinations of low-dose medications can lower blood pressure as well as larger doses of one drug can.

If you still can't meet your blood pressure goal, your doctor may prescribe additional medications:

- **Alpha blockers.** These medications — including doxazosin (Cardura) and prazosin (Minipress) — prevent muscle contractions in smaller arteries and reduce the effects of naturally occurring body chemicals that narrow blood vessels.

- **Alpha-beta blockers.** These drugs, such as carvedilol (Coreg) and labetalol (Trandate), combine the effects of alpha blockers and beta blockers.
- **Central-acting agents.** These medications, such as clonidine (Catapres) and methyldopa, prevent your brain from signaling your nervous system to increase your heart rate and narrow your blood vessels.
- **Direct vasodilators.** These medications include minoxidil, hydralazine and diazoxide (Proglycem). They work directly on the muscles in your artery walls, preventing them from tightening and your arteries from narrowing.

## What you can do

The best strategy for preventing or controlling high blood pressure is to adopt healthy habits.

- **Eat a nutritious diet.** Emphasize fruits and vegetables, whole grains, and low-fat dairy foods in your diet. These foods limit saturated fat and cholesterol and provide plentiful amounts of fiber, potassium, magnesium and calcium. In addition to helping to lower blood pressure, they promote weight loss. It's also important to limit sodium in your diet. Too much sodium can increase blood pressure in some people. The DASH diet is one effective example of a low-sodium eating plan.

- **Maintain a healthy weight.** If you're overweight, losing as little as 10 pounds may reduce your blood pressure.
- **Keep physically active.** Regular aerobic exercise can lower blood pressure in some people — even when the exercise isn't accompanied by weight loss. Aim for at least 30 minutes of moderately intense exercise most days of the week.
- **Don't smoke.** Smoking can lead to the development of tiny deposits (plaques) in your blood vessels and constrict the flow of blood through the vessels.
- **Limit alcohol and caffeine.** Cutting back to a moderate level of alcohol consumption can lower your systolic pressure by two to four points and your diastolic pressure by about two points. Cutting caffeine also can make a difference.
- **Manage stress.** If you feel stressed, try to simplify your daily schedule and experiment with relaxation techniques.
- **Get plenty of sleep.** When you're refreshed, you're better able to tackle the day's problems, allowing you to better cope with stress.

If you've been diagnosed with high blood pressure, try these additional tips:

- Measure your blood pressure. Home monitoring can help you keep closer tabs on your blood pressure. Ask your doctor how often you should check your blood pressure at home.
- Take your medications properly. If you're bothered by side effects, don't stop taking the medication or reduce the amount. Talk with your doctor.
- See your doctor regularly. It takes a team effort to treat high blood pressure successfully. See your doctor on a regular basis.

# Osteoporosis

Osteoporosis is a disease that causes bones to become weak, brittle and prone to fracture. Until recently, osteoporosis was considered a natural part of aging. But there's nothing natural about it.

## The basics

Reduced levels of calcium, phosphorus and other minerals are generally what cause your bones to weaken. With less minerals, bone strength decreases and your bones lose their internal supporting structure. Weakening of bone also can result from endocrine disorders or excessive use of medications such as corticosteroids.

When you're young, your body produces new bone faster than it breaks down old bone, and as a result your bone mass increases. You reach your peak bone mass in your mid- to late-20s. After that, your bone density remains relatively stable until menopause in women or older age in men, when you begin to lose slightly more bone mass than you gain. Not getting enough vitamin D and calcium in your diet can accelerate bone loss.

At menopause, when estrogen levels drop, bone loss in women accelerates to about 1 to 3 percent a year. Bone loss in men also accelerates later in life, though generally not as rapidly. By the time a woman reaches older age — her 70s or 80s — she may have lost up to a third of her bone mass. A man, meanwhile, may lose up to 20 percent of his bone mass.

In the early stages of bone loss, there are generally no symptoms. But once bones have become weakened by osteoporosis, signs and symptoms may occur. They include:

- Back pain after fracture of a vertebra
- Loss of height over time, with an accompanying stooped posture
- Fracture of the vertebrae, wrists, hips or other bones

## Risk factors

Risk factors for osteoporosis include:

- **Sex.** Fractures from osteoporosis are about twice as common in women as in men. But by age 70, women and men lose bone mass at about the same rate.
- **Age.** Your bones become weaker as you age.
- **Race.** You're at greatest risk of osteoporosis if you're white or of Asian descent.
- **Family history.** Having a parent or sibling with osteoporosis puts you at greater risk.
- **Frame size.** People who are exceptionally thin or have small body frames are at higher risk because they often have reserved less bone mass to draw from as they age.
- **Tobacco use.** Smoking disrupts calcium absorption and bone formation.
- **Lifetime exposure to estrogen.** The greater your lifetime exposure to the hormone estrogen, the lower

your risk of osteoporosis. You have a higher risk of osteoporosis if you experienced early menopause or began menstruating at a later than average age.

- **Medications.** Long-term use of steroid medications damages bone. Too much thyroid hormone to treat an underactive thyroid (hypothyroidism) also can cause bone loss. Some diuretic medications also can cause your kidneys to excrete more calcium. Long-term use of the blood-thinning medication heparin, the drug methotrexate, some anti-seizure medications and aluminum-containing antacids also can cause bone loss.
- **Inadequate calcium and vitamin D.** Not getting enough of these bone-building nutrients, especially when you're young, lowers your peak bone mass and increases your risk of fractures later in life.
- **Sedentary lifestyle.** People who spend a lot of time sitting have a higher risk of osteoporosis. Bone health begins in childhood. Children who are the most physically active often grow up to have the greater bone density.
- **Chronic alcoholism.** Excess consumption of alcohol reduces bone formation and interferes with the body's ability to absorb calcium.

## Treatment

Hormone replacement therapy (HRT) may be used to prevent osteoporosis in women. But HRT can result in serious side effects and health risks and is less commonly used today than it once was. To help slow bone loss and possibly even increase bone density, there are other prescription drugs you can take. They include:

- **Bisphosphonates.** Like estrogen, bisphosphonates — including alendronate (Fosamax), risedronate (Actonel), ibandronate (Boniva) and others — can inhibit bone breakdown, preserve bone mass, increase bone density, and decrease risk of spine, hip and other fractures.
- **Raloxifene.** Raloxifene (Evista) is approved only for women. It mimics estrogen's beneficial effects on bone density, without some of the risks associated with estrogen. However, you shouldn't take raloxifene if you have a history of blood clots.
- **Teriparatide.** This medication (Forteo) directly increases bone building. You receive it via daily, self-administered injections in your thigh or abdomen.
- **Calcitonin.** This medication (Fortical, Miacalcin) reduces bone resorption and it keeps bone density

stable. It may also prevent spine fractures. It's generally used to treat people at high risk of fracture who can't take bisphosphonates or other medications.

- **Denosumab.** Compared with bisphosphonates, denosumab (Prolia) produces similar reduction in fractures while targeting a different step in the bone resorption process. It's delivered with a shot under the skin every six months.

## What you can do

Some bone loss is inevitable with age. But there are ways to reduce your risk of osteoporosis or prevent your bones from becoming weaker:

- **Get adequate calcium and vitamin D.** Postmenopausal women ages 51 to 70 should consume at least 1,200 milligrams (mg) of calcium and 600 international units (IU) of vitamin D every day. Men in this same age range should consume 1,000 mg of calcium and 600 IU of vitamin D every day. Both men and women older than 70 should get 1,200 mg of calcium and 800 IU of vitamin D daily.
- **If you don't get enough calcium in your diet, try calcium supplements.**

They're effective, inexpensive and generally well tolerated.

- **Exercise.** It can help you build strong bones and slow bone loss. Combine strength training exercises (weightlifting) with weight-bearing exercises, such as walking, jogging or stair climbing.
- **Don't smoke.** Smoking increases bone loss, perhaps by decreasing the amount of estrogen a woman's body makes and reducing the absorption of calcium in your intestine.
- **Avoid excessive alcohol.** For healthy adults this means no more than one drink a day for women of all ages and men older than age 65, and up to two drinks a day for men age 65 and younger.

# Sexual disorders in women

Pleasurable and satisfying sexual activity is usually an important part of health and well-being throughout life. Women may experience different types of sexual difficulties at different stages of their lives. Often, these are temporary problems that resolve on their own. But sometimes, they persist and cause distress.

## The basics

Sexual dysfunction refers to a persistent or recurrent problem that affects any aspect of the sexual experience, and which concerns or distresses you.

Sexual dysfunction can occur in women of all ages, but as many as half of all postmenopausal women — or even more — may experience sexual changes that bother them at some point.

Doctors and therapists generally divide sexual dysfunction in women into four categories:

- **Low sexual desire.** You have low libido, or lack of interest in sex, and are distressed by it. This is the most common type of sexual disorder among women.
- **Sexual arousal disorder.** You don't experience arousal during sexual activity, which can be related to lack of sensation or other factors.
- **Orgasmic disorder.** You have persistent or recurrent difficulty experiencing an orgasm, even after sufficient stimulation. If you've never experienced an orgasm, the disorder is termed primary orgasmic disorder. If you previously experienced orgasms but no longer can, it's called secondary orgasmic disorder.
- **Sexual pain disorder.** You have pain with sexual activity, which might involve pain on the outside of the vagina (vulva) or inside the vagina. Genital pain associated with intercourse is called dyspareunia. If you have painful, involuntary spasms of the muscles surrounding the entrance to the vagina, when trying to have intercourse, the condition is called vaginismus.

If you have a sexual problem that's distressing to you, see your doctor. Sexual problems are treatable. If your doctor is unable to determine the cause of your problem and help you find approaches that are effective, you may be referred to a specialist for further evaluation and care.

## Risk factors

Several factors may cause or contribute to sexual dysfunction in women. They generally fall into three categories:

- **Physical.** There are numerous physical conditions that may cause or contribute to sexual problems, including diabetes, cardiovascular disease, neurological problems, cancer, urinary or bowel difficulties and arthritis. Fatigue is a well-recognized factor. Certain medications, including some anti-depressants, blood pressure medications, sedatives and antihistamines, can decrease sexual desire, reduce lubrication or reduce your ability to experience orgasm.

- **Hormonal.** Low estrogen levels after menopause may lead to changes in your genital tissue and in your sexual response. The folds of skin that cover your genital region (labia) shrink and become thinner, exposing more of the clitoris. This increased exposure may reduce the sensitivity of the clitoris, or may cause an unpleasant prickling sensation. In addition, vaginal lubrication is reduced in the absence of estrogen and arousal usually takes longer. The opening to your vagina can become narrower and the inside less elastic. These factors can lead to difficult or painful intercourse (dyspareunia). In addition, experiencing orgasm may take longer or may be difficult to reach.

- **Psychological and social.** Stress, anger, anxiety or depression can contribute to sexual problems. Your feelings toward and attraction to your partner, and your view of your own body or your partner's are additional factors that may contribute to sexual problems.

## Treatment

If you have a physical condition that may be contributing to sexual dysfunction, your doctor may recommend treatment of the underlying condition. He or she may also suggest changes in the medications you take to determine whether they're affecting your sexual responsiveness.

If you're postmenopausal and troubled by vaginal dryness, your doctor may recommend vaginal estrogen therapy, which comes in the form of a cream, tablet or flexible vaginal ring. Vaginal estrogen is absorbed directly through the vaginal tissue to counteract vaginal dryness and thinning that can occur with menopause.

If you have a problem with orgasms, your doctor may suggest exercises known as Kegels. These exercises can help you develop the muscles, located in the outer third of your vagina, involved in pleasurable sensations. These same muscles also help control the flow of urine.

Position changes during intercourse also may help. If you've never had an orgasm, learning about your own body's responsiveness may be helpful, as might the use of a vibrator.

For psychological or relationship problems, your doctor may recommend counseling or psychotherapy. Therapy will likely address ways to optimize your emotional as well as sexual intimacy, but often will also address issues that affect other aspects of your relationship.

## What you can do

No matter what your age, it's important not to lose sight of your sexuality. Here are some strategies for enhancing your sexual desire and achieving greater satisfaction:

- **Educate yourself about sexuality.** You may be surprised at how much you can learn about sex — or how much mistaken information you have absorbed over the years.
- **Identify your wishes for sexual activity.** Talk with your partner about your ideas about what is desirable, enjoyable and meaningful sexual activity for the two of you. With good communication and a willingness to try new approaches, you and your partner may find new satisfaction in your sex life.
- **Position for comfort.** Depending on your physical condition and personal preferences, some positions

may be more comfortable for you than others. Talk with your partner about what feels good and what does not. Ask your partner to go slowly as you try different positions.
- **Try vaginal moisturizers or lubricants.** Vaginal moisturizers help moisturize the vagina day to day and can help reduce vaginal atrophy. Lubricants are used to help reduce discomfort during sexual activity.
- **Stay sexually active.** Regular sexual activity can enhance intimacy and improve your relationship with your partner. It also improves vaginal lubrication and helps keep genital tissues more supple.
- **Manage stress.** Learning how to relax can increase desire for sex and arousal during sexual activity.
- **Take care of yourself.** Eating right and getting regular exercise will keep your body finely tuned. This will help keep you ready for sex at any age.

# Sexual disorders in men

For men, one of the most common sexual problems is impotence, also known as erectile dysfunction. Decreased sexual desire also may be a problem for some men.

## Impotence

Three important steps are necessary to produce and sustain an erection.

- The first is sexual arousal, which can come from the senses and from thoughts.
- The second step is the nervous system response, in which the brain communicates sexual arousal to the body's nerves, including the nerves in the penis.
- The third step is a relaxing action of the blood vessels that supply the penis, allowing more blood to flow into the shafts that produce the erection.

If something affects any of these factors or the delicate balance among them, impotence can result.

### The basics

Impotence is a persistent inability to obtain an erection or to keep it long enough for sexual intercourse. Diminished sexual desire or even the loss of sexual desire isn't the same as impotence. Impotence refers to the inability to use the penis for sexual activity even when desire and opportunity are present.

An occasional episode of impotence happens to most men and is perfectly normal. In most cases it's nothing to worry about. As men age, it's also normal to experience changes in erectile function. Erections may take longer to develop, may not be as rigid or may require more direct stimulation to be achieved. Men may also notice that orgasms are less intense, the volume of ejaculate is reduced and recovery time increases between erections.

When impotence becomes a persistent problem, however, it can challenge a man's self-image as well as his sex life. It may also be a sign of a physical or emotional problem that requires help from a professional.

You may view impotence as a personal or embarrassing problem, but it's important to have it evaluated, especially if a physical cause might be to blame. Treating an underlying problem may be enough to reverse erectile dysfunction. Other direct treatments may help, too.

### Risk factors

A wide variety of physical and emotional risk factors can contribute to impotence. They include:

## Decreased desire

Testosterone regulates your sex drive. And although men don't go through menopause, testosterone does decrease gradually over time. This decrease probably accounts for some loss of sexual desire with age.

Some medications, such as those used for depression and high blood pressure, also can decrease sexual desire, as can chronic medical problems such as diabetes or cardiovascular disease. If you're under a lot of emotional stress, you may also lose interest in sex.

If you're concerned about decreased sexual desire, talk with your doctor.

- **Physical diseases and disorders.** Chronic diseases of the lungs, liver, kidneys, heart, nerves, arteries or veins can lead to impotence. So can endocrine system disorders, particularly diabetes. The accumulation of deposits (plaques) in your arteries (atherosclerosis) also can prevent adequate blood from entering the penis. And in some men, impotence may be caused by low levels of the hormone testosterone (male hypogonadism).
- **Surgery or trauma.** Surgery for prostate or colorectal cancer may result in problems with impotence, as may radiation treatment for cancer. Injury to the pelvic area or spinal cord also may cause problems, particularly if the injury damages the nerves that control erections.
- **Medications.** A wide range of drugs — including antidepressants, antihistamines, and medications to treat high blood pressure, pain and prostate cancer — can cause impotence by interfering with nerve impulses or blood flow to the penis. Tranquilizers and sleeping aids also may pose a problem.
- **Substance abuse.** Chronic use of alcohol, marijuana or other drugs often causes impotence and decreased sexual drive.
- **Stress, anxiety or depression.** Psychological conditions also contribute to some cases of impotence.

## Treatment

Treatment for impotence includes everything from medications and simple mechanical devices to surgery and psychological counseling. The treatment your doctor recommends will depend on the cause and severity of your condition:

- **Psychological counseling.** If stress, anxiety or depression is the cause of your impotence, your doctor may suggest that you, or you and your partner, visit a psychologist or psychiatrist with experience in treating sexual problems.
- **Oral medications.** These drugs — including tadalafil (Cialis), vardenafil (Levitra) and sildenafil (Viagra) — enhance the effects of nitric oxide, a chemical messenger that relaxes smooth muscles in the penis. This increases blood flow and allows a natural sequence to occur — an erection in response to sexual stimulation. Although these medications can help many people, not all men can or should take them to treat impotence.
- **Alprostadil.** Alprostadil (Caverject, Edex, others) helps relax smooth muscle tissue in the penis, enhancing blood flow needed for an erection. There are two ways to use alprostadil. With needle-injection therapy, you inject the drug into the base or side of your penis. With intraurethral therapy, you use an applicator to insert a medication pellet through the penis' tip.
- **Hormone replacement therapy.** If you're among the small number of men whose impotence is related to hormone deficiencies, synthetic hormones may help.
- **Vacuum devices.** These involve using a manual hand pump to create a vacuum that pulls blood into the penis. To maintain the erection, you slip a tension ring around the base of your penis.
- **Surgery.** Surgical options may be considered if other treatments fail. Various types of penile implants are available.

## What you can do

These steps may help decrease the likelihood of impotence:

- Limit or avoid the use of alcohol and other similar drugs.
- Stop smoking.
- Exercise regularly.
- Reduce stress.
- Get enough sleep.
- Deal with anxiety or depression.
- Communicate honestly and openly with your partner.
- Consider seeking counseling as a couple.

# Stroke

In the United States, stroke is the fourth-leading cause of death and the leading cause of adult disability. Only heart disease, cancer and chronic respiratory disease cause more deaths annually.

The good news is that fewer Americans die of strokes today than was the case 20 or 30 years ago. Improvement in the control of major risk factors — smoking and high blood pressure — is likely responsible for the decline.

## The basics

Stroke is a common name for several disorders that occur within seconds or minutes after blood supply to the brain is disturbed. A stroke occurs when blood flow to your brain is blocked or blood spills into the brain or surrounding tissues. Within a few minutes to a few hours, brain cells begin to die.

About 80 percent of strokes are ischemic strokes. They occur when blood clots or other particles block arteries to your brain and cause severely reduced blood flow (ischemia). Less common is a hemorrhagic stroke. This type of stroke occurs when a blood vessel in your brain leaks or ruptures.

The most common signs and symptoms of stroke include:

- Sudden numbness, weakness, or paralysis of the face, arm or leg — usually on one side of the body
- Loss of speech, or trouble talking or understanding speech
- Sudden blurred, double or decreased vision
- Dizziness, loss of balance or loss of coordination
- Confusion or problems with memory, spatial orientation or perception
- A sudden, severe headache or an unusual headache, which may be accompanied by a stiff neck, facial pain, vomiting or altered consciousness

For most people, a stroke gives no obvious warning. But one possible sign of an impending stroke is what's called a transient ischemic attack (TIA).

A TIA — also called a ministroke — is a temporary interruption of blood flow to a part of your brain. The signs and symptoms of TIA are the same as for a stroke, but they appear for a short period and then disappear, often in less than five minutes. A TIA doesn't leave lasting symptoms because the blockage is temporary.

If you experience any warning signs of a stroke or TIA, get help right away. The quicker you're diagnosed and treated, the better the outcome will be.

## Risk factors

Many factors can increase your risk of stroke. They include:

- **Age.** Your risk of stroke doubles each decade past age 35.
- **Sex.** Stroke affects men and women about equally. But women are more likely to die of stroke than are men.
- **Race.** Blacks are at greater risk of stroke than are people of other races.
- **Family history.** Your risk is slightly greater if a parent or sibling has a history of stroke or TIA.
- **High blood pressure.** High blood pressure (hypertension) can weaken and damage blood vessels in and around your brain and increase the chance of plaque formation (atherosclerosis), causing narrowed or blocked arteries. It can also increase the risk of hemorrhage from a weakened artery.
- **Undesirable blood cholesterol levels.** High levels of low-density lipoprotein (LDL, or "bad") cholesterol and low levels of high-density lipoprotein (HDL, or "good") cholesterol increase your risk of narrowed or blocked arteries, including those leading to your brain.
- **Smoking.** If you smoke, your risk of a stroke may be two to three times greater than if you don't.
- **Diabetes.** This condition may increase accumulation of plaque in your arteries, and it interferes with your body's ability to break down blood clots.
- **Sedentary lifestyle.** Lack of regular physical activity increases the risk of stroke.
- **Cardiovascular disease.** Congestive heart failure, a previous heart attack, heart valve disease or an irregular heart rhythm (atrial fibrillation) can increase your risk of stroke.
- **Previous stroke or TIA.** If you've already had a stroke and you're older than age 45, your risk of having another one increases by about 10 to 20 times. If you've had a TIA, your risk of a stroke increases significantly.

## Treatment

To treat an ischemic stroke, doctors must remove the obstruction and restore blood flow to the brain. Several drugs may be of benefit:

- **Anti-platelet medications.** These drugs reduce the tendency of blood to clot by preventing blood platelets from sticking together as they pass through narrowed arteries.
- **Anticoagulants.** The drug low-molecular-weight heparin works immediately and may be injected to reduce clotting. Warfarin (Coumadin) also helps prevent blood clots, but it takes several days to become fully effective.
- **Tissue plasminogen activator (TPA).** This clot-busting medication may prevent or minimize damage to your brain by dissolving a blood clot and restoring blood flow. However, it's most effective when used within 4.5 hours of stroke onset. It also increases the risk of bleeding in your brain. Before receiving TPA, you will undergo a computerized tomography (CT) scan to detect any existing bleeding.

After an ischemic stroke, you may need surgery or balloon therapy to clear your carotid artery to prevent another stroke. Your doctor may also recommend medications to reduce the likelihood of another clot forming, and to manage any treatable risk factors.

Treatment for hemorrhagic stroke typically involves controlling blood pressure and limiting fluids, and possible medication to minimize brain tissue swelling. Surgery or other interventions may be necessary to repair the cause of the artery rupture.

## What you can do

To reduce your risk of stroke, develop good health habits.

- **Eat a brain-healthy diet.** Foods that may offer some protection against stroke include fruits, vegetables, oatmeal, beans, soy products and foods rich in omega-3 fatty acids, such as fatty fish.
- **Eat less cholesterol and saturated fat.** If you can't control your cholesterol with dietary changes, talk to your doctor about medications that can help.
- **Maintain a healthy weight.** Being overweight contributes to other risk factors for stroke.
- **Exercise regularly.** It can lower your blood pressure, increase your level of "good" cholesterol and improve the overall health of your blood vessels and heart.
- **Drink alcohol in moderation, if at all.** Heavy alcohol consumption increases your risk of high blood pressure and stroke.

- **Control diabetes and high blood pressure.** Eat right, exercise, control your weight and take your medications as directed.
- **Quit smoking.** There are counseling services and medications that can help you stop if you're unable to quit on your own.
- **Manage stress.** Stress can cause a temporary spike in your blood pressure. It can also increase your blood's tendency to clot, which may elevate your stroke risk.

# Urinary disorders

Bladder-related problems can limit your lifestyle. But treatment often can help you control the problem, or at least cope better.

A common condition that affects women in older age is urinary incontinence. A common condition among men is benign prostatic hyperplasia (BPH).

## Urinary incontinence

Urinary incontinence is much more common in women than in men. The disorder is often associated with aging, but it isn't a normal condition of age.

### The basics

Urinary incontinence refers to the inability to keep urine in your bladder until you go to the bathroom, resulting in an accident. There are five different types.

- With stress incontinence, you leak urine when you cough or sneeze because your pelvic muscles and tissues are too weak to withstand the pressures in the bladder.
- With urge incontinence, your bladder muscle contracts involuntarily, causing urine to leak.
- Mixed incontinence means having more than one type, typically stress and urge incontinence.
- Overflow incontinence stems from the inability to completely empty your bladder, often because your urethra is blocked in some way or because your bladder muscles don't contract forcefully or often enough to maintain normal urination.
- Functional incontinence is the inability to make it to the bathroom in time because of an illness, impairment or disability that's unrelated to your urinary system.

If you're having trouble with urinary incontinence, don't let embarrassment get the better of you. See your doctor. In many cases, incontinence can be eliminated. Even if it can't be treated completely, modern devices and ways of managing urinary incontinence can ease your discomfort and help you regain confidence.

## Risk factors

Many different factors can contribute to urinary incontinence. Some are temporary and can be reversed with treatment or lifestyle changes. These rick factors include:

- **Excessive fluid intake.** This increases the amount of urine your bladder has to deal with and may result in an occasional accident.
- **Inadequate fluid intake.** This can cause wastes to become concentrated in your urine, which can cause urinary urgency and increased frequency.
- **Excessive consumption of bladder irritants.** Carbonated drinks, tea, coffee, citrus fruits and juices, and artificial sweeteners are all common culprits.
- **Excessive alcohol or caffeine intake.** As diuretics, caffeine and alcohol cause your bladder to fill quickly, triggering an urgent and sometimes uncontrollable need to urinate.
- **Urinary tract infection.** This common condition can cause bladder irritation and sudden onset of incontinence. Urinary tract infections can be treated, and your doctor may have advice on steps to help prevent them.
- **Medications.** Sedatives, water pills (diuretics), muscle relaxants and antidepressants can cause or increase incontinence. Some high blood pressure, heart and cold medicines also can affect bladder function.
- **Stool impaction.** A hard mass of stool in your rectum can obstruct the flow of urine at the bottom of the bladder, leading to overflow incontinence, or may cause increased bladder contractions, causing urge incontinence.
- **Obesity.** Being significantly overweight puts constant, increased pressure on your bladder and surrounding structures, weakening them and allowing urine to leak out when you cough or sneeze.
- **Lack of physical fitness.** When you're out of shape, your pelvic floor muscles may be somewhat weak, which may contribute to incontinence.
- **Smoking.** Longtime smokers often have a severe chronic cough, which can aggravate the symptoms of stress incontinence.

Other risk factors for urinary incontinence are uncontrollable. They include:

- **Age.** As you get older, your bladder and urethra muscles lose strength, your bladder walls become less elastic and your pelvic floor muscles become weaker, all of which can contribute to incontinence.
- **Menopause.** With less estrogen after menopause, the tissues lining the urethra become drier and thinner and lose some of their elasticity. This can cause you to leak urine when you cough, laugh or sneeze.
- **Previous surgery or radiation treatment.** Hysterectomy, prostate surgery or surgery for colorectal cancer may damage the muscles and nerves of the urinary tract, which can lead to urinary incontinence. Radiation therapy for gynecologic, urologic or colorectal cancer may make your bladder wall somewhat stiff. This loss of elasticity sometimes results in urinary incontinence.
- **Medical conditions.** Congestive heart failure, diabetes and neurological disorders such as multiple sclerosis, Parkinson's disease, stroke and Alzheimer's disease can all cause urinary incontinence.

### Treatment

In many cases, you can regain bladder control by treating the underlying cause or modifying your daily habits. Your doctor may advise special exercises to strengthen the pelvic area or bladder training techniques such as timed urination. Sometimes, simple adjustments in your daily routine, such as remembering to go to the bathroom regularly or limiting fluids before bedtime, can make the difference.

If urinary incontinence persists, medications, medical devices or surgery may help manage the problem. For symptoms of urge incontinence, medications called anticholinergics may help relax your bladder and prevent involuntary contractions.

Most medical devices to treat urinary incontinence are designed for women, but a few external devices are also available for men. A pessary is a mechanical device, which comes in many shapes and sizes. It's placed in a woman's vagina and helps support the pelvic organs to prevent leakage. A urethral insert is a small, removable plug inserted into the urethra to prevent urine leakage. When you need to urinate, you simply remove the device. For men, a foam rubber clamp may be worn around the penis to temporarily stop the flow of urine.

If these treatments don't help, surgery may be an option to consider. For some men, a urologist may recommend a surgically implanted artificial urinary sphincter. This device allows you to control its open (voiding) and closed (continent) settings.

The most popular surgery for women with stress incontinence is the sling procedure. During this procedure, a surgeon places strips of abdominal tissue or synthetic material under the urethra. These strips act like a hammock, compressing the urethra to prevent urine leakage.

### What you can do

There are a number of practical, self-care strategies for dealing with incontinence.

- **Shed extra pounds.** Studies suggest that losing 5 to 10 percent of your body weight can help improve signs and symptoms of incontinence.
- **Avoid or limit foods and drinks that seem to irritate your bladder.** Caffeine is a common culprit.
- **Try to drink eight 8-ounce glasses of fluid each day.** More than that may make you urinate more frequently, but less may cause wastes to become concentrated in your urine, which can cause urinary urgency and frequency.
- **Add more fiber to your diet.** Fiber can help prevent constipation, which can be a cause of incontinence. This may mean fiber-rich foods or fiber supplements.
- **Exercise most days of the week.** Physical activity can strengthen your pelvic floor muscles, reduce your risk of prostate enlargement and help you maintain your mobility, all of which can reduce your risk of urinary incontinence.
- **Don't smoke.** Smoking can lead to a severe chronic cough, which can aggravate the symptoms of stress incontinence.
- **If you tend to leak urine during sex, try a different position.** For women, being on top generally gives you better control of your pelvic muscles. Also avoid drinking fluids for an hour or so beforehand and empty your bladder immediately before you begin.
- **Try to maintain a positive outlook.** Achieving bladder control may be difficult, but once you do it, you'll find renewed confidence in yourself and your abilities.

## Benign prostatic hyperplasia

Benign prostatic hyperplasia (BPH) is common. If affects about half of men in their 60s and 90 percent of men in their 80s.

## The basics

The prostate gland tends to enlarge with age, beginning at about age 50. As tissues in the gland enlarge, they often compress the urethra and partially block urine flow. By age 75, about half of men report some symptoms.

The severity of symptoms varies and may include:

- Weak urine stream
- Difficulty starting urination
- Stopping and starting again while urinating
- Dribbling at the end of urination
- A frequent or urgent need to urinate
- Increased urination at night (nocturia)
- Inability to completely empty the bladder
- Blood in the urine (hematuria)
- Urinary tract infection

If you're experiencing urinary problems, seek medical advice. Your doctor can help determine whether you have BPH and whether your symptoms warrant treatment.

## Risk factors

The main risk factor for BPH is increasing age. The older you are, the more likely the condition is to occur. Other risk factors include:

- **Heredity.** A family history of prostate enlargement can increase the odds of developing problems from prostate enlargement.
- **Ethnicity.** BPH is more common in American and European men than in Asian men.
- **Marital status.** For reasons that are unknown, married men are more likely to experience prostate enlargement than are single men.

## Treatment

Treatment for BPH depends on its severity and your preference of options.

If your symptoms are mild and they don't bother you, you and your doctor may decide that watchful waiting is appropriate. Your doctor should periodically evaluate your symptoms to see whether they stay the same or worsen.

Drug therapy is the most common method for controlling moderate symptoms of BPH. Alpha blockers (Cardura, Flomax, others) improve the flow of urine by relaxing muscles in the area of the prostate gland. These are usually the most effective drugs to relieve signs and symptoms.

Another class of drugs called 5-alpha-reductase inhibitors, which includes finasteride (Proscar) and dutasteride

(Avodart), shrinks the prostate gland by suppressing certain hormones that stimulate prostate growth.

If drug therapy fails to provide relief or you develop complicating factors, such as urine retention, bleeding through the urethra or stones in the bladder, surgery may be an option. The most common surgical procedure for BPH is transurethral resection of the prostate (TURP). During this procedure, the surgeon removes excess prostate tissue. TURP is effective and relieves symptoms quickly.

Several less invasive techniques also may be used to destroy prostate tissue. Microwave therapy uses computer-controlled heat in the form of microwave energy to destroy the central part of the enlarged gland. Another treatment uses radio waves to heat and destroy prostate tissue. The radio waves are transmitted through needles inserted into the prostate gland. Electrical therapy uses a metal instrument that emits a high-frequency electrical current to cut and vaporize excess tissue. Laser therapy produces concentrated light that heats and destroys the tissue.

### What you can do

A few lifestyle changes can often help control the symptoms of an enlarged prostate and prevent your condition from worsening. Consider these steps:

- **Stop drinking water and other beverages after 7 p.m.** This will reduce your need to go to the bathroom at night. In particular, avoid beverages that contain caffeine. They'll increase urine production, cause bladder irritation and aggravate your symptoms.
- **Urinate all that you can each time you go to the bathroom.** For some men, sitting on the toilet is more effective than standing. Try following a daily time schedule for urinating.
- **Limit alcohol consumption.** Alcohol increases urine production and irritates your bladder.
- **Be careful with over-the-counter decongestants.** They can cause the band of muscles that control urine flow from your urethra (urethral sphincter) to tighten, making urination more difficult.
- **Keep active.** Even a small amount of exercise can reduce urinary problems caused by an enlarged prostate.
- **Stay warm.** Cold weather can lead to urine retention and increase your urgency to urinate.

# Index

## A

AARP, 43
A1C test, 289
aches/pains, exercise and, 197–200
advance directives, 319–324
    durable power of attorney, 321–322
    living will, 322–323
aerobic exercise, 168–173
age
    exercise and, 154
    retirement, 29
    strength and, 176
    wisdom of, 55
aging
    causes of, 64–65
    as individual process, 88
    questions, 12–18
    rate of, 63
alcohol, excessive use
    health risks, 99–100
    limiting, 66, 69, 81, 85, 100, 150, 388, 400, 406
    supplements and, 241
    where to start change, 101
Alzheimer's disease, 342–345
    causes of, 342–343
    family genes and, 106
    prevention and, 131
    resilience to, 132
    risk factors, 343
    treatment, 343–344
    what you can do, 344–345

anti-aging therapies, 262
antioxidants, 205, 253
anxiety
    and exercise, 160
    and friendships, 120
    about retirement, 40
    as stress risk, 95
    *See also* depression
arthritis
    exercise and, 165
    rheumatoid, 346
    risk factors, 345–346
    treatment, 346–347
    what you can do, 347–348
attitude, 11–24

## B

balance exercises, 184–193
benign prostatic hyperplasia (BPH), 404–406
blessings, counting, 116
blood cholesterol test, 283–284
blood pressure measurement, 284–285
body mass index (BMI), 213, 216
bone density
    loss of, 79
    measurement of, 285–286
    *See also* osteoporosis
brain
    aging and, 132–133
    challenging, 67, 131–152
    changes in, 66–67
    cross–training, 143–145

    disease risk, 66
    training resources, 145
    *See also* memory
breast cancer, 348–351

## C

calcium, 253–254, 390, 391
calendar system, 133–138
calories
    burned by exercise, 174
    empty, 214
    serving sizes and, 218–226
    source of, 214
cancer
    breast, 106, 126–127, 286–288, 348–351
    colon, 106, 288–290
    exercise and, 165
    lung, 352–354
    ovarian, 107
    prostate, 293, 354–357
    skin, 294
    as smoking risk, 101
canes, 331–333
car keys, giving up, 329
carbohydrates
    calories and, 206, 214
    serving sizes, 223
    whole grains, 206
cardiovascular disease
    defined, 163
    exercise and, 161–162
    as genetic risk, 107
    as smoking risk, 101–104
    as stress risk, 95
    as stroke risk factor, 399

cardiovascular system
    changes in, 67–69
    components of, 67
    disease, 68–69
    family history and, 69
    heart, 67
    inactivity and, 68
cataracts, 86
cellphones, 330
chronic obstructive pulmonary
    disease (COPD), 101
chronic stress, 150
colon cancer
    genetics in, 106
    as inactive lifestyle risk, 90
    screening, 288–289
constipation, 72, 382–383
COPD. *See* chronic obstruc-
    tive pulmonary disease
core stability training, 177-181
coronary artery disease,
    357–362
creativity
    as ageless, 14
    expressing, 57
cross-training, brain, 143–145
curiosity, 146

## D

daily needs devices, 326–328
daily servings, 217–226
dairy products
    in healthy diet, 207
    serving sizes, 224
dental changes, 69–70
dental checkups, 288–289

depression, 362–366
diabetes
    exercise and, 162–163
    risk factors, 367
    screening, 289–290
    signs and symptoms,
      366–367
    treatment, 367–368
    types, 162, 366
    what you can do, 368–369
diarrhea, 380–382
digestive changes, 71–73
doctors, 274–276
driving
    assistive devices, 333
    giving up, 329
durable power of attorney for
    health care, 321–323

## E

early retirement, 41
e-readers, 331
exercise(s)
    aches/pains, avoiding,
      197–200
    action plan, 195–197
    aerobic, 168–173
    age and, 154
    balance, 184–193
    before beginning, 163
    benefits, 154–167, 200
    calories burned by, 174
    core stability training,
      177–181
    danger signs, 178
    endurance, 155

    exertion scale, 166
    flexibility, 182–184
    getting started, 167–168
    goals, 160, 195
    guide, 185–192
    importance of, 92–93
    motivation, 193–197
    recommended amounts,
      167–168
    sleep and, 86, 159
    strength training, 175–177
    warming up/cooling down,
      172
    warning signs, 200
    *See also* physical activity
expenses
    estimating, 30–31
    home upkeep, 36
eyes
    changes in, 86–88
    exams of, 87–88, 290–291
    *See also* vision changes

## F

family and friends, 56–57,
    122, 146
family health history, 109
fats
    calories and, 214
    good vs. bad, 208
    in moderation, 208
    serving sizes, 225
    types of, 209
fiber, 72, 73, 383
financial planning, 29–35
    expenses calculation, 30